Fibrosis Research

METHODS IN MOLECULAR MEDICINE™

John M. Walker, SERIES EDITOR

125. **Myeloid Leukemia:** *Methods and Protocols,* edited by *Harry Iland, Mark Hertzberg, and Paula Marlton, 2006*
124. **Magnetic Resonance Imaging:** *Methods and Biological Applications,* edited by *Pottumarthi V. Prasadi, 2006*
123. **Marijuana and Cannabinoid Research:** *Methods and Protocols,* edited by *Emmanuel S. Onaivi, 2006*
122. **Placenta Research Methods and Protocols:** *Volume 2,* edited by *Michael J. Soares and Joan S. Hunt, 2006*
121. **Placenta Research Methods and Protocols:** *Volume 1,* edited by *Michael J. Soares and Joan S. Hunt, 2006*
120. **Breast Cancer Research Protocols**, edited by *Susan A. Brooks and Adrian Harris, 2005*
119. **Human Papillomaviruses:** *Methods and Protocols,* edited by *Clare Davy and John Doorbar, 2005*
118. **Antifungal Agents:** *Methods and Protocols,* edited by *Erika J. Ernst and P. David Rogers, 2005*
117. **Fibrosis Research:** *Methods and Protocols,* edited by *John Varga, David A. Brenner, and Sem H. Phan, 2005*
116. **Inteferon Methods and Protocols**, edited by *Daniel J. J. Carr, 2005*
115. **Lymphoma:** *Methods and Protocols,* edited by *Timothy Illidge and Peter W. M. Johnson, 2005*
114. **Microarrays in Clinical Diagnostics**, edited by *Thomas O. Joos and Paolo Fortina, 2005*
113. **Multiple Myeloma:** *Methods and Protocols,* edited by *Ross D. Brown and P. Joy Ho, 2005*
112. **Molecular Cardiology:** *Methods and Protocols,* edited by *Zhongjie Sun, 2005*
111. **Chemosensitivity:** *Volume 2, In Vivo Models, Imaging, and Molecular Regulators,* edited by *Rosalyn D. Blumethal, 2005*
110. **Chemosensitivity:** *Volume 1, In Vitro Assays,* edited by *Rosalyn D. Blumethal, 2005*
109. **Adoptive Immunotherapy:** *Methods and Protocols,* edited by *Burkhard Ludewig and Matthias W. Hoffman, 2005*
108. **Hypertension:** *Methods and Protocols,* edited by *Jérôme P. Fennell and Andrew H. Baker, 2005*
107. **Human Cell Culture Protocols,** *Second Edition,* edited by *Joanna Picot, 2005*
106. **Antisense Therapeutics,** *Second Edition,* edited by *M. Ian Phillips, 2005*
105. **Developmental Hematopoiesis:** *Methods and Protocols,* edited by *Margaret H. Baron, 2005*
104. **Stroke Genomics:** *Methods and Reviews,* edited by *Simon J. Read and David Virley, 2004*
103. **Pancreatic Cancer:** *Methods and Protocols,* edited by *Gloria H. Su, 2004*
102. **Autoimmunity:** *Methods and Protocols,* edited by *Andras Perl, 2004*
101. **Cartilage and Osteoarthritis:** *Volume 2, Structure and In Vivo Analysis,* edited by *Frédéric De Ceuninck, Massimo Sabatini, and Philippe Pastoureau, 2004*
100. **Cartilage and Osteoarthritis:** *Volume 1, Cellular and Molecular Tools,* edited by *Massimo Sabatini, Philippe Pastoureau, and Frédéric De Ceuninck, 2004*
99. **Pain Research:** *Methods and Protocols,* edited by *David Z. Luo, 2004*
98. **Tumor Necrosis Factor:** *Methods and Protocols,* edited by *Angelo Corti and Pietro Ghezzi, 2004*
97. **Molecular Diagnosis of Cancer:** *Methods and Protocols, Second Edition,* edited by *Joseph E. Roulston and John M. S. Bartlett, 2004*
96. **Hepatitis B and D Protocols:** *Volume 2, Immunology, Model Systems, and Clinical Studies,* edited by *Robert K. Hamatake and Johnson Y. N. Lau, 2004*
95. **Hepatitis B and D Protocols:** *Volume 1, Detection, Genotypes, and Characterization,* edited by *Robert K. Hamatake and Johnson Y. N. Lau, 2004*
94. **Molecular Diagnosis of Infectious Diseases,** *Second Edition,* edited by *Jochen Decker and Udo Reischl, 2004*
93. **Anticoagulants, Antiplatelets, and Thrombolytics,** edited by *Shaker A. Mousa, 2004*
92. **Molecular Diagnosis of Genetic Diseases,** *Second Edition,* edited by *Rob Elles and Roger Mountford, 2004*
91. **Pediatric Hematology:** *Methods and Protocols,* edited by *Nicholas J. Goulden and Colin G. Steward, 2003*
90. **Suicide Gene Therapy:** *Methods and Reviews,* edited by *Caroline J. Springer, 2004*
89. **The Blood–Brain Barrier:** *Biology and Research Protocols,* edited by *Sukriti Nag, 2003*
88. **Cancer Cell Culture:** *Methods and Protocols,* edited by *Simon P. Langdon, 2003*
87. **Vaccine Protocols,** *Second Edition,* edited by *Andrew Robinson, Michael J. Hudson, and Martin P. Cranage, 2003*
86. **Renal Disease:** *Techniques and Protocols,* edited by *Michael S. Goligorsky, 2003*

METHODS IN MOLECULAR MEDICINE™

Fibrosis Research

Methods and Protocols

Edited by

John Varga, MD

Feinberg School of Medicine, Northwestern University, Chicago, IL

David A. Brenner, MD

College of Physicians and Surgeons, Columbia University, New York, NY

Sem H. Phan, MD, PhD

University of Michigan Medical School, Ann Arbor, MI

HUMANA PRESS ✱ TOTOWA, NEW JERSEY

999 Riverview Drive, Suite 208
Totowa, New Jersey 07512
humanapress.com

This publication is printed on acid-free paper. ∞
ANSI Z39.48-1984 (American Standards Institute) Permanence of Paper for Printed Library Materials.

Production Editor: C. Tirpak and Melissa Caravella
Cover design by Patricia F. Cleary

Cover Illustration: From Fig. 4 in Chapter 10, "Morphological Methods for Assessment of Fibrosis," by Rakesh K. Kumar and Fig. 1 in Chapter 12, "Approaches to Evaluation of Fibrogenic Pathways in Surgical Lung Biopsy Specimens," by Cory M. Hogaboam, Kristin J. Carpenter, Holly Evanoff, and Steven L. Kunkel.

For additional copies, pricing for bulk purchases, and/or information about other Humana titles, contact Humana at the above address or at any of the following numbers: Tel: 973-256-1699; Fax: 973-256-8341; E-mail: orders@humanapr.com; or visit our Website: www.humanapress.com

Printed in the United States of America. 10 9 8 7 6 5 4 3 2 1
eISBN 1-59259-940-0

Library of Congress Cataloging-in-Publication Data

Fibrosis research : methods and protocols / edited by John Varga, David A. Brenner, Sem H. Phan.
p. ; cm. -- (Methods in molecular medicine ; 117)
Includes bibliographical references and index.
ISBN 1-58829-479-X (alk. paper)
1. Fibrosis. 2. fibrosis–Research–Methodology.
[DNLM: 1. Fibrosis. 2. Cultured Cells. 3. Extracellular
Matrix–metabolism. 4. Models, Animal. QZ 150 F4436 2005]
I. Varga, John.
II. Brenner, David, 1953-
III. Phan, Sem Hin, 1949- IV. Series.
RB150.F52F54 2005
616.7'42–dc22

2005006567

Preface

Fibrosis or scar, defined pathologically as inappropriate repair by connective tissue, is increasingly recognized as an important feature of many chronic diseases (Table 1), and as such, represents an enormous health burden. The United States government estimates that 45% of deaths in the United States can be attributed to fibrosing disorders. Fibrosis can affect virtually every tissue and organ system. Traditionally, fibrosis has been viewed as the irreversible, end-stage sequel to a multitude of diverse disease processes (Table 2). Excessive scarring following physical, thermal, metabolic, ischemic, infectious, inflammatory, or immunological injury can occur in any part of the body, and can cause destruction of the affected structures. Fibrotic tissue is characterized by a loss of normal architecture, paucity of stromal cells, and replacement of blood vessels and other essential parenchymal structures by dense, homogeneous, and increasingly stable extracellular matrix. The scar is composed primarily of type I collagen, but types III and IV collagens, proteoglycans, fibronectin, glycoproteins, and matricellular proteins are also prominent. The process leads to progressive distortion of tissue architecture with consequent dysfunction and ultimate failure of fibrotic organs. Many of the key morphological features of fibrosis are common to scarring affecting the lungs, the liver, the kidneys, the heart, or the skin.

Fibrosis is the "dark side" of normal tissue repair. Following injury, a complex and tightly orchestrated repertoire of cellular responses is called into play, and normally the wound is rapidly and efficiently repaired. This process is spatially and temporally self-limited. In contrast, under some conditions repair is excessive, resulting in pathological scar formation. The pathogenesis of fibrosis remains poorly understood. Fibrosis involves a "fibrogenic cascade" integrating multiple molecular pathways and cellular targets. Historically, the link between inflammation and fibrosis has been emphasized, providing the rationale for anti-inflammatory or immunosuppressive therapies for fibrosis. It has become increasingly evident that these types of interventions are generally ineffective. The lack of effective treatments, and the high mortality and increasing morbidity attributed to chronic fibrotic diseases, has stimulated an explosion of research into the cellular, molecular, and genetic basis of fibrosis.

Recent research progress has led to new and evolving concepts regarding the mechanisms that drive the process of fibrosis. Novel insights include the identification and characterization of an increasingly large panel of molecules

Table 1
Selected Diseases Where Fibrosis Is a Major Cause of Morbidity or Mortality

Organ-specific

- Lung fibrosis (idiopathic and drug-induced pulmonary fibrosis, asthma, sarcoidosis, COPD)
- Liver fibrosis (alcoholic cirrhosis, posthepatitis C cirrhosis, schistosomiasis, primary biliary cirrhosis, sclerosing cholangitis)
- Kidney fibrosis (diabetic nephropathy, lupus glomerulossclerosis)
- Heart fibrosis (post-MI scar)
- Vascular fibrosis (postangioplasty arterial restenosis, atherosclerosis
- Skin fibrosis (burn scar, hypertrophic scar, keloid, nephrogenic fibrosing dermatopathy)
- Eye fibrosis (retro-orbital fibrosis, postcataract surgery, proliferative vitreoretinopathy)
- Bone marrow (idiopathic and drug-induced myelofibrosis)
- Other (Peyronie's disease, thyroid, Dupuytren's contracture, dermatomyositis)

Systemic

- Systemic sclerosis
- Chronic graft vs host disease

Table 2
Association of Fibrosis With Types of Injury: Representative Examples

Burn	Skin and soft tissue scarring and contraction
Physical	Hypertrophic scar, keloid, postangioplasty vascular restenosis
Radiation	Pulmonary fibrosis; skin fibrosis; myelofibrosis
Surgery	Adhesions of visceral organs
Metabolic	Alcoholic cirrhosis, diabetic nephropathy, dialysis-related fibrosing dermatopathy
Ischemic	Post-MI cardiac fibrosis, post-stroke brain scarring
Autoimmune	Systemic sclerosis, myositis, lupus nephritis, chronic graft vs host disease
Inflammatory	Retroperitoneal fibrosis, asthma, sarcoidosis, atherosclerosis, primary biliary cirrhosis
Infectious	Hepatitic C-associated cirrhosis, schistosomal cirrhosis, HIV-associated lymphoid fibrosis
Malignant	Myelofibrosis

that mediate abnormal deposition of extracellular matrix, as well as the cellular constituents that produce and/or react to these molecules. Significant unanswered issues involve basic cellular and molecular mechanisms related to cell proliferation, motility, differentiation, and gene expression. For instance, recent discoveries on the heterogeneity of fibroblast populations in fibrotic lesions have relevance to understanding cellular differentiation and program of gene expression that determines cell phenotype. The demonstration of epithelial–mesenchymal transdifferentiation as a key element in the pathogenesis of renal fibrosis illustrates the need for further research into basic mechanisms to advance the field. The importance of the myofibroblastic phenotype requires improvement in current understanding of how activation and/or transdifferentiation is regulated in the context of progressive fibrosis. Elucidation of mechanisms involved in the regulation of extracellular matrix production and degradation is critical for understanding the basis for the abnormal deposition of connective tissue elements that is the hallmark of fibrosis. The advent of powerful techniques for global assessment of gene expression in cells and tissues should prove an impetus for rapid progress in this area. At the tissue and organismal level, improvement in methods for evaluating the extent, severity, and activity of fibrosis is essential for more precise and less invasive diagnostic and prognostic assessment, as well as for monitoring of therapeutic efficacy.

It is now widely appreciated that the diverse fibroproliferative diseases, be they immunological, metabolic, inflammatory, genetic, or iatrogenic in nature, all have important pathogenetic features in common. That is to say, despite their differing anatomic distribution and clinical manifestations, etiology and natural history, the pathogenesis of these disorders appears to be related. Thus, regardless of whether fibrosis involves the lung parenchyma or airways, the renal glomerulus or interstitium, the parenchyma or biliary tree of the liver, the gastrointestinal tract, the heart, the dermis or tendons, or the eye, in each case secretion and activation of profibrotic cytokines, particularly transforming growth factor (TGF)-β, expansion and activation of mesenchymal cell populations, and extracellular matrix synthesis and organization similarly result in progressive destruction of normal tissue (Table 3).

Fibrosis research is an emerging field. The challenges facing investigators engaged in fibrosis research are many: to describe and annotate the full repertoire of fibrotic mediators and effector cells involved in the fibrotic response, and characterize their deregulation in pathological fibrosis; to identify genes and their variants linked to fibrosis, and define their role in pathogenesis; to recognize shared pathogenetic themes that are common to distinct forms of fibrosis; and ultimately, to translate these insights into the development of specific

Table 3
Underlying Pathophysiologic Processes Common to Different Fibrotic Diseases

Genetic susceptibility
Inflammation
- T-cell activation, Th2 polarization; macrophage activation; eosinophil and mast cell chemotaxis; cytokine and chemokine production
- Vascular injury, endothelial adhesion molecule upregulation

Mesenchymal cell activation
- Increased synthesis of extracellular matrix
- Secretion and activation of TGF-β, other fibrotic cytokines, autocrine stimulation and amplification
- Migration

Cell differentiation
- Myofibroblast transdifferentiation
- Epithelial–mesenchymal transition
- Bone marrow-derived mesenchymal progenitor cell influx and differentiation

Scar formation and persistence; tissue destruction
- Connective tissue contraction
- Blood vessel obliteration, defective vasculogenesis, tissue hypoxia
- Matrix stabilization, collagen crosslinking
- Defective matrix remodeling and degradation

and sensitive diagnostic tools and safe and effective therapies to slow, prevent, and reverse organ fibrosis. For this undertaking to succeed, interactions between laboratory researchers and clinical investigators and clinicians from many different specialities is a must, since fibrosis impacts all fields of Medicine. The 22 chapters of *Fibrosis Research: Methods and Protocols* highlight the interdisciplinary nature of fibrosis research, and emphasize the broad applicability of these experimental methodologies to all areas of fibrosis research.

The book is divided into four parts. Part 1 features a brief introduction to the problem of fibrosis, with clinical overviews of pulmonary and renal fibrosis as examples illustrative of the many fibrosing disorders listed in Table 1, and a bird's-eye view of TGF-β as a paradigm profibrotic mediator. Part 2 focuses on widely used research methodologies utilizing cultured cells to model various aspects of the fibrotic response in vitro. The isolation, characterization, and propagation of mesenchymal cells are described, highlighting similarities and differences between methods that are appropriate for different types of fibroblasts. Chapters 7 to 10 discuss approaches for studying collagen gene regulation and TGF-β production. Part 3 focuses on experimental methodologies utilizing animal models to study the pathogenesis of fibrosis, discussing the advantages and limitations of each. Part 4 covers the evolving genetic approaches to identifying "fibrosis genes" or allelic polymorphisms in human populations, microarray studies for describing global patterns of gene expression associated with fibrosis, and proteomic approaches to the same.

As editors of this new and innovative book, *Fibrosis Research: Methods and Protocols*, we hope that it will reach a broad audience, and prove to be helpful to investigators studying any aspect of pathological fibrosis. It is our further hope that the book will stimulate discussion and promote interdisciplinary research collaborations, with the goal of understanding the daunting problem of fibrosis.

We wish to acknowledge Francesco Ramirez, Sergio Jimenez, Humphrey Gardner, William Schnaper, Partricia Greenwel, Steven Ackerman, and the many other colleagues who have provided helpful suggestions and stimulating discussion in preparation of this book.

John Varga, MD
David A. Brenner, MD
Sem H. Phan, MD, PhD

Contents

Contributors

CAROLYN J. BAGLOLE • *Department of Environmental Medicine, University of Rochester, Rochester, NY*

RAMÓN BATALLER • *Liver Unit, Hospital Clinic, IDIBAPS, University of Barcelona School of Medicine, Catalunya, Spain*

JOHN A. BELPERIO • *Division of Pulmonary and Critical Care Medicine, David Geffen School of Medicine at University of California, Los Angeles, CA*

MARY BIRCH • *School of Biological Sciences, University of Manchester, Manchester, UK*

DAVID A. BRENNER • *Department of Medicine, College of Physicians and Surgeons, Columbia University, New York, NY*

LAURANELL H. BURCH • *Division of Pulmonary, Allergy, and Critical Care Medicine, Duke University Medical Center, Durham, NC*

KRISTIN J. CARPENTER • *Department of Pathology, University of Michigan Medical School, Ann Arbor, MI*

YAN CHEN • *Departments of Cell Biology and Medicine, New York University School of Medicine, New York, NY*

YOUKYUNG HWANG CHOI • *Department of Medicine, Emory University School of Medicine, Atlanta, GA*

CHRISTOTHEA CONSTANDINOU • *Liver Research Group, University of Southampton, Southampton General Hospital, Southampton, UK*

BRANKA DABOVIC • *Departments of Cell Biology and Medicine, New York University School of Medicine, New York, NY*

NILESH B. DAVÉ • *Dorothy P. & Richard P. Simmons Center for Interstitial Lung Disease, Pulmonary, Allergy, and Critical Care Medicine, University of Pittsburgh Medical Center, Pittsburgh, PA*

CHRISTOPHER PAUL DAY • *School of Clinical Medical Sciences (Hepatology), University of Newcastle and Freeman Hospital, Newcastle Upon Tyne, UK*

HOLLY EVANOFF • *Department of Pathology, University of Michigan Medical School, Ann Arbor, MI*

STEVEN E. FELDON • *Department of Ophthalmology, University of Rochester, Rochester, NY*

GARY J. FISHER • *Department of Dermatology, University of Michigan, Ann Arbor, MI*

MARK W. J. FERGUSON • *School of Biological Sciences, University of Manchester, Manchester, UK*

MEHRNAZ GHARAEE-KERMANI • *Department of Internal Medicine, University of Michigan Medical School, Ann Arbor, MI*

RONALD H. GOLDSTEIN • *The Pulmonary Center, Boston University School of Medicine, The Boston VA Medical Center, Boston, MA*

AXEL M. GRESSNER • *Institute of Clinical Chemistry and Pathobiochemistry, University Hospital Aachen, Aachen, Germany*

CURT H. HAGEDORN • *Department of Medicine, Emory University School of Medicine, Atlanta, GA*

NEIL HENDERSON • *MRC Center for Inflammation Research, Edinburgh University, Edinburgh, UK*

CORY M. HOGABOAM • *Department of Pathology, University of Michigan Medical School, Ann Arbor, MI*

JOHN P. IREDALE • *Liver Research Group, University of Southampton, Southampton General Hospital, Southampton, UK*

VLADIMIR JURUKOVSKI • *Department of Biochemistry and Cell Biology, SUNY at Stony Brook, Stony Brook, NY*

RAGHU KALLURI • *Center for Matrix Biology, Department of Medicine, Beth Israel Deaconess Medical Center and Harvard Medical School, Boston, MA*

NAFTALI KAMINSKI • *Dorothy P. & Richard P. Simmons Center for Interstitial Lung Disease, Pulmonary, Allergy, and Critical Care Medicine, University of Pittsburgh Medical Center, Pittsburgh, PA*

NORIFUMI KAWADA • *Department of Hepatology, Graduate School of Medicine, Osaka City University, Osaka, Japan*

MICHAEL P. KEANE • *Division of Pulmonary and Critical Care Medicine, David Geffen School of Medicine at University of California, Los Angeles, CA*

PING-PING KUANG • *The Pulmonary Center, Boston University School of Medicine, The Boston VA Medical Center, Boston, MA*

RAKESH K. KUMAR • *Department of Pathology, School of Medical Sciences, University of New South Wales, Sydney, Australia*

STEVEN L. KUNKEL • *Department of Pathology, University of Michigan Medical School, Ann Arbor, MI*

JOSEPH P. LYNCH, III • *Division of Pulmonary and Critical Care Medicine, David Geffen School of Medicine at University of California, Los Angeles, CA*

ALAIN MAUVIEL • *INSERM U697, Hopital Saint-Louis, Paris, France*

ROBIN J. MCANULTY • *Center for Respiratory Research, Department of Medicine, University College London, London, UK*

Sem H. Phan • *Department of Pathology, University of Michigan Medical School, Ann Arbor, MI*
Richard P. Phipps • *Department of Environmental Medicine, University of Rochester, Rochester, NY*
Stephen J. Pollock • *Department of Environmental Medicine, University of Rochester, Rochester, NY*
Sireesha Y. Reddy • *Department of Obstetrics and Gynecology, University of Rochester, Rochester, NY*
Daniel B. Rifkin • *Departments of Cell Biology and Medicine, New York University School of Medicine, New York, NY*
Richard A. Rippe • *Division of Gastroenterology and Hepatology, University of North Carolina Chapel Hill, Chapel Hill, NC*
David C. Rishikof • *The Pulmonary Center, Boston University School of Medicine, The Boston VA Medical Center, Boston, MA*
Laure Rittié • *Department of Dermatology, University of Michigan, Ann Arbor, MI*
Bernd Schnabl • *Department of Internal Medicine I, University of Regensburg, Regensburg, Germany*
H. William Schnaper • *Department of Pediatrics, Northwestern University, Children's Memorial Research Center, Chicago, IL*
David A. Schwartz • *Division of Pulmonary, Allergy, and Critical Care Medicine, Duke University Medical Center, Durham, NC*
Patricia J. Sime • *Division of Pulmonary and Critical Care Medicine, University of Rochester, Rochester, NY*
Terry J. Smith • *Division of Molecular Medicine, Harbor-UCLA Medical Center, Torrence, CA*
Mary A. Soubasakos • *Center for Matrix Biology, Department of Medicine, Beth Israel Deaconess Medical Center and Harvard Medical School, Boston, MA*
Branko Stefanovic • *Division of Gastroenterology and Hepatology, University of North Carolina Chapel Hill, Chapel Hill, NC*
Robert M. Strieter • *Division of Pulmonary and Critical Care Medicine, Department of Pathology and Laboratory Medicine, David Geffen School of Medicine at University of California, Los Angeles, CA*
Mangalalaxmy Subramanian • *The Pulmonary Center, Boston University School of Medicine, The Boston VA Medical Center, Boston, MA*
Yao Sun • *Division of Cardiovascular Diseases, Department of Medicine, University of Tennessee Health Science Center, Memphis, TN*
Vesna Todorovic • *Departments of Cell Biology and Medicine, New York University School of Medicine, New York, NY*

ANNETTE TOMLINSON • *School of Biological Sciences, University of Manchester, Manchester, UK*

MATTHEW ULLENBRUCH • *Department of Pathology, University of Michigan Medical School, Ann Arbor, MI*

JOHN VARGA • *Feinberg School of Medicine, Northwestern University, Chicago, IL*

KARL T. WEBER • *Division of Cardiovascular Diseases, Department of Medicine, University of Tennesse Health Science Center, Memphis, TN*

RALF WEISKIRCHEN • *Institute of Clinical Chemistry and Pathobiochemistry, University Hospital Aachen, Aachen, Germany*

MICHAEL ZEISBERG • *Center for Matrix Biology, Department of Medicine, Beth Israel Deaconess Medical Center and Harvard Medical School, Boston, MA*

DAVID A. ZISMAN • *Division of Pulmonary and Critical Care Medicine, David Geffen School of Medicine at University of California, Los Angeles, CA*

I

The Clinical Scope of Fibrosis

1

Pulmonary Fibrosis

David A. Zisman, Michael P. Keane, John A. Belperio, Robert M. Strieter, and Joseph P. Lynch, III

Summary

Idiopathic pulmonary fibrosis (IPF) is a chronic fibrosing lung disease limited to the lungs and associated with the histologic appearance of usual interstitial pneumonia (UIP) on surgical lung biopsy. The estimated prevalence in the United States is between 35,000 and 55,000 cases, and evidence suggests that the prevalence is increasing for IPF. Risk factors associated with pulmonary fibrosis include smoking, environmental exposures, gastroesophageal reflux disease, commonly prescribed drugs, diabetes mellitus, infectious agents, and genetic factors. The diagnosis requires a careful history and physical examination, characteristic physiological and radiological studies, and, in some cases, a surgical lung biopsy. The natural history of IPF is not known, but evidence supports the concept of a continuum of idiopathic interstitial pneumonias that may overlap in time. Most patients with IPF succumb to respiratory failure, cardiovascular disease, lung cancer, pulmonary embolism, infection, and other health problems. The median survival time for patients with IPF is less than 3 yr. Factors that predict poor outcome include older age, male gender, severe dyspnea, history of cigarette smoking, severe loss of lung function, appearance and severity of fibrosis on radiological studies, lack of response to therapy, and prominent fibroblastic foci on histopathologic evaluation. Conventional therapy (corticosteroids, azathioprine, cyclophosphamide) provides only marginal benefit. Lung transplantation should be considered for patients with IPF refractory to medical therapy. In light of the poor prognosis and lack of response to available anti-inflammatory therapy, alternative approaches to therapy are being pursued. Emerging strategies to treat patients with IPF include agents that inhibit epithelial injury or enhance repair, anticytokine approaches, agents that inhibit fibroblast proliferation or induce fibroblast apoptosis, and other novel approaches.

Key Words: Idiopathic pulmonary fibrosis; pulmonary fibrosis; interstitial lung disorders; idiopathic interstitial pneumonias; diffuse interstitial pneumonia; occupational lung disease; hypersensitivity pneumonitis; cryptogenic fibrosing alveolitis; connective tissue disorders and lung involvement.

1. Introduction

The diagnosis and management of idiopathic interstitial pneumonias (IIPs) remains a challenge to the clinician. Recently, there have been substantial

From: *Methods in Molecular Medicine, Vol. 117: Fibrosis Research: Methods and Protocols*
Edited by: J. Varga, D. A. Brenner, and S. H. Phan © Humana Press Inc., Totowa, NJ

changes in our understanding and approach to theses diseases. With greater comprehension of the clinical relevance of the different histopathological subgroups that make up the idiopathic interstitial pneumonias, the term idiopathic pulmonary fibrosis (IPF) is now reserved to patients with idiopathic usual interstitial pneumonia (UIP) on surgical lung biopsy. The following review will provide an updated discussion of the epidemiology, risk factors, diagnosis, natural history, morbidity and mortality, prognosis, and conventional therapy of IPF, as well as emerging strategies for the treatment of patients with this disease.

2. Epidemiology

The true prevalence of IPF, also known as cryptogenic fibrosing alveolitis (CFA), is unknown. Despite the poor quality of the data and the changes in diagnostic criteria and classification, there is evidence suggesting that IPF is increasing *(1)*. There are approx 3 to 20.2 cases of IPF per 100,000 in the general population *(1–5)*. The prevalence increases with older age, history of smoking, and male gender *(3,4,6)*. In a population-based study in Bernalillo County, New Mexico, the prevalence for adults from age 35 to 44 yr was 2.7 per 100,000, but surpassed 175 per 100,000 for individuals older than 75 yr *(3)*. The prevalence of IPF is higher in men (20.2 cases per 100,000) than in women (13.2 cases per 100,000) *(3)*. The estimated prevalence in the United States is between 35,000 and 55,000 cases *(3)*.

The incidence of IPF is estimated at 10.7 cases per 100,000 per year for males and 7.4 cases per 100,000 per year for females *(3)*.

Vital statistics figures are limited and incomplete. In 1988, there were 30,000 hospitalizations and 4851 deaths in the United States owing to pulmonary fibrosis (compared with 665,000 hospitalizations owing to chronic obstructive pulmonary disease and asthma). In Japan, the mortality rate for IPF per 100,000 population was estimated to be 3.3 in men and 2.5 in women, with an overall rate of 3.0 in both sexes *(4)*. In the United Kingdom, the annual number of deaths from IPF increased twofold between 1979 and 1988. The age-adjusted rate of pulmonary fibrosis among deceased in the United States increased from 48.6 per 100,000 in 1979 to 50.9 per 100,000 in 1991 in males, and from 21.4 per 100,000 in 1979 to 27.2 per 100,000 in 1991 in females *(7)*. Pulmonary fibrosis listed as a cause of death increased from 40% in 1979 to 56% in 1991. In the United States, the age-adjusted mortality rates are highest in the western and southwestern states and lowest in the midwest and northeast. In the United Kingdom, highest mortality rates are found in industrialized areas of England and Wales *(7,8)*.

3. Risk Factors

3.1. Smoking

In case-control studies, smoking has been identified as a possible risk factor for IPF with an odds ratio (OR) of 1.6 (95% confidence interval [CI] 1.1–2.4) for ever-smoking, and 1.9 (95% CI 1.3–2.9) for former-smokers ***(4,9,10)***. Smokers of 21 to 40 pack-years have an OR of 2.3 (95% CI 1.3–3.8) for pulmonary fibrosis ***(9)***. In a recent study in Japan, the adjusted odds ratio for cigarette smoking was estimated at 5.40 (95% CI 2.30–12.66) ***(11)***. Interestingly, three studies reported improved survival among current or former smokers with UIP compared to never-smokers ***(12–14)***. However, others found no such effect ***(15–17)***. It is possible that the apparent protective effect of cigarette smoking may relate to the following: lead time bias; alterations in the balance of proteinases and antiproteinases that would influence net deposition of extracellular matrix in the lung; or inhibitory effects of cigarette smoke on lung fibroblast proliferation and chemotaxis ***(12,18)***.

3.2. Gastroesophageal Reflux

Instillation of acid in several animal models results in aspiration-induced lung injury and pulmonary fibrosis ***(19)***. Clinical data suggest that a high percentage of patients with IPF have clinically silent gastroesophageal reflux disease (GERD) ***(19,20)***. Small tracheobronchial aspirations of gastric acid may play a role in the pathogenesis of IPF; however, a causal relationship has not been established ***(19,20)***. Investigators at the University of Washington Medical Center are conducting an ongoing prospective study of 65 patients with IPF. Interim results indicate that the prevalence of IPF patients with GERD is 95%, with only 40% of patients reporting symptoms ***(19)***. However, the perpherial pattern of UIP in the lung would be unusual if GERD was truly the cause, as compared with an association.

3.3. Commonly Prescribed Drugs

In one case–control study, IPF was associated with exposure to antidepressants with an OR of 1.79 (95% CI 1.09–2.95), and specifically to imipramine (OR of 4.79 [95% CI 1.50–15.3]), dothiepin OR of 2.37 [95% CI 0.99–5.69]), and mianserin OR of 3.27 [95% CI 1.11–9.61]). These associations were independent of smoking and occupational dust exposure. The authors concluded that exposure to antidepressants may be responsible for approx 10% of cases of IPF seen in their population. No significant association was noted between IPF and the other drug groups tested (anticonvulsants, β-blockers, antibiotics, and nonsteroidal anti-inflammatory drugs [NSAIDs]) *(21)*.

3.4. Diabetes Mellitus

In a recent study, clinical and demographic data were extracted from medical records of 65 consecutive patients with IPF admitted to a Japanese hospital. IPF was associated with diabetes mellitus (DM) with and OR of 4.06 (95% CI 1.80–9.15). The authors concluded that DM might be a risk factor for IPF *(11)*.

3.5. Environmental Exposures

The etiology of IPF is unknown, but environmental factors may play a causative role. Metal and wood dust environments may be important risk factors for pulmonary fibrosis. In one study, metal dust exposure was identified as a risk factor with an odds ratio (OR) of 1.11 (95% CI 1.06–1.16), and wood dust exposure with an OR of 1.12 (95% CI 1.02–1.24). In that study, metal and wood dust exposure may have caused up to 13% and 10% of pulmonary fibrosis cases, respectively. Dust containing brass, lead, cobalt, aluminum, zinc, cadmium, mercury, and pine dusts were associated with pulmonary fibrosis *(10)*.

Certain occupations may predispose to pulmonary fibrosis. In one study, farming was identified as a potential risk factor with and OR of 1.6 (95% CI 1.0–2.5) and exposure to livestock was associated with an OR of 2.7 (95% CI 1.3–5.5). Hairdressing was linked to pulmonary fibrosis with an OR of 4.4 (95% CI 1.2–16.3), metal dust exposure with an OR of 2.0 (95% CI 1.0–4.0), raising birds with an OR of 4.5 (95% CI 1.6–14.1), stone cutting/polishing with an OR of 3.9 (95% CI 1.2–12.7), and vegetable/animal dust exposure with an OR of 4.7 (95% CI 2.1–10.4) *(22)*.

3.6. Infectious Agents

A number of viruses have been associated with pulmonary fibrosis, but true cause-effect relationships remain unproven. A serological survey found an association between active Epstein-Barr virus (EBV) infection and IPF *(23)*. Egan and colleagues reported immunohistochemical evidence of EBV-productive cycle antigens in type II alveolar epithelial cells in IPF *(24)*. Subsequently, these investigators detected EBV DNA by polymerase chain reaction (PCR) in the lung tissue of patients with IPF *(25)*. Further study demonstrated that productive EBV replication is common in IPF and it is not associated with immunosuppressive therapy *(26)*. Tang and co-workers detected one or more of four herpesviruses (cytomegalovirus [CMV], EBV, human herpesvirus 7 [HH-7], and human herpesvirus 8 [HHV-8]) in 97% of patients with IPF and 36% of controls, suggesting that a herpesvirus could be a source of chronic antigenic stimulation in IPF ***(27)***. Relatively high prevalence of serum antibodies to hepatitis C was demonstrated in patients with pulmonary fibrosis, but this finding was not confirmed in other studies ***(28–30)***. Adenovirus DNA was found in transbronchial lung biopsies (TBBx) from patients with IPF, and it was more prevalent in IPF patients treated with corticosteroids (67%) than in those who were not (10%), suggesting that this virus may newly infect or reactivate following corticosteroid therapy ***(31)***. A higher incidence of influenza ***(32–34)***, parainfluenza ***(35,36)***, CMV ***(37)***, human immunodeficiency virus (HIV)-1 ***(38)***, measles ***(39)***, herpes simplex virus-6, Mycoplasma, and Legionella has been reported in IPF ***(23,24,30,40)***.

In a recent study, human T-lymphtropic virus type I (HTVL-I) positive IPF patients had more affected lung parenchyma, demonstrated traction bronchiectasis with honeycomb change, and exhibited increased levels of specific cytokines that correlated with activated T-cells in the bronchoalveolar lavage fluid (BALF). These findings suggested that HTLV-I infection might contribute to the development of IPF via activation of T-cells ***(41)***. The latent nature together with episodic reactivation of many of these viruses may provide a scenario for the concept of "multiple hits" host defense followed by repair that these patients may experience during the course of their disease.

3.7. Genetic Factors

The genetics of familial IPF have not been elucidated. An autosomal dominant trait with variable penetrance may account for approx 70% of cases; there is no clear mode of transmission in the remaining 30% ***(2,42)***. Investigators have linked IPF to an increase in MZ phenotype for α1-antitrypsin inhibition on chromosome 14 ***(43–45)***. Using a candidate gene approach, researchers identified surfactant protein C gene mutations in large familial pulmonary fibrosis kindred, including adults with UIP and children with nonspecific interstitial pneumonia (NSIP) ***(46)***. In a separate study, Selman and co-workers demonstrated that Surfactant protein A and B genetic variants predispose to IPF ***(47)***. Genetic polymorphisms for interleukin-1 receptor antagonist (IL-1ra) and tumor necrosis factor (TFN)-α appear to be important in determining risk ***(48)***. In contrast, transforming growth factor (TGF)-β polymorphisms do not predispose to IPF, but these polymorphisms may affect the course of the disease ***(49)***.

It is unknown what proportion of IPF is familial, but it is estimated that 0.5 to 2.2% of cases have a genetic basis ***(42)***. Thirty-eight families affected by pulmonary fibrosis have been identified and are currently under active investigation. The familial aggregation in those families is consistent with a genetic basis in at least a subset of patients with IPF ***(50)***.

4. Diagnosis

IPF is a specific form of chronic fibrosing interstitial pneumonia limited to the lungs and associated with the histological pattern of UIP on surgical lung biopsy *(2)*. Many earlier studies included various other idiopathic interstitial pneumonias under the term idiopathic pulmonary fibrosis, but the clinical term IPF is now reserved to patients with idiopathic UIP.

4.1. History and Physical Examination

The diagnostic approach to any patient with diffuse lung disease must include a thorough history and physical examination with attention to symptoms or signs suggestive of a connective tissue disease, occupational or environmental exposures, use of fibrogenic drugs, and family history of pulmonary fibrosis. Patient age at disease onset is generally between 50 and 70 yr of age and IPF is more common in males than females. IPF typically presents insidiously, with gradual onset of a nonproductive cough and dyspnea *(2)*. Patients are often treated for other conditions such as congestive heart failure, "walking pneumonia," bronchitis, or asthma before the diagnosis is made. The physical examination in most patients (>80%) reveals fine bibasilar inspiratory crackles ("Velcro rales"), and clubbing is noted in up to 50% of patients *(51,52)*. Signs of right heart failure are evident in advanced cases *(2)*.

4.2. Laboratory and Serological Tests

Laboratory abnormalities are mild and nonspecific. One early study described "autoimmune factors" in blood of 8 patients (4 of whom had autoimmune-associated diseases) among 17 patients with diffuse fibrosing alveolitis *(53)*. A positive rheumatoid factor occurred in 3 of 20 patients with unexplained pulmonary fibrosis and positive antinuclear factor in the serum (ANA) *(54)*. A later study examined serum specimens from 122 patients with IPF and compared them with specimens from age- and sex-matched controls; ANAs were present in 21% of patients with IPF and in 6% of the control subjects *(55)*. Positive circulating ANAs or rheumatoid factor occur in 10% to 20% of patients with IPF, but titers are rarely high *(2,53,54,56)*. An elevated erythrocyte sedimentation rate, lactate dehydrogenase, or hypergammaglobulinemia may be found in patients with IPF, but are nondiagnostic *(2)*. Serological findings do not correlate with extent or severity of disease, and have no prognostic value *(2,57)*. In the absence of symptoms of connective tissue disease, the presence of autoantibodies does not imply an underlying systemic disorder. Recently, investigators reported the occurrence of low fasting triglyceride and high free fatty acid levels in patients with pulmonary fibrosis. Because insulin-like growth factor (IGF)-I is known to lower triglycerides and increase free fatty acids, the authors hypothesized that the reported increased production of IGF-I in patients with IPF may explain such findings ***(58)***.

4.3. Radiological Studies

4.3.1. Chest Radiograph

Classic chest radiographic findings in IPF include a basal predominant reticular, or reticulonodular, pattern associated with decreased lung volumes, and in later stages, cystic areas representing honeycomb (HC) lung ***(2,59–61)***. When a "confident" diagnosis of IPF is made on the basis of the chest radiograph, it is correct in 48 to 87% of cases ***(60,62,63)***. Most patients with IPF will have an abnormal chest radiograph but, rarely, patients may present with a normal plain film ***(2)***. It is important to review all previous chest films to assess the rate of change in disease activity. In addition, radiographs are indicated if clinical deterioration occurs in order to identify superimposed infection or malignancy ***(2,64)***. Pleural effusions, upper lobe predominant disease, air-bronchograms, or prominent lymphadenopathy should suggest an alternative diagnosis.

4.3.2. High-Resolution Chest Computed Tomography

Typical high-resolution chest computed tomography (HRCT) features of IPF/UIP include patchy, predominantly peripheral, subpleural, and symmetrical bibasilar honeycombing, reticular abnormalities, and limited "ground-glass" opacities (GGO) ***(65–68)***. Several studies have shown that experienced radiologists can make a "confident" diagnosis of UIP with specificity greater than 95%, provided CT features are typical ***(65,69–72)***. Although a characteristic HRCT is highly specific for IPF/UIP, "typical" HRCT identifies only 37 to 67% of patients with histological UIP; therefore, a surgical lung biopsy (SLB) is recommended when clinical and radiological information result in an uncertain diagnosis ***(14,65,70,73)***. One study evaluated the proficiency of physicians with expertise in interstitial lung diseases to identify accurately the HRCT scans from patients with biopsy-proven IPF/UIP. When these investigators made a "confident" diagnosis of IPF based on HRCT scan and clinical data, they were right in more than 80% of the cases. However, more than half of the patients with IPF had an uncertain diagnosis on the basis of HRCT and clinical assessment ***(70)***. In a subsequent analysis of these data, investigators identified HRCT features associated with a pathological diagnosis of UIP. On multivariate analysis, lower lobe honeycombing (OR, 5.36), and upper-lung irregular lines (OR, 6.28) were the only independent predictors of UIP. When they combined those two factors, a diagnosis of UIP was established with a sensitivity of 74%, a specificity of 81%, and a positive predictive value of 85%

(65). Interestingly, in that study, adenopathy was observed in 55% and 21% of patients with UIP and without UIP, respectively. This finding suggests that patients with IPF generate a marked lymphoproliferative response to an unknown antigen or antigens; we believe that this observation requires further investigation as it may provide important clues to further our understanding of the pathogenesis the disease. In a separate study, two radiologists independently assessed CT scans from a cohort of patients with either UIP. CT features were "typical" for UIP in only 37% patients, and all of them had histological UIP on SLB. Typical CT features of UIP are associated with advanced, late-stage disease. Among patients with earlier phases of UIP, CT features may be atypical *(74)* or indeterminate *(69)*.

Extensive GGO is not a major feature of UIP, and suggests an alternative diagnosis such as desquamative interstitial pneumonia (DIP), NSIP, lymphocytic interstitial pneumonia (LIP), cryptogenic organizing pneumonia (COP), hypersensitivity pneumonia (HP), or pulmonary alveolar proteinosis (PAP) *(75)*. In contrast, honeycomb change is a cardinal feature of UIP, and is rare in other IIPs *(71,76)*.

4.4. Physiological Studies

4.4.1. Pulmonary Function Testing

Pulmonary function tests (PFTs) characteristically reveal a restrictive ventilatory defect with impaired gas exchange; however, smokers may have preserved lung volumes or airflow obstruction in the initial stages of the disease *(2,77,78)*. Impairments in gas exchange (i.e., carbon monoxide diffusing capasity [DL_{CO}]) and oxygenation may be evident early in the course of the disease, even when spirometry and lung volumes are normal *(79)*. The most appropriate and simple tests are vital capacity and DL_{CO}; these are most useful for assessing the extent and monitoring the progression of the disease *(80)*.

4.4.2. Exercise Testing

Cardiopulmonary exercise testing (CPET) demonstrates hypoxemia, widened A-a O_2 gradient, submaximal exercise endurance, reduced oxygen consumption (VO_2), high respiratory frequency, low tidal volume (V_T) breathing pattern, increased dead space (V_D/V_T), increased minute ventilation for the level of VO_2, and a low O_2 pulse *(80–82)*. Arterial desaturation and abnormal widening of A-a O_2 gradient with exercise may be elicited with relatively simple tests, such as the 6-min walk test *(83,84)*.

4.5. Bronchoalveolar Lavage Fluid

BALF may play a role in the diagnosis of inorganic dust diseases, suspected malignancy, infections, some hematological disorders, drug-induced diseases, pulmonary alveolar proteinosis, Langerhans' cell histiocytosis, and alveolar hemorrhage ***(85)***. BALF is useful in research studies but of limited clinical application when evaluating IIPs ***(85)***. Increases in polymorphonuclear leukocytes, eosinophils, mast cells, alveolar macrophages, and countless cytokines are noted in BALF from patients with IPF/UIP; lymphocyte numbers are usually normal ***(2)***. BALF neutrophilia is present in 67 to 90% of patients with IPF/CFA ***(86,87)***, but does not predict prognosis or therapeutic responsiveness. Elevations in BALF eosinophils were associated with more severe clinical impairment ***(86,87)***, but BALF eosinophil counts do not correlate consistently with prognosis ***(86,87)***. By contrast, the presence of BALF lymphocytosis, found in fewer than 15% of cases, was associated with a greater responsiveness to corticosteroid therapy, a more cellular biopsy, and less honeycombing ***(86,87)***. Data compiled from two studies documented favorable responses to corticosteroids in 12 of 13 patients exhibiting BALF lymphocytosis, but in only 4 of 37 without lymphocytosis ***(86,87)***. Because the studies citing BALF lymphocytosis in steroid-responsive patients with IPF ***(87)*** or CFA ***(86)*** antedated the description of NSIP, it is possible that BALF lymphocytosis reflects disorders distinct from UIP (such as cellular NSIP). Nevertheless, in a recent study, researchers hypothesized that BALF findings may distinguish between UIP and NSIP; BALF total and differential cell counts were not different between the two groups, and in neither group, were BALF findings predictive of survival or changes in lung function ***(88)***.

4.6. Biopsy

The American Thoracic Society (ATS) and the European Respiratory Society (ERS) in collaboration with American College of Chest Physicians (ACCP) published an international consensus statement on the diagnosis and treatment of IPF. This statement stated that the definite diagnosis of IPF requires an SLB showing the UIP pattern. However, an SLB is not recommended in patients with suspected IPF in whom the clinical or radiographic information are stereotypical of IPF/UIP. It has been suggested that, in the absence of an SLB, the presence of all four major diagnostic criteria and at least three minor criteria increases the likelihood of an accurate diagnosis of IPF/UIP ***(2)***. However, these criteria have not been prospectively validated.

An SLB, preferably by video-assisted thoracoscopy (VATS), is recommended in patients with suspected IPF in whom the clinical or radiographic information are not typical of IPF/UIP ***(2)***. Given the patchy and heterogeneous nature of the UIP lesion, a large piece of lung tissue is required and TBBx are used mainly to rule out other disorders that mimic IPF. However, emerging data suggest that TBBx findings may be more useful in diagnosing UIP than previously recognized; characteristic histological features of UIP (interstitial fibrosis with fibroblastic foci [FF] and/or HC change) can be appreciated even in a small sample obtained by TBBx; these findings in a patient with characteristic clinical and radiographic features may indicate a diagnosis of UIP. However, these findings require prospective validation ***(89)***.

Significant advances have been made in our understanding of the idiopathic interstitial pneumonias (IIPs). The most important advancement has been the greater appreciation of the clinical relevance of the different histopathological subgroups that make up the IIPs. Until recently, inflammatory or fibrotic lung disorders of unknown etiology were "lumped" under the term IPF ***(2,75,90)***. However, with the advent of VATS lung biopsies and the greater availability and quality of surgical specimens, pathologists have recognized the heterogeneous nature of these disorders and described specific histopathological patterns that predict response to therapy and survival ***(74,91,92)***. IPF/UIP is the most common of the IIPs, comprised of 47 to 71% of the cases ***(76,91,93,94)***. The UIP lesion is characterized by temporal and geographic heterogeneity, with areas of old scar and HC change, admixed with granulation tissue and normal lung; the lesion has predilection for the subpleural and basilar regions of the lung, there is scant inflammation, and prominent aggregates of fibroblast and myofibroblasts, so-called "fibroblastic foci," which actively secreting extracellular matrix ***(75,92,95)***. Additional features include smooth muscle hypertrophy, metaplasia and hyperplasia of type II pneumocytes, destroyed and disrupted alveolar architecture, traction bronchiectasis and bronchioloectasis, and secondary pulmonary hypertension changes ***(75,92,95)***.

Other categories of IIP that must be distinguished from IPF/UIP include NSIP, DIP, respiratory bronchiolitis-associated interstitial lung disease (RBILD), acute interstitial pneumonia (AIP), COP, and LIP ***(75)***. NSIP is observed in approx 25% of patients with IIP ***(75)***. This provisional category is used to describe a temporally homogeneous lesion with varying degrees of inflammation and fibrosis with favorable response to therapy and prognosis. NSIP can be subdivided into NSIP-cellular and NSIP-fibrotic varieties depending on the degree of inflammation and fibrosis present in the surgical specimen ***(93)***. This subclassification provides important prognostic information; patients with idiopathic NSIP, cellular pattern have a better 5- and 10-yr survival than those with idiopathic NSIP, fibrosing pattern (100% vs 90% and 100% vs 35%, respectively) ***(93)***.

In many patients, however, histological overlap between UIP and NSIP is evident. Flaherty and co-workers reviewed SLBs from 109 patients with IIP who had multiple lobes biopsied and reported histopathological variability between lobes in 26% of patients. Importantly, in that study, UIP in at least one lobe defined prognosis ***(94)***. In a later study, the pathological findings in biopsy and subsequent explant specimens from 20 patients with UIP were reviewed to refine histological criteria and to assess the relationship between UIP and NSIP. The important new finding was that NSIP-like areas were present in the majority of UIP patients (80%) in both biopsy and explants specimens, and in some, these areas were extensive, making accurate diagnosis of UIP difficult (cases were misdiagnosed as NSIP). The most useful feature for diagnosing UIP in difficult cases is the presence of a distinct "patchwork" or variegated pattern of parenchymal involvement *(95)*.

RBILD and DIP comprise approx 15% of IIPs *(75)*. These entities are thought to be smoking-related diseases and, like NSIP, tend to be responsive to anti-inflammatory therapy. This is not surprising, as pathologically, these lesions are characterized by varying degrees of intra-alveolar and/or peribronchial pigmented macrophage infiltration with scant or no fibrosis. AIP is characterized by active fibrosis consisting of proliferating fibroblasts and myofibroblasts with minimal collagen deposition resembling the organizing stage of diffuse alveolar damage (DAD) *(92)*. Finally within the IIPs, some include COP (previously termed bronchiolitis obliterans organizing pneumonia, or BOOP), and LIP. Both are relatively steroid-responsive lesions; pathologically, COP is characterized by the presence of intra-alveolar plugs of granulation tissue, and LIP by lymphocytic infiltration of the alveolar walls. It should be noted, however, that many experts argue that LIP should not be included within the IIPs because it is considered as lymphoproliferative disorder which, in turn, is rarely idiopathic and is mostly observed in association with infections (e.g., HIV) or collagen vascular diseases (CVDs) *(75)*.

5. Natural History

The natural history of the pathogenesis of IPF is not known. The description of temporal heterogeneity for the histopathological entity of UIP would suggest that this process occurs over a significant period of time within the same low-power microscopic field of the lung. Moreover, the description supports the notion that the lesions are not homogeneous for both the timing of the orginal injury and the subsequent response to the injury and repair. In addition, the histopathological entity of UIP is not unique to IPF, and can be found in patients with connective tissue diseases, end-stage asbestosis, and end-stage hypersensitivity pneumonia. Therefore, UIP may represent an end-stage of a "process," not the beginning, intermediate, and end-stage of a disease. The only insight into the natural history of this process comes from two recent studies that suggest the potential concept of a continuum of IIPs that may overlap in time.

In a study of 109 patients whom had multiple lobes biopsied, histological variability was evident in 26% of the patients. Patients concordant for UIP were older (63 ± 9 yr) than those discordant for UIP (57 ± 12 yr) or with fibrotic NSIP (56 ± 11 yr) or cellular NSIP (50 ± 9 yr), suggesting that NSIP may be an early lesion that progresses with time to UIP ***(94)***. In a separate study, investigators found discordant histological diagnoses between lobes in 20% of the patients. NSIP-like reactions were evident in 80% of patients with UIP, suggesting that NSIP may evolve into UIP ***(95)***. In a genetic study, two different histopathological patterns of interstitial pneumonia were found to exist in members of a family who shared protein C gene mutations: adults with UIP and children with NSIP; this supports the notion that NSIP may be a precursor lesion to UIP ***(46)***.

It has been suggested that most patients with IPF progress in a relentless and insidious manner with a median survival of less than 3 yr ***(91)***. This concept was challenged in a recent study of subcutaneous interferon (IFN)-γ1b (200 μg thrice weekly) in 330 patients with mild to moderate IPF (forced vital capacity [FVC] > 50% and DL_{CO} > 30%), where a trend toward lower mortality was seen in IFN-γ1b-treated patients compared with placebo-treated patients ***(96)***. Interestingly, there were no significant differences in lung function or gas exchange between IFN-γ1b-treated and placebo-treated patients at 48 wk of follow-up. In both study groups, 70% of patients remained stable, 25% deteriorated, and the rest improved, suggesting that most patients with mild to moderate IPF remain stable for at least 1 yr on no specific therapy. The so-called "IPF exacerbations" may explain the trend toward lower mortality seen in this study, but this requires further study. IPF exacerbations may be defined as an accelerated deterioration of IPF in the absence of apparent infectious agents and heart failure ***(97,98)***. It is often a terminal event, with features of DAD or organizing pneumonia on lung biopsy or autopsy ***(99,100)***. This syndrome is indistinguishable from idiopathic AIP ***(101)***, and is similar to acute respiratory distress syndrome (ARDS). The factors responsible for this accelerated phase of IPF are unknown, but viral infections, high concentrations of oxygen, or drug reactions are plausible etiological factors ***(101)***.

6. Morbidity and Mortality

Only one study has addressed mechanism of mortality of patients with IPF. Panos and colleagues ***(102)*** found that most patients with IPF succumb to respiratory failure (39%), cardiovascular disease (27%), lung cancer (6–13%), pulmonary embolism (3%), infection (3%), or other health problems (18%) ***(102)***. Although infection would appear unlikely as a cause of mortality in IPF patients, clinically we can only determine the micro-organism cause of community acquired pneumonia in 30% of all patients. Therefore, we do not know the true incidence and prevalence of infection as a cause of mortality in patients with IPF, and perhaps a significant portion of the respiratory failure mortalities had infectious etiologies. With regard to cardiovascular disease, congestive heart failure and coronary artery disease (CAD) account for 30% of deaths ***(102)***. Patients with IPF appear to be at increased risk of developing CAD. In a cross-sectional study of 630 patients referred for lung transplantation, fibrotic lung diseases were associated with an increased prevalence of CAD compared with nonfibrotic diseases after adjustment for traditional risk factors (OR 2.18; 95% CI, 1.17–4.06); the authors theorized that the fibroproliferative process may influence cells beyond the pulmonary compartment, and that mediator molecules produced in these disorders might promote atherogenesis ***(67)***.

Pulmonary arterial hypertension occurs in 70% of patients with advanced IPF and its presence correlates with a vital capacity (VC) below 50% of predicted or a DL_{CO} under 45% of predicted ***(102)***. Left ventricular (LV) dysfunction occurs in less than 10% of patients and it is mostly (66%) a result of coexisting right heart failure. Other causes of LV dysfunction include ischemic and hypertensive heart disease ***(5,102)***. Six to 13% of patients with IPF develop bronchogenic carcinoma. Lung cancer in patients with IPF typically presents as a peripheral squamous cell carcinoma in older male smokers ***(103)***. Predisposing factors include squamous metaplasia, atypical epithelial cells, or occupational exposures ***(13,57,102)***. Hubbard and colleagues, in a population-based cohort in the United Kingdom, studied 890 patients with IPF and 5884 controls. The risk ratio for IPF and lung cancer was 7.31 (95% CI 4.5–11.9). Importantly, adjusting for previous smoking had little effect on this ratio, suggesting that IPF is an independent risk factor for lung cancer ***(104)***.

Pulmonary embolism occurs in approx 3 to 7% of patients; inactivity, heart failure, bronchogenic carcinoma, and possibly corticosteroid therapy predispose patients to thrombosis ***(102)***. Pulmonary infection causes 2 to 4% of deaths in patients with IPF; immunosuppressive therapy, traction bronchiectasis, and possibly GERD are predisposing factors ***(102)***. Pneumothorax occurs in up to 10% of patients with IPF and tends to be less responsive to tube thoracostomy, often necessitating surgical intervention ***(102)***.

6.1. Complications of Therapy

Corticosteroids (CS) can cause a myriad of side effects including myopathy, peptic ulcer disease, cataracts, osteoporosis, compression fractures, fluid and electrolyte abnormalities, adrenal insufficiency, and infection ***(105,106)***. In a cross-sectional study in patients with asthma, chronic obstructive pulmonary disease, or "alveolitis" taking oral corticosteroids (n = 367) vs controls (n = 734), the OR for bone fractures was 1.8 (95% CI 1.3–2.6 [vertebral fracture OR 10, hip fracture OR 6, and ribs or sternum fracture OR 3.2]). Patients taking corticosteroids experienced more cataracts, used more antacids, had more muscle weakness, back pain, bruising, and oral candidiasis, and had fewer teeth compared with controls ***(106)***. One prospective study included 41 patients with IPF; 24 received 100 mg/d of prednisone for 3 mo and 17 received 60 mg/d for 1 mo followed by 40 mg/d for 2 mo. Patients were monitored monthly for steroid-related side effects. All patients experienced at least one side effect. Common side effects included insomnia (76%), cushingoid change (73%), weight gain (71%), irritability (61%), infection (49%), blurred vision (41%), abdominal bloating (34%), glucose intolerance (24%), and fractures or avascular necrosis (10%) ***(105)***.

Cytotoxic agents (cyclophosphamide [CP], azathioprine [AZA]) can cause infections, bone marrow suppression, hepatitis, hemorrhagic cystitis (CP) and/or malignancies ***(107,108)***. In a prospective uncontrolled study, 19 patients with biopsy-proven UIP who were unresponsive or intolerant to CS therapy were treated with oral CP (1–2 mg/kg/d) for 6 mo. Nearly two-thirds of patients reported adverse effects, and 50% of patients discontinued therapy because of intolerable side effects. Common side effects related to CP include nausea/vomiting (26%), anorexia (26%), cytopenias (21%), weight loss (21%), alopecia (10%), infection (Herpes zoster) (10%), and ovarian failure (5%) ***(108)***.

7. Prognosis

Several factors have been shown to predict poor outcome in IPF. These include older age at presentation, male gender, severe dyspnea at presentation, history of cigarette smoking, severe loss of lung function, severity of reticular opacities or honeycomb change on HRCT, characteristic HRCT appearance, lack of response to conventional therapy, and histopathological findings showing prominent FF ***(2,17,69,74,109)***. Investigators from the University of Michigan evaluated the impact of histological diagnosis, baseline clinical, physiological, and radiographical factors on survival in 168 patients with suspected IIP. The presence of histological UIP was the most important risk factor for mortality (risk ratio [RR] of 28.46 [95% CI 5.5–148]), followed by the presence of honeycombing on HRCT, a radiographic feature that was shown to be a good surrogate for histological UIP (sensitivity of 90%, and a specificity of 86%) ***(14)***. The same group evaluated the impact of HRCT appearance on survival in patients with IIP. Patients with histological UIP and stereotypical HRCT appearance of UIP had a shorter survival (median survival 2.08 yr) when compared with patients with histological UIP and indeterminate HRCT scans (median survival 5.76 yr) ***(69)***.

Three studies have shown that a higher HRCT-fibrosis score identify patients with worse prognosis. Gay and colleagues did not find any measure of pulmonary function to be predictive of survival, but did find both the HRCT-fibrosis score and the pathological fibrosis score to be useful in predicting survival *(109)*. Similarly, investigators from the United Kingdom found that baseline percent-predicted DL_{CO} and HRCT-fibrosis score were independent predictors of mortality *(110)*. Japanese investigators demonstrated that the baseline HC score and the rate of HC progression were both predictive of worse survival in patients with IPF *(111)*.

Histopathological findings showing prominent FF identify patients with poor outcome. Nicholson and associates retrospectively studied *(53)* patients with IPF/UIP and analyzed the prognostic significance of four specific microscopic features of UIP. Multivariate analysis revealed that increasing FF and mononuclear cell infiltrate scores were associated with worsening lung function. Higher profusion of FF and a lower DL_{CO} were independent predictors of mortality *(112)*. These results supported the findings by King and co-workers, who also demonstrated that an increase in the number of FF correlated highly with mortality in patients with IPF/UIP *(13)*. In a separate study, expert pathologists reviewed SLB from 108 patients with idiopathic or CVD-associated UIP and assigned a score for FF. Patients with idiopathic UIP had more FF and worse survival compared with patients with CVD-associated UIP *(113)*.

A number of composite scoring systems have been developed with which to predict survival in IPF. King and co-workers studied 238 patients with IPF/UIP and derived a clinical-radiological-physiological (CRP) scoring system using clinical (age, smoking status, clubbing), radiographical (extent of interstitial opacities, presence of pulmonary hypertension on chest radiographs), and physiological parameters (reduced lung volume, abnormal gas exchange during maximal exercise). These investigators demonstrated that the CRP score correlated with important histopathological findings and was helpful in predicting survival in patients with IPF. A second abbreviated CRP scoring system that excluded Pa_{O2} during maximal exercise was inferior in predicting survival *(12,114)*. Similarly, investigators from the Brompton Hospital devised a composite physiological index (CPI) using radiographical and physiological information that predicted mortality more accurately than individual PFT in patients with IPF *(115)*. Even though these composite scoring systems are accurate in their predictive ability, they are expensive and cumbersome to generate in clinical practice. With this in mind, the prognostic value of oxygen desaturation during a 6-min walking test was evaluated in patients with IPF. Desaturation defined as a fall in oxygen saturation to 88% or less during the 6-min walk test identified patients with higher mortality compared with patients who did not desaturate. The 4-yr survival rate of IPF patients who desaturated to that level was 34.5% compared with 69.1% in patients who did not desaturate ***(84)***.

Predicting survival in IPF has been centered on baseline radiographical, pathological, and/or physiological testing. Recently, researchers have focused on the association of serial changes in pulmonary function or radiographical features and prognosis. One study determined that a decrease in FVC (>10% from baseline) during the initial 6 mo of follow-up was associated with increased mortality (hazard ratio 2.06; CI 1.09–3.89) ***(116)***. In a separate study, investigators concluded that at 6 and 12 mo of follow-up, serial pulmonary function trends (change in DL_{CO}, FVC, forced expiratory volume in 1 s [FEV_1], and the CPI) provided important prognostic information in IPF ***(117)***. A third study showed that assessment of changes in clinical and physiological variables (dyspnea score, total lung capacity, thoracic gas volume, FVC, FEV_1, DL_{CO}, p_{O2}, oxygen saturation, and alveolar-arterial oxygen gradient) at 6 and 12 mo provide clinicians with more accurate prognostic information than baseline values alone ***(118)***.

Serum markers and nuclear medicine testing may have a predictive role in IPF. Greene and colleagues found that serum levels of surfactant protein-A (SP-A) were predictive of survival in patients with IPF ***(119)***.

In a prospective study, investigators analyzed the usefulness of inhaled 99m-labeled diethylenetriamine penta-acetic acid ([99m] Tc-DTPA) aerosol clearance and survival in a cohort of 106 patients with UIP. Multiple stepwise Cox regression analysis identified fast clearance as an independent predictor of mortality ***(120)***.

8. Therapy

8.1. Conventional Therapy

Conventional therapy (CS, AZA, or CP) for IPF provides only marginal benefit. Unfortunately, in many studies, diagnoses were not based on the findings of lung biopsies or were not classified by current pathological criteria; thus, there is uncertainty as to the nature of the disease being treated. Two recent meta-analyses searched two large databases for randomized controlled trials (RCT) and controlled clinical trials (CCT) using CS or non-CS agents in patients with histological UIP or who fulfilled all ATS criteria for IPF; the authors could not find RCTs or CCTs evaluating CS alone in IPF and concluded that there are scant good-quality data regarding the efficacy of non-CS agents in IPF ***(121,122)***. The following is a brief discussion of anti-inflammatory (conventional) therapy in the treatment of IPF.

8.1.1. Corticosteroids

CS were the mainstay of therapy for more than four decades, but are of unproven efficacy, and are associated with significant toxicities ***(105,123,124)***. Early studies of patients with IPF/CFA cited response rates of 10 to 30% with CS (alone or combined with immunosuppressive agents), but complete or sustained remissions were rare ***(105,125–127)***. More importantly, many responders likely had IIPs other than UIP (e.g., NSIP or RBILD/DIP).

In recent studies, response rates to CS among patients with histological evidence for UIP are low (0–17%) ***(16,57,74,76,123)***. Large retrospective studies of patients with IPF showed no survival benefit with CS ***(12; 15,123,128)***. In one retrospective study from England, survival was worse among IPF patients treated with CS or CP, although this likely reflects a selection bias ***(15)***. Given the potential severe toxicities associated with CS ***(105,124)***, recent international consensus statements argue that high-dose CS should not be used to treat IPF ***(2,61)***. However, because anecdotal responses to CS are occasionally noted in patients with IPF/UIP ***(14)***, these statements acknowledge that selected patients with clinical or physiological impairment or worsening PFTs should be treated ***(2,61)***. Both statements ***(2,61)*** advocate an individualized approach to treating IPF/UIP. Among patients requiring treatment, both statements recommend combining therapy with either oral AZA or CP plus low-dose prednisone or prednisolone (0.5 mg/kg [lean body weight per d] for 4 wk, then 0.25 mg/kg for 8 wk, then 0.125 mg/kg). This represents a substantial departure from earlier regimens advocating high-dose prednisone (e.g., ≥1 mg/kg/d for ≥6–12 wk) ***(114,125,126)***. Combined therapy should be continued for 6 mo in the absence of adverse effects. Treatment should be continued beyond 6 or 12 mo or later time points only if patients improve or remain stable. It should be emphasized that these recommendations ***(2,61)*** reflect expert opinion, but have *not* been validated in clinical trials. We believe CS should not be given to patients at high risk for adverse effects (e.g., age > 70 yr, osteoporosis, DM, extreme obesity, and so on).

8.1.2. Azathioprine

Two prospective studies evaluated AZA for IPF ***(125,126)***. In both studies, AZA was combined with prednisone. In the first study, 20 patients with progressive IPF were initially treated with prednisone alone for 3 mo ***(125)***. At that point, AZA (3 mg/kg/d) was added and both agents were continued for an additional 9 mo or longer. Twelve patients (60%) responded. The independent effect of AZA was difficult to assess, because all patients received prednisone concomitantly. In a second, double-blind trial, Raghu and associates compared the effect of AZA plus prednisone on lung function with that of prednisone alone in previously untreated patients with IPF (the study population may have included patients with IIP other than UIP). Forty-three percent of patients randomly assigned to AZA plus prednisone died during the 9-yr follow-up period, compared with 77% of patients randomly assigned to prednisone alone. The difference became statistically significant only after adjustment for age (p = 0.02) ***(126)***.

8.1.3. Cyclophosphamide

Two randomized trials evaluated CP for IPF ***(127,129)***. In one 6-mo trial, 28 patients with "mid-course" IPF were randomized to prednisone alone (n = 16); prednisone plus oral CP (1.5 mg/kg/d) (n = 9); or CP alone (n = 5) (129). Mean BALF neutrophil counts declined in the cohort receiving CP, but PFTs did not change in any group. Johnson and colleagues compared the effect of prednisolone alone with that of prednisolone plus CP on breathlessness, radiographic appearance, and lung function in patients with IPF (the study population included patients with CVD and with IIP other than UIP). Initial improvement occurred in 7 of the 22 patients in the prednisolone-only group and in 5 of the 21 patients in the CP plus prednisolone group. However, at 36 mo, only 2 of the 22 patients in the prednisolone-only group remained improved, and only 1 of the 21 patients in the CP-prednisolone group remained improved. Life-table analysis suggested better survival in patients in the CP-prednisolone group, but this was not statistically significant ***(127)***. In a prospective uncontrolled study, Zisman and associates studied the efficacy of CP in 19 patients with biopsy-proven UIP who were unresponsive or intolerant to CS therapy. Only 1 patient improved; 7 remained stable, and 11 deteriorated. Nearly two-thirds of the patients developed drug-related side effects and one half of the patients discontinued therapy due to intolerable side effects ***(108)***. Intermittent, intravenous "pulse" CP, administered every 2 to 4 wk, has been tried for IPF refractory to CS in nonrandomized studies, but benefit was not convincing ***(130–132)***.

8.2. Lung Transplantation

Lung transplantation should be considered for patients with IPF refractory to medical therapy ***(133,134)***. Two-year survival following single lung transplant (SLT) ranges from 60 to 80%; 5-yr survival is 40 to 60% ***(134–136)***. In one study, lung transplantation reduced the risk of death by 75% ***(135)***. In addition, patients surviving lung transplantation appear to achieve considerable improvement in most dimensions of health-related quality of life ***(137–139)***. Unfortunately, owing to a shortage of donor organs, waiting time may be prolonged (up to 2–3 yr) and many patients with IPF die while awaiting transplantation ***(134,135)***. One study evaluated baseline PFT and HRCT fibrosis scores and the relationship to 2-yr survival in patients with IPF younger than 65 yr of age; the optimal points on the receiving operator characteristics (ROC) curves for discriminating between survivors and nonsurvivors corresponded to a combination of DL_{CO} of 39% predicted with HRCT-fibrosis score of 2.25 ***(110)***. In a separate study, investigators reviewed all transplant referrals for IIP that were listed for lung transplantation at their center. The aim of the study was to determine a parameter that would discriminate between patients who survived and patients who died awaiting transplantation. The severity of hypoxemia at rest was the only significant difference between both groups ***(140)***. Unless contraindications exist, patients with severe functional impairment (e.g., FVC <60% predicted, DL_{CO} <40% predicted), oxygen dependency, and a deteriorating course refractory to medical therapy should be listed promptly for transplantation ***(133,134)***.

8.3. Antifibrotic Therapy

Historically, the fibrotic process in IPF has been thought to be preceded by a chronic inflammatory process that injures the lung and modulates fibrogenesis ***(141)***. Conventional management of IPF has been primarily based on the notion that suppressing inflammation may prevent progression to fibrosis. Evidence against the notion that inflammation plays an important role in the pathogenesis of IPF comes from the lack of correlation of most markers of inflammation with disease stage or outcome, and the recognition that inflammation is not a prominent histopathological finding in UIP ***(92,141)***. Additionally, emerging evidence suggests that inflammation is not required for the development of a fibrotic response ***(141)***. In light of the poor prognosis and lack of response to available anti-inflammatory therapy, alternative approaches to the treatment of IPF are being pursued. The following is a brief discussion of antifibrotic therapy and other promising agents in the treatment of IPF.

8.3.1. Colchicine

Colchicine is an alkaloid derivative of the plant *Colchicum autumnale*, which has been used in acute attacks of gout. It is known to bind microtubular proteins necessary for intracellular trafficking and cellular mitosis, thus adversely affecting secretion of proteins from cells and cellular proliferation ***(142,143)***. Its antifibrotic activity was described following the discovery that colchicine inhibits secretion of collagen and other important growth factors necessary for fibroblast proliferation ***(144)***. However, further studies ***(145)*** with or without additional therapeutic agents, such as steroids, failed to document efficacy of colchicine in the treatment of human pulmonary fibrosis. It is thus not currently recommended for use in therapy of IPF.

8.3.2. Penicillamine

The D-isomer of penicillamine has been extensively studied in animal models of fibrosis, in which it has been shown to prevent accumulation of collagen in the lung by interrupting cross-linking of collagen molecules ***(146)***. This observation has led to its use in treating fibrotic lung disease associated with systemic sclerosis with good results ***(147)***. However, its efficacy in the treatment of IPF has been disappointing ***(148)***, and it is known to have toxic and significant adverse effects ***(2)***. Thus it is currently not recommended as therapy for IPF.

8.3.3. Pirfenidone

Pirfenidone is a novel agent with broad-spectrum antifibrotic activity. Numerous in vitro and animal model studies have demonstrated its effectiveness as an antifibrotic agent. In vitro studies have shown that pirfenidone significantly reduced mRNA levels of type I and type III collagen, and may act at the transcriptional or translational level of collagen synthesis ***(149)***. In vivo, it has been shown to inhibit TGF-β1-induced collagen synthesis, decrease extracellular matrix deposition, and suppress the overexpression of TGF-β in the bleomycin model of pulmonary fibrosis ***(150,151)***. Because IPF is becoming increasingly recognized as primarily a fibrotic process, the potential role of pirfenidone as a therapeutic agent is being explored.

In a prospective open-label study, Raghu and colleagues ***(152)*** treated 54 (42 biopsy-proven) consecutive patients with pirfenidone who were either unwilling to receive or unresponsive to conventional therapy. Survival rates of 78% at 1 yr and 63% at 2 yr compared favorably with historical controls. In addition, 83% of patients discontinued prednisone therapy and the remaining 17% were able to reduce their daily dose. All patients treated with immunosuppressive therapy tolerated discontinuation of the drug. Interestingly, patients whose lung function had deteriorated before enrollment appeared to stabilize after beginning pirfenidone. Side effects were relatively common, with patients reporting nausea (44%), fatigue (44%), and photosensitivity (24%). Despite these encouraging observations, the results of this study are difficult to interpret owing to the lack of appropriate controls, incomplete pre-entry and follow-up pulmonary function test data, a small study population, and a bias associated with survivorship effect (pulmonary function data of patients who died were not included in the analysis, and this could have biased the results). Furthermore, the observed steroid- and immunosuppressive-sparing effects of pirfenidone may have simply reflected lack of efficacy of conventional therapy rather than a true effect of pirfenidone. In a second open-label trial, Japanese investigators evaluated oral pirfenidone in eight patients with IPF and two with diffuse lung disease associated with systemic sclerosis; after 1 yr of therapy, there was no change in chest radiographic scores and arterial oxygen tension; the drug was well tolerated ***(153)***. Early treatment with pirfenidone appears to slow the progression of pulmonary fibrosis in patients with Hermansky–Pudlak syndrome ***(154)***. A randomized-controlled trial focusing on early treatment is warranted to test the efficacy and safety of this agent in IPF.

8.3.4. Interferon-γ1b

IFNs play an integral role in the regulation of fibroblast proliferation and collagen synthesis, but the mechanism by which they exert their effect is not clearly understood. Recent observations have shown that IFN-γ has antiproliferative, immunomodulatory, and antifibrotic effects ***(155)***, and thus may play a crucial role in the pathogenesis of IPF. IFN-γ decreases collagen content in the bleomycin model of lung fibrosis by inhibiting TGF-β transcription and subsequent procollagen mRNA production ***(156)***. In addition, IFN-γ inhibits fibroblast proliferation in cultures derived from normal and fibrotic human lung, making an argument that IFN-γ may have therapeutic applications ***(157)***. Lower levels of IFN-γ have been found in patients with IPF compared with patients with less fibrotic diseases such as pulmonary sarcoidosis ***(158)***. Kuroki and associates ***(159)*** measured levels of type III collagen in patients with progressive pulmonary fibrosis and found an inverse correlation with IFN-γ levels, particularly in patients with IPF. These studies suggest that patients with IPF may have a defect in IFN-γ production or function, which predisposes them to develop fibrosis following injury. However, the potential for developing fibrosis is not likely to be dependent on one factor; rather it is likely the result of a complex interplay of fibrotic mediators, differential gene expression, and feedback mechanisms. A study by Shaw and colleagues ***(160)*** showed that alveolar macrophages from patients with interstitial lung disease had increased production of platelet-derived growth factor, which is a potent mitogen for fibroblasts. This increase in platelet-derived growth factor was upregulated following treatment with IFN-γ, suggesting that IFN-γ may act to potentiate fibrosis in certain cellular environments.

Clearly, there is a complex regulatory mechanism in place with regard to whether fibrosis occurs or not, and conflicting in vitro studies must be interpreted with caution. A randomized, prospectively controlled trial was conducted in 18 patients with IPF comparing IFN-γ1b and low-dose prednisolone with prednisolone alone for 12 mo ***(161)***. The results were remarkable in that patients with progressive pulmonary fibrosis treated with IFN-γ1b plus low-dose prednisolone demonstrated improvement in pulmonary function, whereas those who received prednisolone alone experienced further decline in pulmonary function. The authors showed that all patients treated had almost undetectable levels of IFN-γ mRNA, and increased levels of both TGF-β and connective tissue growth factor mRNA in lung tissue. Furthermore, after treatment with IFN-γ1b, transcription of TGF-β and connective tissue growth factor were both significantly decreased. Several concerns have been raised regarding the findings reported by Ziesche and co-workers ***(162)***, particularly the unexpectedly good results with IFN-γ1b. To address some of the issues raised, an outside panel of experts reanalyzed the study data by reviewing each patient's lung function studies, CT scans, and SLBs to assess the clinical course and diagnosis of IPF according to the International Consensus Statement ***(2,163)***. Fifteen of 18 patients had either definite ($n = 9$) or probable ($n = 6$) IPF. The panel reanalyzed treatment response using published criteria and eliminated the patients who definitely did not have IPF. Patients treated with IFN-γ1b plus low-dose prednisolone demonstrated either stability or improvement in pulmonary function and gas exchange after 1 yr of treatment, whereas treatment with prednisolone alone was associated with no improvement in all patients ***(163)***. The observed benefit of IFN-γ1b on lung function has not been reproduced in subsequent studies. In one retrospective uncontrolled observation of 21 patients with IPF treated with IFN-γ1b, only one patient experienced objective improvement, 7 discontinued therapy (owing to lack of perceived benefit), and 11 died after 6 mo of therapy ***(164)***. In a separate study of five patients with IPF treated with IFN-γ1b, only one patient improved, two discontinued treatment owing to adverse effects and decline in lung function, and one died after 3 mo of therapy ***(165)***.

In a recent prospective, randomized, placebo-controlled, double-blind, multicenter phase III clinical trial of subcutaneous IFN-γ1b (200 μg thrice weekly) in 330 patients with mild to moderate idiopathic pulmonary fibrosis (FVC >50% and DL_{CO} >30%), a trend toward lower mortality was seen in IFN-γ1b-treated patients compared with placebo-treated patients. However, there were no significant differences in lung function or gas exchange between IFN-γ1-treated and placebo-treated patients after 48 wk of therapy ***(96)***. A prospective controlled multinational trial is planned to verify the possible survival benefit observed with IFN-γ1b therapy in IPF.

8.3.5. Interferon β-1a

IFN-β is used for the treatment of chronic hepatitis C and multiple sclerosis. In vitro IFN-β1a has been shown to reduce fibroblast proliferation ***(166)***, inhibit collagen production by fibroblasts ***(167)***, increase collagenase mRNA ***(168)***, decrease pro-collagen mRNA ***(169)***, and increase collagenase activity ***(167)***. Further, IFN-β inhibits irradiation-induced pulmonary fibrosis in mice ***(170)***.

A multicenter randomized, double-blind clinical trial examining the efficacy of IFNβ-1a was recently completed. Patients were randomized into four groups: placebo or IFNβ-1a at 15, 30, or 60 μg intramuscularly twice per week for a minimum of 12 mo and up to 2.5 yr. Preliminary results suggest that IFNβ-1a lacks significant efficacy ***(171)***.

8.4. Emerging Strategies

With a dismal response to existing therapy and its accompanied toxicity, the search for additional therapies has intensified in the past decade. The following is an overview of other therapeutic approaches, most of which are undergoing investigation and have not been adequately studied in humans.

8.4.1. Agents That Inhibit Epithelial Injury or Enhance Repair

The prior discussion has centered on fibroblast proliferation and collagen deposition as two areas of therapeutic intervention. It is becoming more apparent that the fibrotic process has multiple pathogenetic mechanisms. One of the fundamental hypotheses of pulmonary fibrosis involves an imbalanced response to injury, in which the capacity of the alveolar epithelium to repair itself is compromised, ultimately leading to fibrosis. Some investigators propose that the alveolar epithelium itself has antifibrotic properties, and that chronic loss of alveolar epithelium leads to an environment conducive to the development of fibrosis ***(172)***. Support for this notion exists in the fact that induction of apoptosis of alveolar epithelium has been shown to occur following administration of bleomycin ***(173)***. Therapies that either inhibit epithelial injury or enhance repair may limit the fibrotic response. In this regard, captopril, an angiotensin-converting enzyme inhibitor widely used in clinical practice, may have a role in the treatment of IPF. In vitro, captopril inhibits fibroblast proliferation, and in models of bleomycin-induced pulmonary fibrosis, it has been shown to reduce alveolar epithelial cell apoptosis and fibroproliferation. In addition, captopril abrogates Fas-induced apoptosis in human alveolar epithelial cells ***(141,174)***. There is currently an ongoing clinical trial at the National Institute of Respiratory Diseases in Mexico testing the efficacy of captopril in patients with IPF ***(141)***.

Another agent that may protect the alveolar epithelium is keratinocyte growth factor (KGF). This class of growth factor stimulates type II cell proliferation with no direct effects on fibroblasts ***(175)***. Keratinocyte growth factor increases surfactant protein gene expression and sodium/potassium adenosine triphosphatase, factors that may protect the alveolar epithelium ***(175)***. In vivo, KGF has been shown to protect animals from injury and subsequent development of fibrosis caused by a variety of insults ***(175)***.

There is evidence that an exaggerated oxidant stress may play a role in the pathogenesis of pulmonary fibrosis by injuring the alveolar epithelial cells. This oxidant burden is thought to be a consequence of both increased levels of reactive oxygen species and a defective antioxidant response. A major protector of oxidant-induced injury of the alveolar epithelium is glutathione, which has been shown to be deficient in the BALF of patients with IPF ***(176)***. Moreover, in vitro studies have shown that *N*-acetylcysteine (NAC), a precursor for glutathione synthesis, may augment the antioxidant defense system and protect the alveolar epithelium from free radical-induced injury ***(177)***. In vivo, Hagiwara and associates ***(178)*** reported a significant inhibition of bleomycin-induced lung fibrosis in mice following aerosolized NAC during the early inflammatory phase of injury. Whether this effect was secondary to NAC inhibition of cellular inflammation, or its role as a scavenger of reactive oxygen species, is not clear. German investigators evaluated oral NAC as a strategy to augment lung glutathione levels in 17 patients with biopsy-proven IPF. Following therapy with NAC, glutathione levels in BALF were significantly increased compared with pretreatment levels ***(177)***. In a separate study, Behr and colleagues ***(179)*** prospectively studied 18 patients with IPF and assessed the redox balance of the lung and changes in lung function following high-dose NAC therapy for 12 wk. They reported an increase in the total and reduced form of glutathione concentration in the BALF, and significant improvement in pulmonary function. The authors suggest that NAC may be considered as an adjunct in the treatment of IPF. Currently, there is a clinical trial in Europe to evaluate the potential benefits of NAC in IPF.

8.4.2. Anticytokine Approaches

As mechanisms of fibrosis at the cellular and molecular level become elucidated, their application to the development of novel therapeutic strategies appears promising. Given the temporal heterogeneity of the UIP lesion, early histopathological abnormalities may be present even in patients with advanced IPF. If early cytokine release is relevant to the initiation of this pathogenic response, then the targeting of early cytokines such as TNF-α should be considered. TNF-α appears to be upregulated soon after bleomycin-induced injury and has been implicated in a variety of inflammatory processes ***(180)***. Sime and colleagues ***(181)*** showed that transient overexpression of TNF-α in rat lung led to fibrosis associated with concomitant TGF-β expression and proliferation of myofibroblasts ***(181)***. Furthermore, upregulation of TNF-α expression has been shown to occur in inbred murine strains that are sensitive to bleomycin-induced lung fibrosis, with similar expression being absent in resistant strains ***(180)***. In addition, Ortiz and colleagues ***(182)*** showed that TNF receptor-deficient mice did not develop pulmonary fibrosis following exposure to bleomycin despite increased TNF expression. Studies of human lung biopsy specimens of patients with IPF have shown an upregulation of TNF-α mRNA and protein ***(183)***. These observations along with other studies in animal models demonstrating abrogation of pulmonary fibrosis following treatment with soluble TNF receptors suggest that TNF-α may play an important role in the pathogenesis of pulmonary fibrosis ***(184)***. Several agents that can block TNF-α are now available for human use ***(185)***. There is currently an ongoing clinical trial evaluating the safety and efficacy of etanercept, a TNF-α receptor antagonist, in patients with IPF.

The expression of TNF-α is inhibited by certain cytokines such as IL-10, which is produced by a variety of cells including T-helper (Th) cells, monocytes, and alveolar macrophages ***(186,187)***. It is conceivable that IL-10 may be useful in blunting the action of increased TNF-α observed following bleomycin-induced lung injury, therefore possibly inhibiting progression to fibrosis. Arai and colleagues ***(188)*** investigated the possible inhibitory effects of IL-10 by introducing the IL-10 gene into mice exposed to bleomycin and found that bleomycin-induced pulmonary fibrosis was suppressed. These results suggest that treatment with IL-10 during the early inflammatory phases of lung injury may be promising and requires further investigation. Concerns regarding the role of this agent in treating pulmonary fibrosis exist in that IL-10 is a type-2 Th (Th2) cytokine that could suppress IFN-γ expression and promote fibrogenesis ***(189)***. A clinical trial to study the effect of this cytokine is now underway in the United States.

The realization that Th cell subsets could be categorized on the basis of cytokine profiles has helped clarify our understanding of chronic cell-mediated immune responses. The type-1 (Th1) cytokines include IFN-γ, IL-2, IL-12, IL-18, and Th2 cytokines include IL-4, IL-5, IL-10, and IL-13. Analysis of subset populations of Th cells within the interstitium of patients with IPF reveal a predominantly Th2-type pattern of cytokine production, suggesting that alterations in T-cell subpopulations of Th1 and Th2 cells and their associated pattern of cytokine production may contribute to progression of IPF ***(190)***. Supporting evidence comes from studies demonstrating that IFN-γ (a Th1 cytokine) has profound antifibrotic effects in IPF possibly because it shifts the balance away from a Th2-dependent profibrotic environment. Thus, it seems reasonable to target therapy to correct the Th imbalance by either favoring a Th1 phenotype or abrogating the predominant Th2 response (e.g., administration of IL-12 to promote IFN-γ expression, or inhibition of IL-4, IL-13, and so on).

TGF-β is a critical cytokine for the promotion of fibrosis. In bleomycin-induced pulmonary fibrosis, passive immunization with neutralizing antibodies against TGF-β reduces collagen deposition ***(191)***. In addition, the overexpression of TGF-β results in a fibrogenic response resembling UIP (i.e., abundant FF) ***(192)***. In patients with IPF, increased expression of TGF-β is localized to bronchiolar epithelial cells, epithelial cells of HC cysts, and hyperplastic type II pneumocytes ***(193)***. It is possible that therapy with neutralizing antibodies against TGF-β1, or utilization of a TGF-β1 inhibitor such as decorin, may become useful in the treatment of IPF ***(194)***.

TGF-β signals through a receptor that activates transcription factors Smad2 and Smad3 promoting TGF-β gene transcription. Interestingly, IFN-γ inhibits the activation of Smad3 and induces the expression of Smad7, an antagonistic molecule that inhibits TGF-β expression. Smad7 can be produced in the laboratory and may become a useful molecule in the treatment of IPF ***(195)***.

Monocyte chemoattractant protein (MCP)-1 is a member of the C-C subfamily of chemokines involved in monocyte/macrophage mediated inflammation ***(196,197)***. In addition, MCP-1 has been shown to stimulate pulmonary fibroblasts, TGF-β synthesis, and collagen production ***(198)***. Analysis of serum, BALF, and lung biopsy specimens from patients with IPF reveal increased levels of this chemokine ***(196,197,199)***. Furthermore, serum MCP-1 levels correlate with clinical course in patients with interstitial lung disease ***(199)***. Further investigation into the clinical significance of MCP-1 and its contribution into the pathogenesis of IPF are necessary, and may provide the groundwork for novel therapies.

Another potential mediator of fibrosis produced in a variety of cells in the lung is the vasoactive peptide endothelin (ET)-1 ***(200,201)***. First thought to be primarily a vasoactive agent, ET-1 has been shown to stimulate fibroblast proliferation, activate monocytes, induce collagen production, and regulate cytokine production ***(202)***. Mutsaers and colleagues ***(203)*** revealed that ET-1 levels are augmented following administration of bleomycin with increased localization of the agent in areas of fibrosis. With increases in ET-1 synthesis following TNF-α and TGF-β stimulation, one may speculate that ET-1 may play an important role in the cascade of events leading to pulmonary fibrosis ***(204,205)***. Additional support for its role in pulmonary fibrosis comes from studies in animals in which fibrosis was attenuated following treatment with bosentan, an ET receptor antagonist ***(206)***. ET-1 has also been associated with pulmonary fibrosis in humans. In a study examining the expression of ET-1 in patients with interstitial lung fibrosis, Giaid and associates ***(200)*** found a striking expression of ET-1 in lung tissue that correlated with parameters of disease activity in patients with IPF. There is currently an ongoing clinical trial evaluating the safety and efficacy of bosentan in patients with IPF.

8.4.3. Other Agents That Inhibit Fibroblast Proliferation or Induce Fibroblast Apoptosis

Some have hypothesized that inducing fibroblast apoptosis may curb progression of fibrosis. Lovastatin is a pharmacological agent widely used in the treatment of hypercholesterolemia that inhibits 3-hydroxy-3-methylglutaryl-coenzyme A, therefore affecting many cellular functions essential for normal cell homeostasis including proliferation and cell survival. Tan and associates showed that clinically achievable concentrations of lovastatin induced apoptosis of human lung fibroblasts in vitro, and in vivo reduced granulation tissue formation and induced fibroblast apoptosis in a guinea pig wound model of fibroproliferation *(207)*. With its known safety profile and potential antifibrotic effect, lovastatin is an attractive candidate in the treatment of IPF.

Suramin is a sulfonated napthylurea that has been used to treat onchocerciasis, acquired immunodeficiency virus, and prostate cancer. In vitro, suramin antagonizes the effects of a number of growth factors that promote fibrogenesis such as TGF-β, insulin-like growth factor-1, platelet-derived growth factor, epidermal-like growth factor, and fibroblast growth factor. In vivo, suramin has been shown to delay wound healing *(175)*.

Relaxin is a protein secreted by the gravid uterus responsible for remodeling of the interpubic ligament and cervix during the later phases of pregnancy. Relaxin inhibits the TGF-β-mediated overexpression of extracellular matrix, stimulates the expression of collagenases by lung fibroblasts in vitro, and has been shown to block bleomycin-induced fibrosis in mice *(141)*.

The eicosanoids are potential candidates for therapeutic intervention. The prostaglandin PGE_2 is a potent inhibitor of fibroblast proliferation and extracellular matrix deposition and may ameliorate the fibrotic process in IPF *(175)*. Indomethacin, an inhibitor of cyclo-oxygenase, has been shown to decrease bleomycin-induced pulmonary fibrosis in an animal model but to our knowledge, it has not been evaluated in human IPF *(175)*. The profibrotic leukotriene B4 has been shown to be increased in BALF and lung tissue of patients with IPF *(175)*. Inhibition of leukotriene production may be an effective adjuvant therapy, and drugs are now available to block leukotriene synthesis.

Gene-specific antisense therapy against proteins known to be important in human lung fibroblast proliferation may become an effective approach in treating IPF patients. In vitro, Chen and associates showed that gene-specific oligonucleotides (oligos) against c-Ki-RAS substantially inhibited the proliferation of human fibroblasts *(141)*.

Beractan is a natural bovine lung extract containing phospholipids, neutral lipids, fatty acids, and surfactant-associated proteins. In vitro, beractan provoked fibroblast apoptosis, induced collagenase-1 expression, and decreased type I collagen ***(141)***.

8.4.4. Other Novel Strategies

Pulmonary fibrosis can be complicated by pulmonary hypertension limiting exercise tolerance and survival. German investigators performed a randomized-controlled, open-label trial in 16 individuals with pulmonary hypertension secondary to pulmonary fibrosis. They compared oral sildenafil with inhaled nitric oxide and infused epoprostenol. A single dose of sildenafil reduced pulmonary vascular resistance by nearly one-third and increased the mean arterial blood oxygen tension by 14 mmHg. The drug was well tolerated with no adverse effects on ventilation-perfusion matching ***(208)***. A clinical trial evaluating sildenafil in patients with IPF and pulmonary hypertension will be conducted soon.

9. Conclusions

In recent years, significant advances have been made in our understanding and management of IPF. However, in order to further our knowledge and make significant progress in the care of these patients, it is critical that we improve our understanding of the natural history and pathogenesis of IPF. In addition, we need to pursue novel imaging and diagnostic technologies to improve earlier diagnosis and we must also educate primary care physicians and pulmonologists to refer patients early to an interstitial lung disease specialist or lung transplant center. Therapeutic strategies must target specific aberrant pathways during the natural history of the pathogenesis of pulmonary fibrosis. Only when these issues are in place will we be able to improve the prognosis of disorders associated with progressive pulmonary fibrosis.

References

1. Hubbard, R., Johnston, I., Coultas, D. B., and Britton, J. (1996) Mortality rates from cryptogenic fibrosing alveolitis in seven countries. *Thorax* **51,** 711–716.
2. American Thoracic Society. (2000) Idiopathic pulmonary fibrosis: diagnosis and treatment. International consensus statement. American Thoracic Society (ATS), and the European Respiratory Society (ERS). *Am. J. Respir. Crit. Care Med.* **161,** 646–664.
3. Coultas, D. B., Zumwalt, R. E., Black, W. C., and Sobonya, R. E. (1994) The epidemiology of interstitial lung diseases. *Am. J. Respir. Crit. Care Med.* **150,** 967–972.
4. Iwai, K., Mori, T., Yamada, N., Yamaguchi, M., and Hosoda, Y. (1994) Idiopathic pulmonary fibrosis. Epidemiologic approaches to occupational exposure. *Am. J. Respir. Crit. Care Med.* **150,** 670–675.
5. Gross, T. J. and Hunninghake, G. W. (2001) Idiopathic pulmonary fibrosis. *N. Engl. J. Med.* **345,** 517–525.

6. Scott, J., Johnston, I., and Britton, J. (1990) What causes cryptogenic fibrosing alveolitis? A case-control study of environmental exposure to dust. *BMJ* **301,** 1015–1017.
7. Mannino, D. M., Etzel, R. A., and Parrish, R. G. (1996) Pulmonary fibrosis deaths in the United States, 1979–1991. An analysis of multiple-cause mortality data. *Am. J. Respir. Crit. Care Med.* **153,** 1548–1552.
8. Johnston, I., Britton, J., Kinnear, W., and Logan, R. (1990) Rising mortality from cryptogenic fibrosing alveolitis. *BMJ* **301,** 1017–1021.
9. Baumgartner, K. B., Samet, J. M., Stidley, C. A., Colby, T. V., and Waldron, J. A. (1997) Cigarette smoking: a risk factor for idiopathic pulmonary fibrosis. *Am. J. Respir. Crit. Care Med.* **155,** 242–248.
10. Hubbard, R., Lewis, S., Richards, K., Johnston, I., and Britton, J. (1996) Occupational exposure to metal or wood dust and aetiology of cryptogenic fibrosing alveolitis. *Lancet* **347,** 284–289.
11. Enomoto, T., Usuki, J., Azuma, A., Nakagawa, T., and Kudoh, S. (2003) Diabetes mellitus may increase risk for idiopathic pulmonary fibrosis. *Chest* **123,** 2007–2011.
12. King, T. E., Jr., Tooze, J. A., Schwarz, M. I., Brown, K. R., and Cherniack, R. M. (2001) Predicting survival in idiopathic pulmonary fibrosis: scoring system and survival model. *Am. J. Respir. Crit. Care Med.* **164,** 1171–1181.
13. King, T. E., Jr., Schwarz, M. I., Brown, K., et al. (2001) Idiopathic pulmonary fibrosis: relationship between histopathologic features and mortality. *Am. J. Respir. Crit. Care Med.* **164,** 1025-32.
14. Flaherty, K. R., Toews, G. B., Travis, W. D., et al. (2002) Clinical significance of histological classification of idiopathic interstitial pneumonia. *Eur. Respir. J.* **19,** 275–283.
15. Hubbard, R., Johnston, I., and Britton, J. (1998) Survival in patients with cryptogenic fibrosing alveolitis: a population-based cohort study. *Chest* **113,** 396–400.
16. Nicholson, A. G., Colby, T. V., du Bois, R. M., Hansell, D. M., and Wells, A. U. (2000) The prognostic significance of the histologic pattern of interstitial pneumonia in patients presenting with the clinical entity of cryptogenic fibrosing alveolitis. *Am. J. Respir. Crit. Care Med.* **162,** 2213–2217.
17. Schwartz, D. A., Helmers, R. A., Galvin, J. R., et al. (1994) Determinants of survival in idiopathic pulmonary fibrosis. *Am. J. Respir. Crit. Care Med.* **149,** 450–454.
18. Nakamura, Y., Romberger, D. J., Tate, L., et al. (1995) Cigarette smoke inhibits lung fibroblast proliferation and chemotaxis. *Am. J. Respir. Crit. Care Med.* **151,** 1497–1503.
19. Raghu, G. (2003) The role of gastroesophageal reflux in idiopathic pulmonary fibrosis. *Am. J. Med.* **115(Suppl 3A),** 60S–64S.
20. Tobin, R. W., Pope, C. E., 2nd, Pellegrini, C. A., Emond, M. J., Sillery, J., and Raghu, G. (1998) Increased prevalence of gastroesophageal reflux in patients with idiopathic pulmonary fibrosis. *Am. J. Respir. Crit. Care Med.* **158,** 1804–1808.
21. Hubbard, R., Venn, A., Smith, C., Cooper, M., Johnston, I., and Britton, J. (1998) Exposure to commonly prescribed drugs and the etiology of cryptogenic fibrosing alveolitis: a case-control study. *Am. J. Respir. Crit. Care Med.* **157,** 743–747.

22. Baumgartner, K. B., Samet, J. M., Coultas, D. B., et al. (2000) Occupational and environmental risk factors for idiopathic pulmonary fibrosis: a multicenter case-control study. Collaborating Centers. *Am. J. Epidemiol.* **152,** 307–315.
23. Vergnon, J. M., Vincent, M., de The, G., Mornex, J. F., Weynants, P., and Brune, J. (1984) Cryptogenic fibrosing alveolitis and Epstein-Barr virus: an association? *Lancet* **2,** 768–771.
24. Egan, J. J., Stewart, J. P., Hasleton, P. S., Arrand, J. R., Carroll, K. B., and Woodcock, A. A. (1995) Epstein-Barr virus replication within pulmonary epithelial cells in cryptogenic fibrosing alveolitis. *Thorax* **50,** 1234–1239.
25. Stewart, J. P., Egan, J. J., Ross, A. J., et al. (1999) The detection of Epstein-Barr virus DNA in lung tissue from patients with idiopathic pulmonary fibrosis. *Am. J. Respir. Crit. Care Med.* **159,** 1336–1341.
26. Kelly, B. G., Lok, S. S., Hasleton, P. S., Egan, J. J., and Stewart, J. P. (2002) A rearranged form of Epstein-Barr virus DNA is associated with idiopathic pulmonary fibrosis. *Am. J. Respir. Crit. Care Med.* **166,** 510–513.
27. Tang, Y. W., Johnson, J. E., Browning, P. J., et al. (2003) Herpesvirus DNA is consistently detected in lungs of patients with idiopathic pulmonary fibrosis. *J. Clin. Microbiol.* **41,** 2633–2640.
28. Irving, W. L., Day, S., and Johnston, I. D. (1993) Idiopathic pulmonary fibrosis and hepatitis C virus infection. *Am. Rev. Respir. Dis.* **148,** 1683–1684.
29. Meliconi, R., Andreone, P., Fasano, L., et al. (1996) Incidence of hepatitis C virus infection in Italian patients with idiopathic pulmonary fibrosis. *Thorax* **51,** 315–317.
30. Ueda, T., Ohta, K., Suzuki, N., et al. (1992) Idiopathic pulmonary fibrosis and high prevalence of serum antibodies to hepatitis C virus. *Am. Rev. Respir. Dis.* **146,** 266–268.
31. Kuwano, K., Nomoto, Y., Kunitake, R., et al. (1997) Detection of adenovirus E1A DNA in pulmonary fibrosis using nested polymerase chain reaction. *Eur. Respir. J.* **10,** 1445–1449.
32. Pinsker, K. L., Schneyer, B., Becker, N., and Kamholz, S. L. (1981) Usual interstitial pneumonia following Texas A2 influenza infection. *Chest* **80,** 123–126.
33. Winterbauer, R. H., Ludwig, W. R., and Hammar, S. P. (1977) Clinical course, management, and long-term sequelae of respiratory failure due to influenza viral pneumonia. *Johns Hopkins Med. J.* **141,** 148–155.
34. Louria, D. B., Blumenfeld, H. L., Ellis, J. T., Kilbourne, E. D., and Rogers, D. E. (1959) Studies on influenza in the pandemic of 1957-1958. II. Pulmonary complications of influenza. *J. Clin. Invest.* **38,** 213–265.
35. Jakab, G. J. (1990) Sequential virus infections, bacterial superinfections, and fibrogenesis. *Am. Rev. Respir. Dis.* **142,** 374–379.
36. Weintrub, P. S., Sullender, W. M., Lombard, C., Link, M. P., and Arvin, A. (1987) Giant cell pneumonia caused by parainfluenza type 3 in a patient with acute myelomonocytic leukemia. *Arch. Pathol. Lab. Med.* **111,** 569–570.
37. Jiwa, M., Steenbergen, R. D., Zwaan, F. E., Kluin, P. M., Raap, A. K., and van der Ploeg, M. (1990) Three sensitive methods for the detection of cytomega-

lovirus in lung tissue of patients with interstitial pneumonitis. *Am. J. Clin. Pathol.* **93,** 491–494.
38. Hartelius, H., Gaub, J., Ingemann Jensen, L., Jensen, J., and Faber, V. (1988) Computed tomography of the lungs in acquired immunodeficiency syndrome. An early indicator of interstitial pneumonia. *Acta Radiol.* **29,** 641–644.
39. Siegel, C., Johnston, S., and Adair, S. (1990) Isolation of measles virus in primary rhesus monkey cells from a child with acute interstitial pneumonia who cytologically had giant-cell pneumonia without a rash. *Am. J. Clin. Pathol.* **94,** 464–469.
40. Tubbs, R. R., Benjamin, S. P., Osborne, D. G., and Barenberg, S. (1978) Surface and transmission ultrastructural characteristics of desquamative interstitial pneumonitis. *Hum. Pathol.* **9,** 693–703.
41. Matsuyama, W., Kawabata, M., Mizoguchi, A., Iwami, F., Wakimoto, J., and Osame, M. (2003) Influence of human T lymphotrophic virus type I on cryptogenic fibrosing alveolitis–HTLV-I associated fibrosing alveolitis: proposal of a new clinical entity. *Clin. Exp. Immunol.* **133,** 397–403.
42. Marshall, R. P., Puddicombe, A., Cookson, W. O., and Laurent, G. J. (2000) Adult familial cryptogenic fibrosing alveolitis in the United Kingdom. *Thorax* **55,** 143–146.
43. Geddes, D. M., Webley, M., Brewerton, D. A., Turton, C. W., Turner-Warwick, M., Murphy, A. H., and Ward, A. M. (1977) Alpha 1-antitrypsin phenotypes in fibrosing alveolitis and rheumatoid arthritis. *Lancet* **2,** 1049–1051.
44. Musk, A. W., Zilko, P. J., Manners, P., Kay, P. H., and Kamboh, M. I. (1986) Genetic studies in familial fibrosing alveolitis. Possible linkage with immunoglobulin allotypes (Gm). *Chest* **89,** 206–210.
45. Hubbard, R., Baoku, Y., Kalsheker, N., Britton, J., and Johnston, I. (1997) Alpha1-antitrypsin phenotypes in patients with cryptogenic fibrosing alveolitis: a case-control study. *Eur. Respir. J.* **10,** 2881–2883.
46. Thomas, A. Q., Lane, K., Phillips, J., 3rd, et al. (2002) Heterozygosity for a surfactant protein C gene mutation associated with usual interstitial pneumonitis and cellular nonspecific interstitial pneumonitis in one kindred. *Am. J. Respir. Crit. Care Med.* **165,** 1322–1328.
47. Selman, M., Lin, H. M., Montano, M., et al. (2003) Surfactant protein A and B genetic variants predispose to idiopathic pulmonary fibrosis. *Hum. Genet.* **113,** 542–550.
48. Whyte, M., Hubbard, R., Meliconi, R., et al. (2000) Increased risk of fibrosing alveolitis associated with interleukin-1 receptor antagonist and tumor necrosis factor-alpha gene polymorphisms. *Am. J. Respir. Crit. Care Med.* **162,** 755–758.
49. Xaubet, A., Marin-Arguedas, A., Lario, S., et al. (2003) Transforming growth factor-beta1 gene polymorphisms are associated with disease progression in idiopathic pulmonary fibrosis. *Am. J. Respir. Crit. Care Med.* **168,** 431–435.
50. Wahidi, M. M., Speer, M. C., Steele, M. P., Brown, K. K., Schwarz, M. I., and Schwartz, D. A. (2002) Familial pulmonary fibrosis in the United States. *Chest* **121,** 30S.
51. Johnston, I. D., Prescott, R. J., Chalmers, J. C., and Rudd, R. M. (1997) British Thoracic Society study of cryptogenic fibrosing alveolitis: current presentation

and initial management. Fibrosing Alveolitis Subcommittee of the Research Committee of the British Thoracic Society. *Thorax* **52,** 38–44.

52. Turner-Warwick, M., Burrows, B., and Johnson, A. (1980) Cryptogenic fibrosing alveolitis: clinical features and their influence on survival. *Thorax* **35,** 171–180.
53. Scadding, J. G. and Hinson, K. F. (1967) Diffuse fibrosing alveolitis (diffuse interstitial fibrosis of the lungs) Correlation of histology at biopsy with prognosis. *Thorax* **22,** 291–304.
54. Nagaya, H., Buckley, C. E., 3rd, and Sieker, H. O. (1969) Positive antinuclear factor in patients with unexplained pulmonary fibrosis. *Ann. Intern. Med.* **70,** 1135–1145.
55. Chapman, J. R., Charles, P. J., Venables, P. J., et al. (1984) Definition and clinical relevance of antibodies to nuclear ribonucleoprotein and other nuclear antigens in patients with cryptogenic fibrosing alveolitis. *Am. Rev. Respir. Dis.* **130,** 439–443.
56. Nagaya, H. and Sieker, H. O. (1972) Pathogenetic mechanisms of interstitial pulmonary fibrosis in patients with serum antinuclear factor. A histologic and clinical correlation. *Am. J. Med.* **52,** 51–62.
57. Lynch, J. P. I., M, W., Flaherty, K., White, E., Martinez, F. J., Travis, W. D., and Raghu, G. (2001) Usual interstitial pneumonia. *Semin. Respir. Crit. Care Med.* **22,** 357–385.
58. Iannello, S., Cavaleri, A., Camuto, M., Pisano, M. G., Milazzo, P., and Belfiore, F. (2002) Low fasting serum triglyceride and high free fatty acid levels in pulmonary fibrosis: a previously unreported finding. *Med. Gen. Med.* **4,** 5.
59. Crystal, R. G., Fulmer, J. D., Roberts, W. C., Moss, M. L., Line, B. R., and Reynolds, H. Y. (1976) Idiopathic pulmonary fibrosis. Clinical, histologic, radiographic, physiologic, scintigraphic, cytologic, and biochemical aspects. *Ann. Intern. Med.* **85,** 769–788.
60. Mathieson, J. R., Mayo, J. R., Staples, C. A., and Muller, N. L. (1989) Chronic diffuse infiltrative lung disease: comparison of diagnostic accuracy of CT and chest radiography. *Radiology* **171,** 111–116.
61. (1999) The diagnosis, assessment and treatment of diffuse parenchymal lung disease in adults. Introduction. *Thorax* **54(Suppl 1),** S1–14.
62. Grenier, P., Valeyre, D., Cluzel, P., Brauner, M. W., Lenoir, S., and Chastang, C. (1991) Chronic diffuse interstitial lung disease: diagnostic value of chest radiography and high-resolution CT. *Radiology* **179,** 123–132.
63. Tung, K. T., Wells, A. U., Rubens, M. B., Kirk, J. M., du Bois, R. M., and Hansell, D. M. (1993) Accuracy of the typical computed tomographic appearances of fibrosing alveolitis. *Thorax* **48,** 334–338.
64. Guerry-Force, M. L., Muller, N. L., Wright, J. L., et al. (1987) A comparison of bronchiolitis obliterans with organizing pneumonia, usual interstitial pneumonia, and small airways disease. *Am. Rev. Respir. Dis.* **135,** 705–712.
65. Hunninghake, G. W., Lynch, D. A., Galvin, J. R., et al. (2003) Radiologic findings are strongly associated with a pathologic diagnosis of usual interstitial pneumonia. *Chest* **124,** 1215–1223.

66. Wells, A. (1998) Clinical usefulness of high resolution computed tomography in cryptogenic fibrosing alveolitis. *Thorax* **53,** 1080–1087.
67. Kizer, J., Zisman, D., Blumenthal, N., et al. (2004) The association between pulmonary fibrosis and coronary artery disease. *Arch. Int. Med.* **164,** 551–556.
68. Johkoh, T., Muller, N. L., Cartier, Y., et al. (1999) Idiopathic interstitial pneumonias: diagnostic accuracy of thin-section CT in 129 patients. *Radiology* **211,** 555–560.
69. Flaherty, K. R., Thwaite, E. L., Kazerooni, E. A., et al. (2003) Radiological versus histological diagnosis in UIP and NSIP: survival implications. *Thorax* **58,** 143–148.
70. Hunninghake, G. W., Zimmerman, M. B., Schwartz, D. A., et al. (2001) Utility of a lung biopsy for the diagnosis of idiopathic pulmonary fibrosis. *Am. J. Respir. Crit. Care Med.* **164,** 193–196.
71. Zisman, D., Kazerooni, E., Flaherty, K., Martinez, F., and Lynch, III, J. P. Idiopathic pulmonary fibrosis: role of high-resolution thin section computed tomographic scanning. In: *Idiopathic Pulmonary Fibrosis* (Lynch, III, J. P., ed.), Marcel Dekker, New York, NY: in press.
72. Swensen, S. J., Aughenbaugh, G. L., and Myers, J. L. (1997) Diffuse lung disease: diagnostic accuracy of CT in patients undergoing surgical biopsy of the lung. *Radiology* **205,** 229–234.
73. Raghu, G., Mageto, Y. N., Lockhart, D., Schmidt, R. A., Wood, D. E., and Godwin, J. D. (1999) The accuracy of the clinical diagnosis of new-onset idiopathic pulmonary fibrosis and other interstitial lung disease: a prospective study. *Chest* **116,** 1168–1174.
74. Daniil, Z. D., Gilchrist, F. C., Nicholson, A. G., et al. (1999) A histologic pattern of nonspecific interstitial pneumonia is associated with a better prognosis than usual interstitial pneumonia in patients with cryptogenic fibrosing alveolitis. *Am. J. Respir. Crit. Care Med.* **160,** 899–905.
75. American Thoracic Society/European Respiratory Society International Multidisciplinary Consensus Classification of the Idiopathic Interstitial Pneumonias. (2002) This joint statement of the American Thoracic Society (ATS), and the European Respiratory Society (ERS) was adopted by the ATS board of directors, June 2001 and by the ERS Executive Committee, June 2001. *Am. J. Respir. Crit. Care Med.* **165,** 277–304.
76. Nagai, S., Kitaichi, M., Itoh, H., Nishimura, K., Izumi, T., and Colby, T. V. (1998) Idiopathic nonspecific interstitial pneumonia/fibrosis: comparison with idiopathic pulmonary fibrosis and BOOP. *Eur. Respir. J.* **12,** 1010–1019.
77. Schwartz, D. A., Merchant, R. K., Helmers, R. A., Gilbert, S. R., Dayton, C. S., and Hunninghake, G. W. (1991) The influence of cigarette smoking on lung function in patients with idiopathic pulmonary fibrosis. *Am. Rev. Respir. Dis.* **144,** 504–506.
78. Nava, S. and Rubini, F. (1999) Lung and chest wall mechanics in ventilated patients with end stage idiopathic pulmonary fibrosis. *Thorax* **54,** 390–395.

79. Dunn, T. L., Watters, L. C., Hendrix, C., Cherniack, R. M., Schwarz, M. I., and King, T. E., Jr. (1988) Gas exchange at a given degree of volume restriction is different in sarcoidosis and idiopathic pulmonary fibrosis. *Am. J. Med.* **85,** 221–224.
80. Flaherty, K. R. and Martinez, F. J. (2000) The role of pulmonary function testing in pulmonary fibrosis. *Curr. Opin. Pulm. Med.* **6,** 404–410.
81. Weissman, I., Lynch III, J., and Martinez, F. (2003) Role of physiologic assessment in advanced lung disease. In: *Management of Non-Neoplastic Advanced Lung Disease* (Maurer, J., ed.), Marcel Dekker, New York.
82. Doherty, M. J., Pearson, M. G., O'Grady, E. A., Pellegrini, V., and Calverley, P. M. (1997) Cryptogenic fibrosing alveolitis with preserved lung volumes. *Thorax* **52,** 998–1002.
83. Sciurba, F. and Slivka, W. (1998) Six-minute walk testing. *Semi. Resp. Crit. Care Med.* **19,** 383–392.
84. Lama, V. N., Flaherty, K. R., Toews, G. B., et al. (2003) Prognostic value of desaturation during a 6-minute walk test in idiopathic interstitial pneumonia. *Am. J. Respir. Crit. Care Med.* **168,** 1084–1090.
85. Costabel, U. and Guzman, J. (2001) Bronchoalveolar lavage in interstitial lung disease. *Curr. Opin. Pulm. Med.* **7,** 255–261.
86. Turner-Warwick, M. and Haslam, P. L. (1987) The value of serial bronchoalveolar lavages in assessing the clinical progress of patients with cryptogenic fibrosing alveolitis. *Am. Rev. Respir. Dis.* **135,** 26–34.
87. Watters, L. C., Schwarz, M. I., Cherniack, R. M., et al. (1987) Idiopathic pulmonary fibrosis. Pretreatment bronchoalveolar lavage cellular constituents and their relationships with lung histopathology and clinical response to therapy. *Am. Rev. Respir. Dis.* **135,** 696–704.
88. Veeraraghavan, S., Latsi, P. I., Wells, A. U., et al. (2003) BAL findings in idiopathic nonspecific interstitial pneumonia and usual interstitial pneumonia. *Eur. Respir. J.* **22,** 239–244.
89. Berbescu, E., Katzenstein, A., Snow, J., and Zisman, D. (2003) Diagnostic Value of Transbronchial Biopsy in Usual Interstitial Pneumonia. Presented at the American Society for Clinical Pathology Annual Meeting, Washington, DC.
90. Ryu, J. H., Colby, T. V., and Hartman, T. E. (1998) Idiopathic pulmonary fibrosis: current concepts. *Mayo Clin. Proc.* **73,** 1085–1101.
91. Bjoraker, J. A., Ryu, J. H., Edwin, M. K., et al. (1998) Prognostic significance of histopathologic subsets in idiopathic pulmonary fibrosis. *Am. J. Respir. Crit. Care Med.* **157,** 199–203.
92. Katzenstein, A. L. and Myers, J. L. (1998) Idiopathic pulmonary fibrosis: clinical relevance of pathologic classification. *Am. J. Respir. Crit. Care Med.* **157,** 1301–1315.
93. Travis, W. D., Matsui, K., Moss, J., and Ferrans, V. J. (2000) Idiopathic nonspecific interstitial pneumonia: prognostic significance of cellular and fibrosing patterns: survival comparison with usual interstitial pneumonia and desquamative interstitial pneumonia. *Am. J. Surg. Pathol.* **24,** 19–33.

94. Flaherty, K. R., Travis, W. D., Colby, T. V., et al. (2001) Histopathologic variability in usual and nonspecific interstitial pneumonias. *Am. J. Respir. Crit. Care Med.* **164,** 1722–1727.
95. Katzenstein, A. L., Zisman, D. A., Litzky, L. A., Nguyen, B. T., and Kotloff, R. M. (2002) Usual interstitial pneumonia: histologic study of biopsy and explant specimens. *Am. J. Surg. Pathol.* **26,** 1567–1577.
96. Raghu, G., Brown, K. K., Bradford, W. Z., et al. (2004) A placebo-controlled trial of interferon gamma-1b in patients with idiopathic pulmonary fibrosis. *N. Engl. J. Med.* **350,** 125–133.
97. Akira, M., Hamada, H., Sakatani, M., Kobayashi, C., Nishioka, M., and Yamamoto, S. (1997) CT findings during phase of accelerated deterioration in patients with idiopathic pulmonary fibrosis. *AJR Am. J. Roentgenol.* **168,** 79–83.
98. Yokoyama, A., Kohno, N., Hamada, H., et al. (1998) Circulating KL-6 predicts the outcome of rapidly progressive idiopathic pulmonary fibrosis. *Am. J. Respir. Crit. Care Med.* **158,** 1680–1684.
99. Kondoh, Y., Taniguchi, H., Kawabata, Y., Yokoi, T., Suzuki, K., and Takagi, K. (1993) Acute exacerbation in idiopathic pulmonary fibrosis. Analysis of clinical and pathologic findings in three cases. *Chest* **103,** 1808–18012.
100. Saydain, G., Islam, A., Afessa, B., Ryu, J. H., Scott, J. P., and Peters, S. G. (2002) Outcome of patients with idiopathic pulmonary fibrosis admitted to the intensive care unit. *Am. J. Respir. Crit. Care Med.* **166,** 839–842.
101. Bouros, D., Nicholson, A. C., Polychronopoulos, V., and du Bois, R. M. (2000) Acute interstitial pneumonia. *Eur. Respir. J.* **15,** 412–418.
102. Panos, R. J., Mortenson, R. L., Niccoli, S. A., and King, T. E., Jr. (1990) Clinical deterioration in patients with idiopathic pulmonary fibrosis: causes and assessment. *Am. J. Med.* **88,** 396–404.
103. Aubry, M. C., Myers, J. L., Douglas, W. W., et al. (2002) Primary pulmonary carcinoma in patients with idiopathic pulmonary fibrosis. *Mayo Clin. Proc.* **77,** 763–770.
104. Hubbard, R., Venn, A., Lewis, S., and Britton, J. (2000) Lung cancer and cryptogenic fibrosing alveolitis. A population-based cohort study. *Am. J. Respir. Crit. Care Med.* **161,** 5–8.
105. Flaherty, K. R., Martinez, F. J., Travis, W. D., and Lynch, J. P. I. (2001) Nonspecific interstitial pneumonia (NSIP) *Semin. Respir. Crit. Care Med.* **22,** 423–433.
106. Walsh, L. J., Wong, C. A., Oborne, J., et al. (2001) Adverse effects of oral corticosteroids in relation to dose in patients with lung disease. *Thorax* **56,** 279–284.
107. Lynch, J. P., 3rd and McCune, W. J. (1997) Immunosuppressive and cytotoxic pharmacotherapy for pulmonary disorders. *Am. J. Respir. Crit. Care Med.* **155,** 395–420.
108. Zisman, D. A., Lynch, J. P., 3rd, Toews, G. B., Kazerooni, E. A., Flint, A., and Martinez, F. J. (2000) Cyclophosphamide in the treatment of idiopathic pulmonary fibrosis: a prospective study in patients who failed to respond to corticosteroids. *Chest* **117,** 1619–1626.
109. Gay, S. E., Kazerooni, E. A., Toews, G. B., et al. (1998) Idiopathic pulmonary fibrosis: predicting response to therapy and survival. *Am. J. Respir. Crit. Care Med.* **157,** 1063–1072.

110. Mogulkoc, N., Brutsche, M. H., Bishop, P. W., Greaves, S. M., Horrocks, A. W., and Egan, J. J. (2001) Pulmonary function in idiopathic pulmonary fibrosis and referral for lung transplantation. *Am. J. Respir. Crit. Care Med.* **164,** 103–108.
111. Nagao, T., Nagai, S., Hiramoto, Y., et al. (2002) Serial evaluation of high-resolution computed tomography findings in patients with idiopathic pulmonary fibrosis in usual interstitial pneumonia. *Respiration* **69,** 413–419.
112. Nicholson, A. G., Fulford, L. G., Colby, T. V., du Bois, R. M., Hansell, D. M., and Wells, A. U. (2002) The relationship between individual histologic features and disease progression in idiopathic pulmonary fibrosis. *Am. J. Respir. Crit. Care Med.* **166,** 173–177.
113. Flaherty, K. R., Colby, T. V., Travis, W. D., et al. (2003) Fibroblastic foci in usual interstitial pneumonia: idiopathic versus collagen vascular disease. *Am. J. Respir. Crit. Care Med.* **167,** 1410–1415.
114. Watters, L. C., King, T. E., Schwarz, M. I., Waldron, J. A., Stanford, R. E., and Cherniack, R. M. (1986) A clinical, radiographic, and physiologic scoring system for the longitudinal assessment of patients with idiopathic pulmonary fibrosis. *Am. Rev. Respir. Dis.* **133,** 97–103.
115. Wells, A. U., Desai, S. R., Rubens, M. B., et al. (2003) Idiopathic pulmonary fibrosis: a composite physiologic index derived from disease extent observed by computed tomography. *Am. J. Respir. Crit. Care Med.* **167,** 962–969.
116. Flaherty, K. R., Mumford, J. A., Murray, S., et al. (2003) Prognostic implications of physiologic and radiographic changes in idiopathic interstitial pneumonia. *Am. J. Respir. Crit. Care Med.* **168,** 543–548.
117. Latsi, P. I., du Bois, R. M., Nicholson, A. G., et al. (2003) Fibrotic idiopathic interstitial pneumonia: the prognostic value of longitudinal functional trends. *Am. J. Respir. Crit. Care Med.* **168,** 531–537.
118. Collard, H. R., King, T. E., Jr., Bartelson, B. B., Vourlekis, J. S., Schwarz, M. I., and Brown, K. K. (2003) Changes in clinical and physiologic variables predict survival in idiopathic pulmonary fibrosis. *Am. J. Respir. Crit. Care Med.* **168,** 538–542.
119. Greene, K. E., King, T. E., Jr., Kuroki, Y., et al. (2002) Serum surfactant proteins-A and -D as biomarkers in idiopathic pulmonary fibrosis. *Eur. Respir. J.* **19,** 439–46.
120. Mogulkoc, N., Brutsche, M. H., Bishop, P. W., et al. (2001) Pulmonary (99m)Tc-DTPA aerosol clearance and survival in usual interstitial pneumonia (UIP) *Thorax* **56,** 916–923.
121. Davies, H. R., Richeldi, L., and Walters, E. H. (2003) Immunomodulatory agents for idiopathic pulmonary fibrosis. *Cochrane Database Syst. Rev.* CD003134.
122. Richeldi, L., Davies, H. R., Ferrara, G., and Franco, F. (2003) Corticosteroids for idiopathic pulmonary fibrosis. *Cochrane Database Syst. Rev.* CD002880.
123. Douglas, W. W., Ryu, J. H., and Schroeder, D. R. (2000) Idiopathic pulmonary fibrosis: Impact of oxygen and colchicine, prednisone, or no therapy on survival. *Am. J. Respir. Crit. Care Med.* **161,** 1172–1178.

124. Douglas, W. W., Ryu, J. H., Bjoraker, J. A., et al. (1997) Colchicine versus prednisone as treatment of usual interstitial pneumonia. *Mayo Clin. Proc.* **72,** 201–209.
125. Winterbauer, R. H., Hammar, S. P., Hallman, K. O., et al. (1978) Diffuse interstitial pneumonitis. Clinicopathologic correlations in 20 patients treated with prednisone/azathioprine. *Am. J. Med.* **65,** 661–672.
126. Raghu, G., Depaso, W. J., Cain, K., et al. (1991) Azathioprine combined with prednisone in the treatment of idiopathic pulmonary fibrosis: a prospective double-blind, randomized, placebo-controlled clinical trial. *Am. Rev. Respir. Dis.* **144,** 291–296.
127. Johnson, M. A., Kwan, S., Snell, N. J., Nunn, A. J., Darbyshire, J. H., and Turner-Warwick, M. (1989) Randomised controlled trial comparing prednisolone alone with cyclophosphamide and low dose prednisolone in combination in cryptogenic fibrosing alveolitis. *Thorax* **44,** 280–288.
128. Nagai, S., Kitaichi, M., Hamada, K., et al. (1999) Hospital-based historical cohort study of 234 histologically proven Japanese patients with IPF. *Sarcoidosis Vasc. Diffuse Lung Dis.* **16,** 209–214.
129. O'Donnell, K., Keogh, B., Çantin, A., and Crystal, R. G. (1987) Pharmacologic suppression of the neutrophil component of the alveolitis in idiopathic pulmonary fibrosis. *Am. Rev. Respir. Dis.* **136,** 288–292.
130. Dayton, C. S., Schwartz, D. A., Helmers, R. A., et al. (1993) Outcome of subjects with idiopathic pulmonary fibrosis who fail corticosteroid therapy. Implications for further studies. *Chest* **103,** 69–73.
131. Baughman, R. P. and Lower, E. E. (1992) Use of intermittent, intravenous cyclophosphamide for idiopathic pulmonary fibrosis. *Chest* **102,** 1090–1094.
132. Kolb, M., Kirschner, J., Riedel, W., Wirtz, H., and Schmidt, M. (1998) Cyclophosphamide pulse therapy in idiopathic pulmonary fibrosis. *Eur. Respir. J.* **12,** 1409–1414.
133. Maurer, J. R., Frost, A. E., Estenne, M., Higenbottam, T., and Glanville, A. R. (1998) International guidelines for the selection of lung transplant candidates. The International Society for Heart and Lung Transplantation, the American Thoracic Society, the American Society of Transplant Physicians, the European Respiratory Society. *J. Heart Lung Transplant.* **17,** 703–709.
134. Arcasoy, S. M. and Kotloff, R. M. (1999) Lung transplantation. *N. Engl. J. Med.* **340,** 1081–1091.
135. Thabut, G., Mal, H., Castier, Y., et al. (2003) Survival benefit of lung transplantation for patients with idiopathic pulmonary fibrosis. *J. Thorac. Cardiovasc. Surg.* **126,** 469–475.
136. Hertz, M. I., Taylor, D. O., Trulock, E. P., et al. (2002) The registry of the international society for heart and lung transplantation: nineteenth official report-2002. *J. Heart Lung Transplant.* **21,** 950–970.
137. Meyers, B. F., Lynch, J. P., Trulock, E. P., Guthrie, T., Cooper, J. D., and Patterson, G. A. (2000) Single versus bilateral lung transplantation for idiopathic pulmonary fibrosis: a ten-year institutional experience. *J. Thorac. Cardiovasc. Surg.* **120,** 99–107.

138. Stavem, K., Bjortuft, O., Lund, M. B., Kongshaug, K., Geiran, O., and Boe, J. (2000) Health-related quality of life in lung transplant candidates and recipients. *Respiration* **67,** 159–165.
139. Lanuza, D. M., Lefaiver, C. A., and Farcas, G. A. (2000) Research on the quality of life of lung transplant candidates and recipients: an integrative review. *Heart Lung* **29,** 180–195.
140. Timmer, S. J., Karamzadeh, A. M., Yung, G. L., Kriett, J., Jamieson, S. W., and Smith, C. M. (2002) Predicting survival of lung transplantation candidates with idiopathic interstitial pneumonia: does PaO(2) predict survival? *Chest* **122,** 779–784.
141. Selman, M., King, T. E., and Pardo, A. (2001) Idiopathic pulmonary fibrosis: prevailing and evolving hypotheses about its pathogenesis and implications for therapy. *Ann. Intern. Med.* **134,** 136–151.
142. Malkinson, F. (1982) Colchicine: new uses of an old drug. *Arch. Dermatol.* **118,** 453–457.
143. Redman, C. M., Banerjee, D., Howell, K., and Palade, G. E. (1975) Colchicine inhibition of plasma protein release from rat hepatocytes. *J. Cell Biol.* **66,** 42–59.
144. Dubrawsky, C., Dubravsky, N., and Withers, H. (1978) The effect of colchicine on the accumulation of hydroxyproline and on lung compliance after irradiation. *Radiat. Res.* **73,** 111–120.
145. Peters, S. G., McDougall, J. C., Douglas, W. W., Coles, D. T., and DeRemee, R. A. (1993) Colchicine in the treatment of pulmonary fibrosis. *Chest* **103,** 101–104.
146. Fedullo, A. J., Karlinsky, J. B., Snider, G. L., and Goldstein, R. H. (1980) Lung statics and connective tissues after penicillamine in bleomycin-treated hamsters. *J. Appl. Physiol.* **49,** 1083–1090.
147. Jimenez, S. and Sigal, S. (1991) A 15-year prospective study of treatment of rapidly progressive systemic sclerosis with D-penicillamine. *J. Rheumatol.* **18,** 1496–1503.
148. Selman, M., Carrillo, G., Salas, J., et al. (1998) Colchicine, D-penicillamine, and prednisone in the treatment of idiopathic pulmonary fibrosis: a controlled clinical trial. *Chest* **114,** 507–512.
149. Lee, B., Margolin, S., and Nowak, R. (1997) Pirfenidone: a novel pharmacological agent that inhibits leiomyoma cell proliferation and collagen production. *J. Clin. Endocrinol. Metab.* **83,** 219–223.
150. Iyer, S., Gurujeyalakshmi, G., and Guri, S. N. (1999) Downregulation of procollagen genes at the transcriptional level in bleomycin hamster model of lung fibrosis. *J. Pharmacol. Exp. Ther.* **289,** 211–218.
151. Iyer, S. N., Gurujeyalakshmi, G., and Giri, S. N. (1999) Effects of pirfenidone on transforming growth factor-beta gene expression at the transcriptional level in bleomycin hamster model of lung fibrosis. *J. Pharmacol. Exp. Ther.* **291,** 367–373.
152. Raghu, G., Johnson, W. C., Lockhart, D., and Mageto, Y. (1999) Treatment of idiopathic pulmonary fibrosis with a new antifibrotic agent, pirfenidone: results of a prospective, open-label Phase II study. *Am. J. Respir. Crit. Care Med.* **159,** 1061–1069.

153. Nagai, S., Hamada, K., Shigematsu, M., Taniyama, M., Yamauchi, S., and Izumi, T. (2002) Open-label compassionate use one year-treatment with pirfenidone to patients with chronic pulmonary fibrosis. *Intern. Med.* **41,** 1118–1123.
154. Gahl, W. A., Brantly, M., Troendle, J., et al. (2002) Effect of pirfenidone on the pulmonary fibrosis of Hermansky-Pudlak syndrome. *Mol. Genet. Metab.* **76,** 234–242.
155. Billiau, A. (1996) Interferon-gamma: biology and role in pathogenesis. *Adv. Immunol.* **62,** 61–130.
156. Gurujeyalakshmi, G. and Giri, S. N. (1995) Molecular mechanisms of antifibrotic effect of interferon gamma in bleomycin-mouse model of lung fibrosis: downregulation of TGF-beta and procollagen I and III gene expression. *Exp. Lung Res.* **21,** 791–808.
157. Narayanan, A. S., Whithey, J., Souza, A., and Raghu, G. (1992) Effect of gamma-interferon on collagen synthesis by normal and fibrotic human lung fibroblasts. *Chest* **101,** 1326–1331.
158. Prior, C. and Haslam, P. L. (1992) In vivo levels and in vitro production of interferon-gamma in fibrosing interstitial lung diseases. *Clin. Exp. Immunol.* **88,** 280–287.
159. Kuroki, S., Ohta, A., Sueoka, N., Katoh, O., Yamada, H., and Yamaguchi, M. (1995) Determination of various cytokines and type III procollagen aminopeptide levels in bronchoalveolar lavage fluid of the patients with pulmonary fibrosis: inverse correlation between type III procollagen aminopeptide and interferon-gamma in progressive patients. *Br. J. Rheumatol.* **34,** 31–36.
160. Shaw, R. J., Benedict, S. H., Clark, R. A., and King, T. E., Jr. (1991) Pathogenesis of pulmonary fibrosis in interstitial lung disease. Alveolar macrophage PDGF(B) gene activation and up-regulation by interferon gamma. *Am. Rev. Respir. Dis.* **143,** 167–173.
161. Ziesche, R., Hofbauer, E., Wittmann, K., Petkov, V., and Block, L. H. (1999) A preliminary study of long-term treatment with interferon gamma-1b and low-dose prednisolone in patients with idiopathic pulmonary fibrosis. *N. Engl. J. Med.* **341,** 1264–1269.
162. King, T. E., Jr. (2000) Interferon gamma-1b for the treatment of idiopathic pulmonary fibrosis. *N. Engl. J. Med.* **342,** 974–975.
163. King, T. J. (September 2000) New Approaches to Managing Idiopathic Pulmonary Fibrosis. Continuing Education Monograph Series. American Thoracic Society, New York.
164. Kalra, S., Utz, J. P., and Ryu, J. H. (2003) Interferon gamma-1b therapy for advanced idiopathic pulmonary fibrosis. *Mayo Clin. Proc.* **78,** 1082–1087.
165. Prasse, A., Muller, K. M., Kurz, C., Hamm, H., and Virchow, J. C., Jr. (2003) Does interferon-gamma improve pulmonary function in idiopathic pulmonary fibrosis? *Eur. Respir. J.* **22,** 906–911.
166. Pfeffer, L. M., Murphy, J. S., and Tamm, I. (1979) Interferon effects on the growth and division of human fibroblasts. *Exp. Cell Res.* **121,** 111–120.
167. Duncan, M. R. and Berman, B. (1989) Differential regulation of glycosaminoglycan, fibronectin, and collagenase production in cultured human dermal fibroblasts by interferon-alpha, -beta, and -gamma. *Arch. Dermatol. Res.* **281,** 11–18.

168. Sciavolino, P. J., Lee, T. H., and Vilcek, J. (1994) Interferon-beta induces metalloproteinase mRNA expression in human fibroblasts. Role of activator protein-1. *J. Biol. Chem.* **269,** 21,627–21,634.
169. Goldring, M. B. (1987) Control of collagen synthesis in human chondrocyte cultures by immune interferon and interleukin-1. *J. Rheumatol.* **14(Spec No),** 64–66.
170. McDonald, S., Rubin, P., Chang, A. Y., et al. (1993) Pulmonary changes induced by combined mouse beta-interferon (rMuIFN-beta) and irradiation in normal mice—toxic versus protective effects. *Radiother. Oncol.* **26,** 212–218.
171. Raghu, G., Bozic, C. R., Brown, K., et al. (2001) Feasibility Of A Trial Of Interferon Beta-1A (IFN- Beta-1A) In The Treatment Of Idiopathic Pulmonary Fibrosis (IPF). Meeting of the American Thoracic Society.
172. Adamson, I. Y., Young, L., and Bowden, D. H. (1988) Relationship of alveolar epithelial injury and repair to the induction of pulmonary fibrosis. *Am. J. Pathol.* **130,** 377–383.
173. Hagimoto, N., Kuwano, K., Miyazaki, H., et al. (1997) Induction of apoptosis and pulmonary fibrosis in mice in response to ligation of Fas antigen. *Am. J. Respir. Cell Mol. Biol.* **17,** 272–278.
174. Wang, R., Ibarra-Sunga, O., Verlinski, L., Pick, R., and Uhal, B. D. (2000) Abrogation of bleomycin-induced epithelial apoptosis and lung fibrosis by captopril or by a caspase inhibitor. *Am. J. Physiol. Lung Cell. Mol. Physiol.* **279,** L143–151.
175. Mason, R. J., Schwarz, M. I., Hunninghake, G. W., and Musson, R. A. (1999) NHLBI Workshop Summary. Pharmacological therapy for idiopathic pulmonary fibrosis. Past, present, and future. *Am. J. Respir. Crit. Care Med.* **160,** 1771–1777.
176. Cantin, A. M., Hubbard, R. C., and Crystal, R. G. (1989) Glutathione deficiency in the epithelial lining fluid of the lower respiratory tract in idiopathic pulmonary fibrosis. *Am. Rev. Respir. Dis.* **139,** 370–372.
177. Meyer, A., Buhl, R., and Magnussen, H. (1994) The effect of oral N-acetylcysteine on lung glutathione levels in idiopathic pulmonary fibrosis. *Eur. Respir. J.* **7,** 431–436.
178. Hagiwara, S. I., Ishii, Y., and Kitamura, S. (2000) Aerosolized administration of N-acetylcysteine attenuates lung fibrosis induced by bleomycin in mice. *Am. J. Respir. Crit. Care Med.* **162,** 225–231.
179. Behr, J., Maier, K., Degenkolb, B., Krombach, F., and Vogelmeier, C. (1997) Antioxidative and clinical effects of high-dose N-acetylcysteine in fibrosing alveolitis. Adjunctive therapy to maintenance immunosuppression. *Am. J. Respir. Crit. Care Med.* **156,** 1897–1901.
180. Phan, S. H. and Kunkel, S. L. (1992) Lung cytokine production in bleomycin-induced pulmonary fibrosis. *Exp. Lung Res.* **18,** 29–43.
181. Sime, P. J., Marr, R. A., Gauldie, D., Xing, Z., Hewlett, B. R., Graham, F. L., and Gauldie, J. (1998) Transfer of tumor necrosis factor-alpha to rat lung induces severe pulmonary inflammation and patchy interstitial fibrogenesis with induction of transforming growth factor-beta1 and myofibroblasts. *Am. J. Pathol.* **153,** 825–832.

182. Ortiz, L. A., Lasky, J., Hamilton, R. F., Jr., et al. (1998) Expression of TNF and the necessity of TNF receptors in bleomycin-induced lung injury in mice. *Exp. Lung Res.* **24,** 721–743.
183. Piguet, P. F., Ribaux, C., Karpuz, V., Grau, G. E., and Kapanci, Y. (1993) Expression and localization of tumor necrosis factor-alpha and its mRNA in idiopathic pulmonary fibrosis. *Am. J. Pathol.* **143,** 651–655.
184. Piguet, P. F. and Vesin, C. (1994) Treatment by human recombinant soluble TNF receptor of pulmonary fibrosis induced by bleomycin or silica in mice. *Eur. Respir. J.* **7,** 515–518.
185. Moreland, L. W., Baumgartner, S. W., Schiff, M. H., et al. (1997) Treatment of rheumatoid arthritis with a recombinant human tumor necrosis factor receptor (p75)-Fc fusion protein. *N. Engl. J. Med.* **337,** 141–147.
186. Wanidworanun, C. and Strober, W. (1993) Predominant role of tumor necrosis factor-alpha in human monocyte IL-10 synthesis. *J. Immunol.* **151,** 6853–6861.
187. Martinez, J. A., King, T. E., Jr., Brown, K., et al. (1997) Increased expression of the interleukin-10 gene by alveolar macrophages in interstitial lung disease. *Am. J. Physiol.* **273,** L676–683.
188. Arai, T., Abe, K., Matsuoka, H., et al. (2000) Introduction of the interleukin-10 gene into mice inhibited bleomycin-induced lung injury in vivo. *Am. J. Physiol. Lung. Cell. Mol. Physiol.* **278,** L914–922.
189. Morita, Y., Yamamura, M., Kawashima, M., et al. (2001) Differential in vitro effects of IL-4, IL-10, and IL-13 on proinflammatory cytokine production and fibroblast proliferation in rheumatoid synovium. *Rheumatol. Int.* **20,** 49–54.
190. Wallace, W. A., Ramage, E. A., Lamb, D., and Howie, S. E. (1995) A type 2 (Th2-like) pattern of immune response predominates in the pulmonary interstitium of patients with cryptogenic fibrosing alveolitis (CFA) *Clin. Exp. Immunol.* **101,** 436–441.
191. Giri, S. N., Hyde, D. M., and Hollinger, M. A. (1993) Effect of antibody to transforming growth factor beta on bleomycin induced accumulation of lung collagen in mice. *Thorax* **48,** 959–966.
192. Sime, P. J., Xing, Z., Graham, F. L., Csaky, K. G., and Gauldie, J. (1997) Adenovector-mediated gene transfer of active transforming growth factor-beta1 induces prolonged severe fibrosis in rat lung. *J. Clin. Invest.* **100,** 768–776.
193. Khalil, N., O'Connor, R. N., Flanders, K. C., and Unruh, H. (1996) TGF-beta 1, but not TGF-beta 2 or TGF-beta 3, is differentially present in epithelial cells of advanced pulmonary fibrosis: an immunohistochemical study. *Am. J. Respir. Cell Mol. Biol.* **14,** 131–138.
194. Peters, H., Noble, N. A., and Border, W. A. (1997) Transforming growth factor-beta in human glomerular injury. *Curr. Opin. Nephrol. Hypertens.* **6,** 389–393.
195. Ulloa, L., Doody, J., and Massague, J. (1999) Inhibition of transforming growth factor-beta/SMAD signalling by the interferon-gamma/STAT pathway. *Nature* **397,** 710–713.
196. Car, B. D., Meloni, F., Luisetti, M., Semenzato, G., Gialdroni-Grassi, G., and Walz, A. (1994) Elevated IL-8 and MCP-1 in the bronchoalveolar lavage fluid of

patients with idiopathic pulmonary fibrosis and pulmonary sarcoidosis. *Am. J. Respir. Crit. Care Med.* **149,** 655–659.

197. Antoniades, H. N., Neville-Golden, J., Galanopoulos, T., Kradin, R. L., Valente, A. J., and Graves, D. T. (1992) Expression of monocyte chemoattractant protein 1 mRNA in human idiopathic pulmonary fibrosis. *Proc. Natl. Acad. Sci. USA* **89,** 5371–5375.
198. Gharaee-Kermani, M., Denholm, E. M., and Phan, S. H. (1996) Costimulation of fibroblast collagen and transforming growth factor beta1 gene expression by monocyte chemoattractant protein-1 via specific receptors. *J. Biol. Chem.* **271,** 17,779–17,784.
199. Suga, M., Iyonaga, K., Ichiyasu, H., Saita, N., Yamasaki, H., and Ando, M. (1999) Clinical significance of MCP-1 levels in BALF and serum in patients with interstitial lung diseases. *Eur. Respir. J.* **14,** 376–382.
200. Giaid, A., Michel, R. P., Stewart, D. J., Sheppard, M., Corrin, B., and Hamid, Q. (1993) Expression of endothelin-1 in lungs of patients with cryptogenic fibrosing alveolitis. *Lancet* **341,** 1550–1554.
201. Yanagisawa, M., Kurihara, H., Kimura, S., et al. (1988) A novel potent vasoconstrictor peptide produced by vascular endothelial cells. *Nature* **332,** 411–415.
202. Teder, P. and Noble, P. W. (2000) A cytokine reborn? Endothelin-1 in pulmonary inflammation and fibrosis. *Am. J. Respir. Cell Mol. Biol.* **23,** 7–10.
203. Mutsaers, S. E., Marshall, R. P., Goldsack, N. R., Laurent, G. J., and McAnulty, R. J. (1998) Effect of endothelin receptor antagonists (BQ-485, Ro 47-0203) on collagen deposition during the development of bleomycin-induced pulmonary fibrosis in rats. *Pulm. Pharmacol. Ther.* **11,** 221–225.
204. Saleh, D., Furukawa, K., Tsao, M. S., et al. (1997) Elevated expression of endothelin-1 and endothelin-converting enzyme-1 in idiopathic pulmonary fibrosis: possible involvement of proinflammatory cytokines. *Am. J. Respir. Cell Mol. Biol.* **16,** 187–193.
205. Barnes, P. J. (1994) Endothelins and pulmonary diseases. *J. Appl. Physiol.* **77,** 1051–1059.
206. Park, S. H., Saleh, D., Giaid, A., and Michel, R. P. (1997) Increased endothelin-1 in bleomycin-induced pulmonary fibrosis and the effect of an endothelin receptor antagonist. *Am. J. Respir. Crit. Care Med.* **156,** 600–608.
207. Tan, A., Levrey, H., Dahm, C., Polunovsky, V. A., Rubins, J., and Bitterman, P. B. (1999) Lovastatin induces fibroblast apoptosis in vitro and in vivo. A possible therapy for fibroproliferative disorders. *Am. J. Respir. Crit. Care Med.* **159,** 220–227.
208. Ghofrani, H. A., Wiedemann, R., Rose, F., et al. (2002) Sildenafil for treatment of lung fibrosis and pulmonary hypertension: a randomised controlled trial. *Lancet* **360,** 895–900.

2

Renal Fibrosis

H. William Schnaper

Summary

The kidney has unique attributes that are related to its complex structure and that affect the nature of fibrogenesis in this organ. It is divided into functional units, called nephrons, that have both a filtering and a reabsorbing component. Sclerosis may initiate in the sites of either of these components but ultimately involves both. The epidemiology and clinical manifestations of renal fibrosis suggest complex genetic and environmental influences on the development of fibrosis. Further, the different structures in the kidney manifest different mechanisms of fibrogenesis. These are determined by a combination of differences in the biology of the affected cells and the physical effects of nephron failure. Although therapy for renal fibrosis remains somewhat problematic, new insights into the mechanisms of the underlying diseases offer the promise of improved approaches to treatment.

Key Words: Kidney; fibrosis; TGF-β; glomerulosclerosis; nephron; basement membrane.

1. Introduction

The kidney serves a variety of functions essential to our physiology. The characteristic renal function that, when lost, requires replacement with dialysis or transplantation involves the cleansing of water-soluble impurities from the blood through the production of urine, and of maintenance of proper fluid and electrolyte homeostasis. In addition, the kidney regulates acid–base balance in tandem with the lung, controls bone metabolism through its roles in phosphate excretion and the metabolic activation of vitamin D, stimulates bone marrow function through the production of erythropoietin, and serves as a site for gluconeogenesis. Fibrosis of the kidney, whether it is a primary pathological process or the ultimate manifestation of organ involution and loss, can affect all of these functions, and thus remains an important clinical problem in both developed countries and the developing nations. In the United States in 2001, more than 400,000 patients were receiving treatment for chronic kidney failure, and the cost of treating this problem was approx $22.8 billion *(1)*.

From: *Methods in Molecular Medicine, Vol. 117: Fibrosis Research: Methods and Protocols*
Edited by: J. Varga, D. A. Brenner, and S. H. Phan © Humana Press Inc., Totowa, NJ

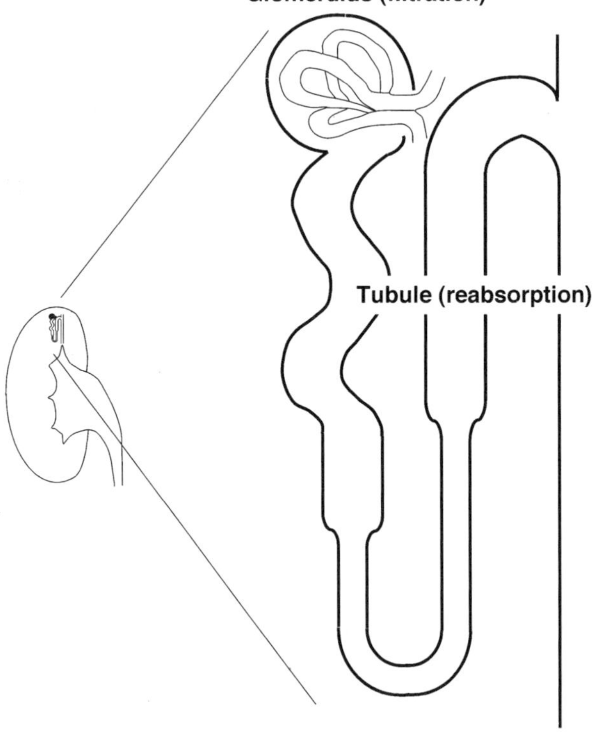

Fig. 1. Schematic depiction of the nephron. Water and small molecular solute pass from the glomerular capillaries into the urinary space, whereas most of the protein normally is restricted from passing through the filter. Ninety-nine percent of the filtrate is reabsorbed in the renal tubule. Reproduced from **ref.** ***37***, with permission.

Understanding renal fibrosis requires some sense of the functional anatomy of the kidney. It is a complex organ with highly specialized structures, each of which undergoes fibrosis in a unique way. The functional anatomy of the kidney is depicted schematically in **Fig. 1**. The major unit of the kidney is the *nephron*, which in turn is comprised of the filtering apparatus, the *glomerulus*, and an apparatus that regulates fluid and electrolyte homeostasis, the *tubule*. Although the glomerulus occupies only 3 to 5% of the renal mass, it is the initial site at which many acute and chronic inflammatory processes involve the kidney and has attracted a large share of the mechanistic analysis of renal fibrogenesis. The tubulointerstitium, however, is the site of significant inflammation and plays a role in the progression of chronic kidney disease. Fibrogenesis at both of these locations will be considered here.

The glomerulus is comprised of a ball (glomus) of capillaries surrounded by a cup of epithelial cells that serve as the beginning of the tubule. The approx 1,000,000 glomeruli in the kidneys filter the entire body water about five times per day. Ninety-nine percent of this filtrate is reabsorbed by the tubule emanating from each glomerulus, permitting precise regulation of fluid and electrolyte homeostasis. A fine balance between glomerular and tubular function prevents dehydration from occurring. This is effected through regulation of perfusion, hydrostatic pressure and filtration surface area in the glomerulus. A diagram of a cross-section of a capillary tuft within the glomerulus is shown in **Fig. 2A**. Several capillaries are draped over a stalk of *mesangial cells*, which have similarities to both macrophages and vascular smooth muscle cells. In this view, blood flow runs through the capillaries in a direction perpendicular to the plane of the page. The capillaries are comprised of an inner lining of fenestrated endothelial cells that permit the passage of solvent (water) and solute (electrolytes and other small molecules). An outer support structure is comprised of visceral epithelial cells that spread interdigitating process across the external surface of the capillary. The appearance of these interdigitating structures has led to their being called foot processes, and the unique cells from which they arise are termed *podocytes*. Because both the endothelial cells and the podocytes lay down a basement membrane, the result is a glomerular basement membrane (GBM) that is trilaminar, with a relatively electron-dense lamina densa between the lamina rara interna and lamina rara externa (**Fig. 2B**). Water and solute are extruded from the capillary space into the urinary space. Because of striking electrostatic properties (negative charge) as well as the role of the capillary membranes in filtering the plasma water, immune complexes often are trapped in the GBM or form *in situ* from circulating antibodies and glomerular antigens. This process activates the complement cascade or other inflammatory pathways, leading to the development of *glomerulonephritis*. If these events are sufficiently chronic to lead to scar formation, the process is known as *glomerulosclerosis*. In addition to inflammation, glomerulosclerosis can result from other diseases of a structural, functional, or genetic nature, or it may be idiopathic.

Filtered antigens, biologically active proteins, or lipids are trapped by the renal tubular cells in the process of pinocytosis. At times, these antigens or biologically active molecules may change the structure of the renal tubular cells or are themselves chemokinetic, initiating an inflammatory process in which macrophages are recruited and exacerbate the degree of tubular damage. This inflammation generates *tubulointerstitial nephritis* (TIN). TIN, too, may become chronic, leading to tubulointerstitial fibrosis *(2)*. TIN may result from toxic or allergenic effects of drugs, viral infections, genetic abnormalities of the tubulointerstitium, or metabolic activation of the tubular epithelia.

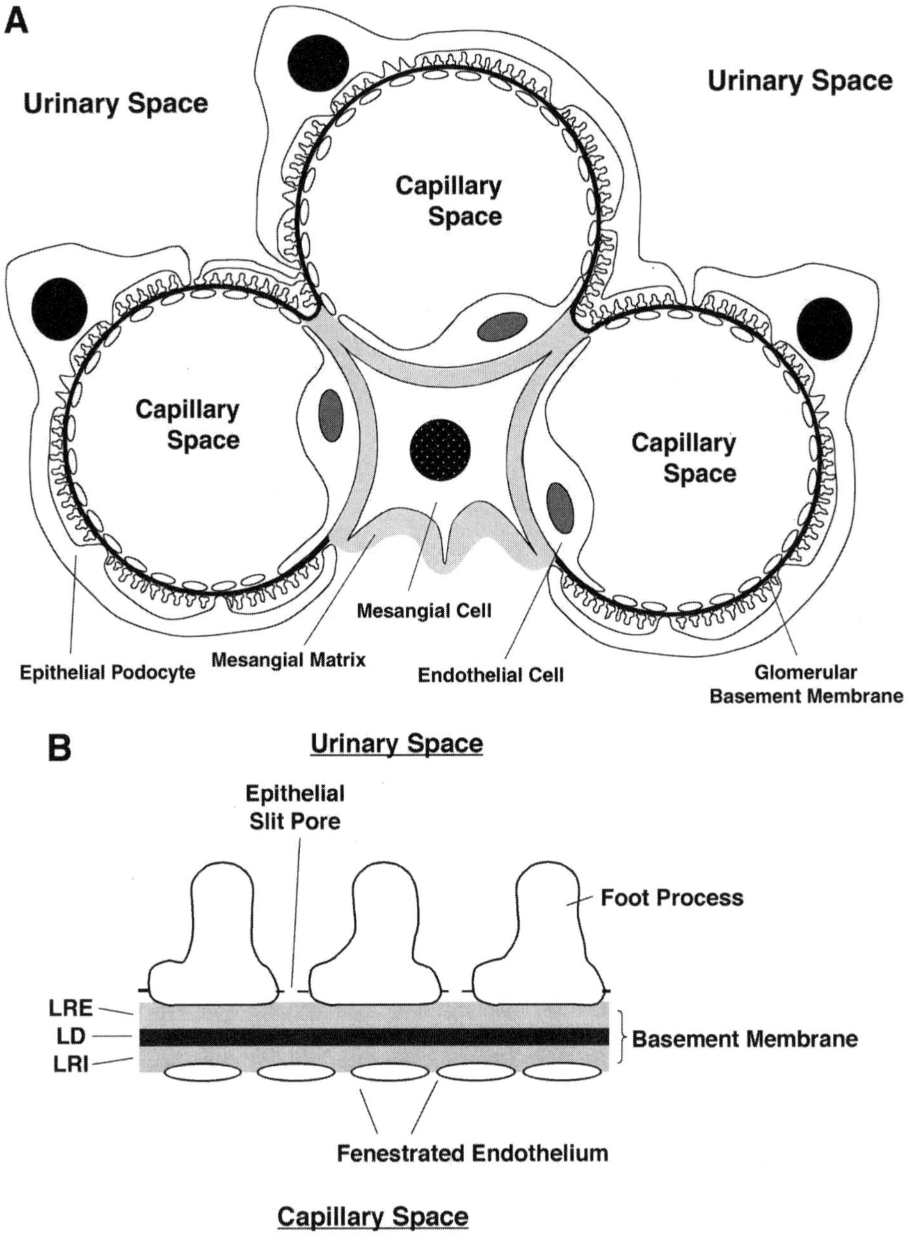

Fig. 2. Microscopic structure and ultrastructure of the glomerulus. **(A)** A cross-section of a glomerular tuft, with the blood flow running perpendicular to this page. Filtration occurs from the capillaries into the urinary space. A fenestrated endothelium lines the capillaries. The podocyte provides external support, while its interdigitations provide sufficient space for the passage of filtrate. A basement membrane is adjacent

2. Kidney Diseases Causing Fibrosis

Any disease that leads to chronic kidney damage may result in fibrosis. Given the complexity of renal structure, the compartmentalization delineated by normal basement membranes is essential for maintaining the functional integrity of the nephron. Thus, in conditions involving acute toxicity, the ability of the renal tubular epithelial cell to rapidly regenerate assures that recovery can occur as long as the tubular basement membrane remains intact. However, if this, too, is destroyed, then the likelihood of regeneration of a normal nephron may decrease. Therefore, the factors regulating both the balance and timing of extracellular matrix (ECM) turnover are critical *(3)*. For example, in some models of inflammatory glomerulonephritis, infiltrating macrophages produce proteolytic enzymes that destroy the structure *(4)*. In contrast, in the rat anti-Thy1 nephritis model, an injected antibody against a thymic antigen cross-reacts with a similar antigen in the rat mesangial cell. The resulting disease involves mesangiolysis and ECM accumulation that is self-limited, with resolution beginning to occur by 1 wk. Interestingly, resolution is preceded by increased expression of matrix metalloproteinase (MMP)-2 *(5)*, suggesting that this ECM protease activity is, in this case, important for resolving a potential scar rather than for the degree of damage it might cause to glomerular structures.

Human diseases associated with fibrosis can be divided roughly into three categories. As described previously, a number of glomerular diseases, such as those associated with inflammation of the basement membrane or cells comprising the filter (glomerulonephritis), or diabetes mellitus, can lead to scarring of the glomerulus *(6)*. In addition, *idiopathic focal segmental glomerulosclerosis* (FSGS) is a disease in which scarring of this filter occurs in a focally distributed pattern and without any apparent antecedent cause *(7)*. **Figure 3** illustrates three different types of glomerular disease to emphasize the importance of structural considerations in the type of fibrosis that occurs. The first shows a glomerulus from a kidney with membranous nephropathy (MN). Immune complexes trapped in the glomerular filter cause a thickening of the capillary wall, leading to an accentuation of the capillary loops. Whereas the epithelial and endothelial cell likely contribute to this thickened membrane, the process clearly is different from that in FSGS. In FSGS, the central location

---

Fig. 2. *(continued)* to all of the cells (black line for glomerular basement membrane [GBM], gray shading for mesangial matrix). **(B)** Ultrastructure of the capillary basement membrane. Note the trilaminar structure of the GBM and the pores in the epithelial slit diaphragm that are the ultimate determinant of steric selectivity for the filtration of macromolecules. LRE, lamina rara externa; LD, lamina densa; LRI, lamina rara interna. Reprinted with permission from **ref. *37***.

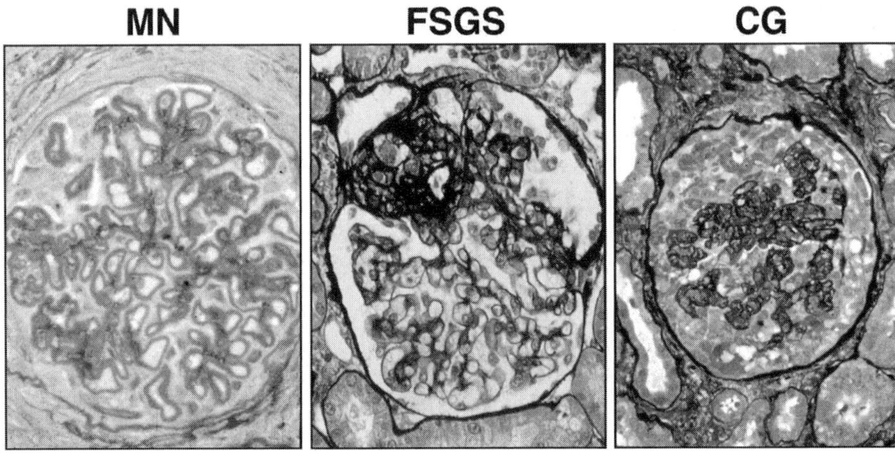

Fig. 3. Glomeruli from patients with membranous nephropathy (MN), focal segmental glomerulosclerosis (FSGS), or collapsing glomerulopathy (CG). The darkest areas show staining for collagen. MN shows thickened basement membranes; FSGS involves the segmental accumulation of collagen; and CG manifests similar accumulation of collagen with collapsed capillary structures. Microphotographs courtesy of Drs. Charles Alpers and Stuart Shankland, University of Washington.

of ECM accumulation and the segmental appearance of the lesion contrast with the diffuse, finely structured involvement of the capillary loops in MN. The likely source of this ECM is the mesangial cell. In collapsing glomerulopathy (CG), FSGS is accompanied by additional events involving the podocyte, leading to a different pattern of matrix accumulation. Thus, the nature of the glomerular scar is likely determined by the structural pattern of the cells that are involved.

A third form of renal fibrosis starts in the tubulointerstitium. In its most common form, diseases like chronic recurrent kidney infections combine with reflux of urine into the renal parenchyma to stimulate fibrogenesis, even in the glomeruli. Another example is the sclerosing effect of chronic tubular toxins. It is important to emphasize that glomerular and tubular processes cannot be entirely distinguished as a cause of end-stage kidney disease. For example, loss of nephrons as a result of tubular damage from reflux or of certain progressive genetic disorders of the tubule causes involution of the glomeruli that are at the proximal portion of the same tubules. Conversely, progression of FSGS is predicted by the identification of lymphocytic infiltration of the tubulointerstitium *(8)*, suggesting that excessive delivery of serum components to the tubule initiates an inflammatory cascade that plays an important part in nephron loss and fibrogenesis. Even in diseases that typically have been thought of as glomerular (such as protein-overload proteinuria, in which repeated intraperitoneal injections of albumin into rats eventually causes glomerulosclerosis), the critical pathogenetic event in the progression towards end-stage disease may be increased expression of tissue inhibitor of metalloproteinase (TIMP)-1 in the peritubular space *(9)*. Together, glomerulosclerosis and tubulointerstitial fibrosis may be the necessary twin hallmarks of ECM accumulation and scarring in progressive kidney disease.

3. Epidemiology and Genetics of Renal Fibrosis

Several factors suggest an interplay of environmental factors and genes in the advent of renal fibrosis. The incidence of FSGS, which already is the most common acquired cause of chronic renal failure in children, is increasing in both children and adults *(7)*. FSGS has been associated with numerous syndromes and a number of sibling pairs have been reported to have the disease *(6)*. A striking aspect of this familial incidence is that cases may be clustered temporally within families, suggesting that a genetic predisposition was present in those families and that a common event precipitated the disease.

Recently, a series of genes has been identified whose mutations define apparently Mendelian inheritance patterns for FSGS. The Wilms tumor suppressor gene, *WT1*, is one such gene. Mutation of exons 8 or 9, which encode the zinc finger region of the protein, has been associated with two syndromes *(10)*. Denys–Drash syndrome includes congenital nephrotic syndrome (massive proteinuria leading to severe edema), XY pseudohermaphroditism, and Wilms tumor *(11)*. The histopathology in these patients is diffuse mesangial sclerosis, characterized by increased ECM production and cellular proliferation in the mesangium. Other patients with *WT1* mutations have Frasier syndrome *(12)*. These patients manifest histopathology more like that of FSGS, in which the cellularity of the glomerulus is unaffected and ECM accumulation has a characteristic focal and segmental (rather than diffusely distributed) pattern. They also have associated gonadal abnormalities. It is striking that the nature and severity of clinical findings may vary even among family members *(13)*, suggesting the important influence of additional genes or environmental factors.

Single-gene mutations for glomerulosclerosis have been identified in *NPHS1*, *NPHS2*, or *ACTN4*. All of these genes encode for podocyte structural proteins. *NPHS1* is the gene for nephrin, a protein that helps form the epithelial slit diaphragm that is the final restrictive component regulating the size of molecules permitted to pass through the glomerular filtration barrier. It is mutated in congenital nephrotic syndrome of the Finnish type *(14)*, a progressive and treatment-resistant condition in which infants are born with massive proteinuria. *NPHS2* is the gene for podocin *(15)*, a protein that is found in the foot-processes of the podocyte. Homozygous and single-allele mutations have been found in some cases of FSGS in children who manifest a variety of clinical presentations ***(16)***. *ACTN4* is the gene for α-actinin4, a protein that helps mediate attachments between the cytoskeleton and adhesion molecules on the surface of the podocyte. Mutations inherited in an autosomal dominant pattern are found most commonly in patients who present with FSGS in early adulthood ***(17)***.

An intriguing consideration in the genetics of renal fibrosis is the possible existence of a so-called "renal failure gene." Conjecture regarding such a gene is based on two considerations. One is the observation that patients in families with renal disease are much more likely than those in the general population to require dialysis for end-stage kidney disease ***(18)***. The second consideration is the increased incidence of end-stage renal disease ***(19)***, or more aggressive rates of the progression of fibrosis ***(20)***, in African-American patients compared with Caucasians. This increased incidence in African-Americans has been attributed to hypertension but, in the families with a high incidence of close relatives on dialysis, most of the cases were not the result of hypertensive kidney disease. These observations of familial and racial predilections may intersect in the classic studies of the Pima Indian tribe in the American southwest. This group has an extremely high incidence of type 2 diabetes mellitus, but not all of the patients have progressive kidney disease. Instead, there is a familial distribution of severe renal involvement ***(21)***, suggesting that the genetic trait responsible for the renal failure may be distinct from that for the type 2 diabetes.

The nature of such a genetic trait remains a subject of considerable interest. Areas of potential study include gene polymorphisms that might lead to overexpression of molecules that exacerbate the physical factors contributing to glomerulosclerosis, molecules that represent hormonal mediators that enhance renal scarring, and molecules for which no obvious connection to sclerosis exists. In order to understand how such targets might be selected, it is appropriate to first consider the physical and biochemical factors that have been associated with renal scarring.

4. Pathophysiology of Renal Disease

4.1. Animal Models

The first clues regarding the causes of progressive kidney disease were derived from studies of animal models, largely in the rat. These models examine the effects of excessive nephron load or mechanical injury, toxic/metabolic stimuli of fibrosis, genetic predilection (hypertensive or diabetic rats and mice, Samoyed dogs) or, most recently, gene overexpression or deletion studies. Nephron overload has been accomplished either by repeated injections of bovine serum albumin (BSA) to cause excessive glomerular filtration of protein *(22)*, or ablation of renal mass to cause a compensatory response in remaining nephrons *(23)*. In both models, proteinuria is accompanied by sclerosis of both the glomeruli and the tubulointerstitium. In particular, the subtotal nephrectomy model has been used to study the hemodynamic factors that contribute to renal scarring *(24)*. Another form of injury is that involved with unilateral ureteral obstruction *(25)*. Together, these models can be conceptualized as involving insults delivered primarily to the glomerulus (subtotal nephrectomy), the tubule (obstruction), or both (overload), yet the effect is to stimulate fibrosis in both sites.

Biochemical stimuli of fibrogenesis include treatment with puromycin aminonucleoside *(26)* or doxorubicin (Adriamycin) *(27)*, a model felt to have some elements of FSGS but also to show tubulointerstitial changes. Other common models of fibrosis in animals include immune complex diseases *(28)*, and diabetes mellitus *(29)*. Rats rendered hyperlipidemic by diet or other manipulations also develop glomerulosclerosis *(30)*. Hyperlipidemia from genetically inherited traits also leads to kidney fibrosis *(31)*. Another genetic trait that has been associated with glomerulosclerosis in the rat is hypertension *(32)*. Finally, just as there may be a "renal failure" gene in humans, different strains of rodents show differential susceptibility to the induction of renal fibrosis. For example, mice with the ragged oligosyndactyly pintail background show enhanced susceptibility to a variety of stimuli of renal fibrosis compared with those lacking this background *(33)*.

Finally, a number of transgenic mouse models develop glomerulosclerosis. Two involve the disruption of podocyte genes that are identical to those identified in relation to human disease, *ACTN4* (34) and nephrin *(35)*. Mice with deficient expression of the podocyte structural protein CD2AP, which interacts with nephrin, develop a disease that histologically approximates FSGS and die at an early age *(36)*, again supporting the importance of effective podocyte structure and cell–cell interactions in maintaining normal ECM expression. For other transgenic or knockout models, however, the relationship is less direct. Thus, overexpression of growth hormone, interleukin-6, or a portion of the human immunodeficiency virus genome in mice leads to glomerulosclerosis. All of these genes likely enhance glomerular cell activation or inflammation (reviewed in **ref.** *37*). Less clear is the role of the peroxisomal protein Mpv-17; glomerulosclerosis develops in mice lacking this gene *(38)*.

4.2. Physical Factors That Contribute to Glomerulosclerosis

Clinical observations have suggested that hypertension may accelerate the progression of renal fibrosis *(39)*. However, the majority of investigators now believe that the critical parameter is not systemic hypertension, but rather intraglomerular hypertension *(39)*. It is possible that this reflects not just the level of pressure within the glomerulus, but a degree of glomerular hyperfiltration *(40)*. Thus, when the renal mass is reduced, the remaining nephrons may hypertrophy and assume the work of the lost nephrons, leading to possible nephron overload *(41)*. In humans with a mild reduction in renal mass, no significant deleterious effects are encountered *(42)*. However, severe reductions in renal mass are frequently associated with glomerular scarring and further nephron loss *(41)*, and even milder degrees of renal ablation can accelerate progression when superimposed upon other lesions *(43)*.

One potential explanation of this phenomenon is that, in the remnant kidney, nephron overload causes increased passage of proteins and biologically active molecules across the glomerular filter to the tubule, with resulting activation of tubulointerstitial fibrosis as described above. In this case, nephron overload has similar effects to those of proteinuria induced by recurrent albumin injections. However, it also has been suggested that reactive hypertrophy directly causes the progressive fibrosis *(43)*. By this model, the same signals that lead to growth of the cellular elements of the nephron also could stimulate fibrogenesis. In support of this possibility, glomerular fibrosis in FSGS often is presaged by enlargement of otherwise normal-appearing glomeruli *(44)*. Regardless of the primary cause, the reactive inflammation and fibrogenesis are exacerbated by alterations in the local physiology. Biologically active lipids stimulate immune responses *(45)* and the production of inflammatory eicosanoids. Activation of the podocytes and the extrusion of plasma proteins leads to adhesion of the glomerular tuft to the surrounding epithelium *(46)*. This may permit extrusion of plasma proteins into the interstitium, instead of the urinary space, triggering an inflammatory reaction.

4.3. Humoral and Cellular Mechanisms

A variety of cytokines and soluble mediators have been implicated in renal fibrosis. Angiotensin II, which plays a critical role in regulating intraglomerular hydrostatic pressure, also stimulates hypertrophy by glomerular cells and the production of additional growth factors. Insulin, growth hormone, and insulin-like growth factor (IGF)-1 stimulate both cellular hypertrophy and ECM accumulation *(47)*. An important mediator of fibrogenesis in the glomerulus and the tubulointerstitium is transforming growth factor (TGF)-β. This pleiotrophic cytokine enhances ECM synthesis and decreases ECM degradation *(48)*, and also stimulates the expression of connective tissue growth factor (CTGF), another profibrotic cytokine *(49)*. Mechanisms of TGF-β action will be discussed later. Other peptides that are expressed locally during renal fibrogenesis include basic fibroblast growth factor (bFGF) ***(50,51)***, epidermal growth factor (EGF) ***(52)***, platelet-derived growth factor (PDGF) ***(53)***, endothelin-1 ***(54)***, tumor necrosis factor (TNF)-α ***(55)***, osteopontin ***(56)***, and leptin ***(57)*** (for a more extensive review of agents that contribute to renal fibrosis, see **ref.** ***37***). Some of these factors contribute directly by stimulating ECM accumulation, whereas others activate cells, stimulate inflammation or angiogenesis, and induce hypertrophy.

Not all of the cells of the kidney produce all of the mediators required for fibrogenesis. Significant paracrine interactions likely contribute to ECM accumulation. For example, most of the genes for which mutations have been linked to FSGS are expressed specifically in the podocyte, and podocyte abnormalities such as defective structure and apoptosis have been associated with progressive sclerosis. However, ECM accumulation is most often prominent in the mesangium, leading to the segmental appearance of the lesion. Thus, either the podocyte manifests pathological production of cytokines that stimulate mesangial cell fibrogenesis, or the structural changes that occur in the glomerulus as a result of podocyte abnormalities stimulate profibrotic mechanisms in the mesangial cell. The latter possibility could reflect a change in the normal balance of signals that are exchanged among the podocyte, endothelial cell, and mesangial cell to maintain physiological homeostasis. Alternatively, it may reflect changes in physical forces on the cell that occur with the loss of the support structure provided by the podocytes. The resulting stretching could be similar to that observed with intraglomerular hypertension.

An important aspect of cellular responses is the role of epithelial-to-mesenchymal transition (EMT). Although fibroblasts clearly contribute to interstitial fibrosis, increasing evidence supports the notion that at least some of the ECM accumulation is derived from cells that originate in the tubular epithelium. The nephron forms initially from interaction between the branching ureteric bud and nests of mesenchymal cells that condense around the leading edge of the bud. These cells switch from a migratory phenotype to a quiescent, epithelial phenotype (**Fig. 4**) in the process of mesenchymal-to-epithelial transition (MET). This differentiated phenotype is maintained by a combination of cytokines/growth factors, cell adhesion to a basement membrane, and cell–cell interactions that lead to polarity and thus support the transport functions of the tubule. As a consequence of the disease process inflammation, TGF-β expression and the loss of cell–ECM adhesion and cell polarity stimulate the cell to de-differentiate back to a matrix-accumulating phenotype that is defined, although not necessarily determined, by the expression of smooth muscle α-actin (αSMA) ***(58)***. This cell migrates into the interstitium where it has similar properties to those of the native or infiltrating fibroblast. A similar phenom-

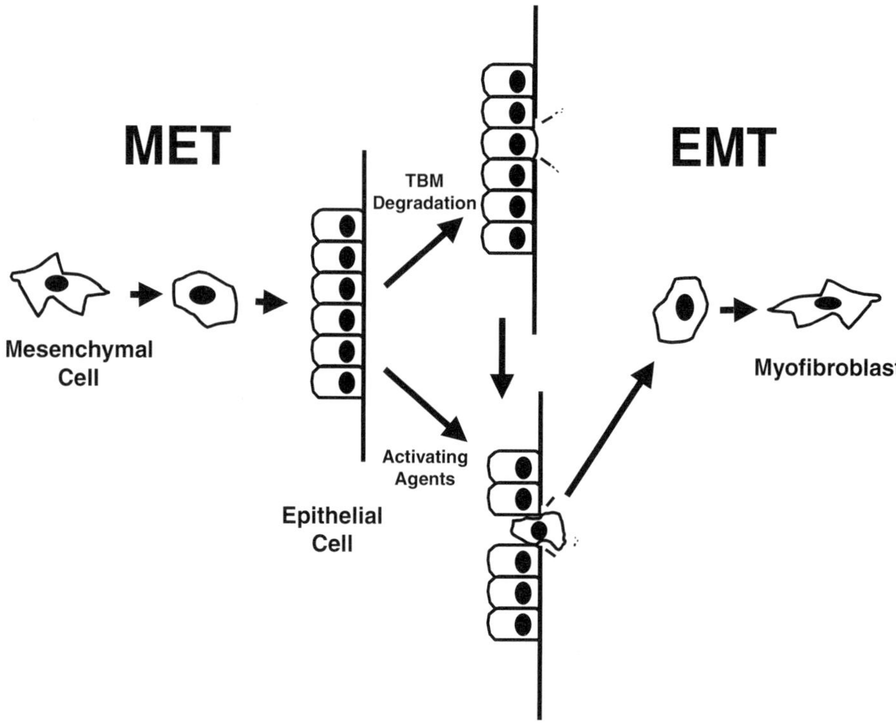

Fig. 4. Differentiation and de-differentiation of the renal tubular epithelial cell. Mesenchymal cells condense during nephrogenesis by the process of mesenchyme-to-epithelial transition (MET) to form a polarized epithelial barrier with tight junctions that permit selectivity of transport. With loss of anchorage and/or degradation of the tubular basement membrane (TBM), the cells become myofibroblasts by undergoing epithelial-to-mesenchymal transition (EMT). Alternatively, activating agents such as growth factors and cytokines may stimulate phenotypic changes that directly cause TBM degradation. In either case, the resulting loss of cell–cell or cell–matrix adhesion generates cells that likely contribute to tubulointerstitial fibrosis.

enon could occur with podocytes, and in the mesangial cell the fibrogenic response in disease *(59)* and to TGF-β *(60)* is associated with increased αSMA expression.

4.4. Molecular Mechanisms in Renal Fibrogenesis

As with other systems, the critical determinant of ECM accumulation in the kidney is the balance between ECM synthesis and its degradation. The constituents of this balance in the kidney have been characterized. The glomerular

ECM surrounding the mesangial cell and that in the GBM between the endothelial cells and the podocytes differ in the isoforms of type IV collagen that are found: α3(IV), α4(IV), and α5(IV) in the GBM *(61)*, but α1(IV) and α2(IV) in the mesangium. The mesangial matrix is relatively unique in that it is not a basement membrane in the true sense but still contains basement membrane collagens rather than interstitial collagens. The glomerulus also includes s-laminin, a kidney-specific laminin *(62)*. The kidney-specific ECM proteins are critical for normal glomerular development; in Alport's disease, where α1/2(IV) chains are incorporated into an abnormal GBM *(63)*, structural abnormalities may manifest as the gradual development of renal disease *(64)*. Alternatively, abnormal glomerular ECM may impair development sufficiently that a proper glomerulus is not formed *(65)*. The tubular basement membrane and the small amount of interstitial matrix in the tubulointerstitium are more typical of other matrices in the body.

The major ECM proteases are expressed in the kidney: MMPs such as gelatinase A (MMP-2) *(66)* and meprin *(67)*, and plasminogen activators urokinase (uPA) and tissue-type plasminogen activator *(4)*. The regulators of these ECM proteases, the TIMPs *(68)* and the plasminogen activator inhibitors (PAIs) *(69)* also are present. Under normal conditions, the balance among the proteases, their inhibitors, and the synthesis of ECM proteins is tightly regulated. However, in disease, the regulation of the expression of these proteins, and the timing of this regulation, is crucial. For example, as described above under **Subheading 2.**, ECM proteases could play an important role in the resolution of the acute model of anti-Thy-1 nephritis *(5)*, but it may have a critical negative effect on basement membrane integrity in the initiation phase of other diseases *(70)*. Similarly, TIMP-1 expression appears important in the progression of several models of renal fibrosis *(71)*, and PAI-1 appears to have an important role in the ECM accumulation of diseases mediated by TGF-β *(72)*. Notably, however, mice deficient in TIMP-1 do not show a decrease in rates of disease progression *(23)*; this could reflect the redundancy of TIMP-related systems that are available to counter the effects of proteases.

Studies of the regulation of this balance have centered on models of kidney diseases that are mediated by TGF-β or by diabetes-related effects of high glucose and insulin. TGF-β effects have been related to the Smad signaling pathway. In the mesangial cell, collagen I expression is mediated by Smad3 and Smad4 interacting with the *COL1A1/2* promoters *(73)*. Phosphorylation of Smad3 is enhanced by activity of the extracellular signal regulated kinase (ERK) mitogen-activated protein (MAP) kinase *(74)* and is further dependent on other mediators including protein kinase C (PKC) δ *(75)* and phosphatidylinositol-3-kinase *(76)*. TGF-β also stimulates cytoskeletal rearrangement in the mesangial cell *(60)*, an event associated with increased Ca^{2+} flux *(77)*. Nuclear activity of the Smad complex requires the Sp1 transcription factor binding to its sites on the collagen promoter *(78)*. Type IV collagen expression also is activated by TGF-β through Smad signaling. Phosphodiesterases appear to play a role in this process *(79)*. Finally, laminin-γ1 expression is regulated in mesangial cells by several transcription factors, including the basic helix-loop-helix/leucine zipper transcription factor, TFE3 *(80)*, and the gut-enriched Kruppel-like factor (GKLF) that bind to the bcn-1 element on the *LAMC1* gene *(81)*, in a manner that requires synergy with Sp1. Although some of these studies have not yet been linked with TGF-β stimulation, experiments in other systems indicate that TGF-β/Smad signaling may interact with and/or activate these transcription factors.

Although many of the same pathways mediate collagen expression in renal tubular cell culture, there are some important differences. One is that the activation of ERK MAP kinase decreases collagen expression in the renal tubular epithelium. Although there may be opposite effects of ERK on Smad signaling in renal tubular epithelial cells *(82)*, the main mechanism by which collagen expression is inhibited may be the blockage of EMT by ERK in these cells *(83)*; this is a much more complex response than direct activation of collagen genes, and the effects of ERK may therefore be more subtle or complicated. Regardless of the effects on specific events, fibrosis in the kidney is clearly Smad-mediated, since Smads show signs of activation in the kidneys of diabetic mice *(84)*. Further, diabetic nephropathy *(85)* and obstructive uropathy *(86)*, both of which have major tubulointerstitial components, are ameliorated in Smad3-null mice.

In diabetes, in addition to TGF-b/Smad signaling, other pathways have been demonstrated to play a role in fibrogenesis. Insulin activates the signaling pathway mediated by Janus kinase (JAK) and signal transducers and activators of transcription (STAT). High local glucose concentrations also activate JAK/STAT signaling in mesangial cells, leading to cell activation and the production of TGF-β and fibronectin *(87)*. Antisense to JAK2 blocks angiotensin II-stimulated type IV collagen expression *(88)*. Because angiotensin II may stimulate TGF-β production, and JAK is upstream of TGF-β expression, the role of JAK2 could relate to an effect mediated by TGF-β. However, it is possible that JAK/STAT directly signals ECM expression as well. In studies with significance for type II diabetes mellitus, excess insulin has been found to phosphorylate the protein translation repressor 4E-BP1, an eIF4E-binding protein, in renal epithelial cells. The result is enhanced translation of laminin proteins that could explain the paradox of decreased laminin mRNA expression but increased laminin protein expression in db/db mice, a model of type II diabetes *(89)*. Finally, the peroxisome proliferator-activated receptors (PPARs) may have diverse roles in fibrogenesis *(90)*. PPARγ is an insulin-sensitizing agent that also affects the kidney. Troglitazone, a PPARγ agonist of the thiazolidinedione family, reduces collagen I production by mesangial cells in response to hyperglycemia ***(91)***, and PPARγ agonists also may ameliorate non-diabetic glomerulosclerosis ***(92)***. PPARα may have deleterious effects on the kidney through its effects on lipid metabolism. Direct effects on renal scarring currently are a subject of investigation.

5. Treatment of Renal Fibrosis

The present therapy for kidney fibrosis is comprised of three approaches: strategies to combat inflammation, treatments directed at the physiology of fibrosis, and more novel therapies that have been identified by empirical means. The only accepted therapies directed at the disease process as it is traditionally understood involve anti-inflammatory strategies. Patients whose disease responds to such treatment usually have a better prognosis than those who do not respond. Thus, very high-dose corticosteroids have been used to treat FSGS in children ***(93)*** and long-term oral treatment with high-dose corticosteroids has been reported to be efficacious in adults ***(94)***. A more standard approach to FSGS is the use of cyclosporine ***(95)***. This is the only treatment that has been shown to be efficacious with controlled, prospective trial ***(96)***. A significant side effect of cyclosporine is nephrotoxicity, so its long-term use requires cautious monitoring of renal function. Anecdotal reports indicating that other anti-inflammatory drugs such as FK506 (tacrolimus) or mycophenolate mofetil have not yet been tested in larger studies.

To address the physiology of chronic renal disease, clinicians have sought to decrease intraglomerular hypertension or hyperfiltration. Thus, inhibition of angiotensin-converting enzyme (ACE) or blockade of the angiotensin II receptor has been used to delay the progression of diabetic nephropathy ***(97)***. Although ACE inhibition has been utilized in other diseases as well, the results have not been as clear-cut. Nonsteroidal anti-inflammatory agents have been used to reduce glomerular filtration rate in order to reduce proteinuria, although such reports are anecdotal and the treatment is potentially nephrotoxic. Studies in rats indicate that severe protein restriction, likely causing decreased glomerular filtration, also may slow the progression of renal failure. Multicenter clinical trials of protein restriction in humans have met with equivocal results ***(98,99)***. Anticoagulants or antiplatelet agents also have been tried as treatments for some forms of chronic glomerulonephritis ***(100)***, although this approach has not proven broadly successful. It should be noted that some investigators believe that ACE inhibition or angiotensin receptor blockade affects the biology of kidney cells directly, in addition to its hemodynamic effects. Angiotensin II stimulates TGF-β expression by several renal cell types ***(101)***, suggesting that it stimulates autocrine fibrogenic pathways. Moreover, angiotensin II expression has been related to glomerular hypertrophy. Thus, inhibition of this mediator could retard disease progression through multiple mechanisms. Finally, in diabetes mellitus, the best "therapy" is tight control of glucose levels to prevent the deleterious effects of hyperglycemia.

Recently identified empirical treatments are under study in animal models and human trials. Pirfenidone may suppress growth factor production, signal transduction, or reactive oxygen species propagation ***(102)*** and presently is in clinical trials. Heparinoids such as pentosan polysulfate bind to growth factors and prevent progression in rats that have experimental reductions in renal mass to stimulate fibrogenesis ***(103)***. These properties were originally identified in heparin and were determined to reflect effects on growth factor activity, not the coagulation pathway ***(104)***. Other treatments that have been used experimentally in animal models with less clear effects include anti-oxidants and estrogens.

6. New Directions for the Study of Renal Fibrosis

Significant challenges remain in the study of renal fibrosis. Two critical issues in the pathogenesis of fibrosis are the process of ECM organization and the mechanism(s) by which physiological events such as intraglomerular hypertension modulate signal transduction pathways to effect scarring. With regard to matrix organization, in vitro and in vivo studies have demonstrated that integration of collagens into a stable basement membrane requires ascorbic acid. Indeed, in scorbutic mesangial cell cultures, collagen protein can be remarkably short-lived, with more than 80% of recently synthesized collagen degraded within 2 h ***(105)***. ECM organization is directed largely by the cells that are adjacent to the matrix, in a process that requires integrin binding ***(106)***. Although it is established that the diabetic milieu may make the ECM more resistant to degradation by proteolytic enzymes ***(107)***, in general the issue of how organization and stability of the renal ECM are accomplished has not been addressed.

A second issue is that of relating the physiological events to the cell and molecular biology of renal fibrogenesis. How does the replacement of α3/4/5(IV) collagen with α1/2(IV) collagen lead to the development of kidney disease in patients with Alport's syndrome? How does glomerular hypertension accelerate the progression of glomerular sclerosis? What are the specific proteins, delivered to the tubule via pathological filtration of proteins through the glomerulus, that stimulate tubulointerstial fibrosis? Are some of these proteins critical effectors of EMT, and, if so, how do they stimulate this process? Understanding how physiology relates to biochemistry will be an important step in understanding how to prevent the loss of kidney function.

The development of new treatments, informed by our improved understanding of disease pathogenesis, remains the ultimate challenge. Given the structural complexity of the nephron and the functional complexity of fibrogenic signals, the elucidation of essential stimuli regulating the development and maintenance of nephron integrity will provide one key to treatment. Another will depend upon the identification of critical nodes of interaction between signaling pathways; interrupting signals at these points will be the most effective way of interrupting disease progression. Finally, several agents have been identified as blocking specific cellular responses to fibrogenic signals. Thus, hepatocyte growth factor (HGF) antagonizes renal tubular cell EMT ***(82)***, and bone morphogenetic protein (BMP)-7 similarly antagonizes EMT ***(108)*** and perhaps other effects of TGF-β/Smad signaling, as it activates an alternative Smad pathway to that activated by TGF-β ***(109)***. Recent studies suggest that a construct expressing the anti-Smad, Smad7, can be delivered directly to the kidney by infusion and focused ultrasound pulses ***(25)***. In addition to gene therapy, the efficacy of biochemical inhibitors related to newer insights regarding fibrogenesis is under study. Thus, because reactive oxygen species have been determined to play a role in at least some models of kidney disease ***(110)***, the use of anti-oxidants such as ascorbic acid, α-tocopheryl (vitamin) E, and selenium may be of benefit. Given the broad number of avenues for investigation and potential treatments, the future can be regarded with significant optimism.

Acknowledgments

Supported in part by Grant R01-DK49362 from the National Institute of Diabetes, Digestive, and Kidney Diseases.

References

1. United States Renal Data System (2003) *2003 Annual Data Report.* Division of Kidney, Urologic and Hematologic Diseases, NIDDK/NIH, Department of Health and Human Services, Bethesda, MD.
2. Eddy, A. A. (1994) Experimental insights into the tubulointerstitial disease accompanying primary glomerular lesions. *J. Am. Soc. Nephrol.* **5**, 1273–1287.
3. Schnaper, H. W. (1995) Balance between matrix synthesis and degradation: a determinant of glomerulosclerosis. *Pediatr. Nephrol.* **9**, 104–111.
4. Baricos, W. H. (2002) Protease mediated tubular injury: a new direction in acute renal failure? *Kidney Int.* **61**, 1174–1175.
5. Lovett, D. H., Johnson, R. J., Marti, H. P., Martin, J., Davies, M., and Couser, W. G. (1992) Structural characterization of the mesangial cell type IV collagenase and enhanced expression in a model of immune complex-mediated glomerulonephritis. *Am. J. Pathol.* **141**, 85–98.

6. Schnaper, H. W. (2001) Focal segmental glomerulosclerosis. In: *Immunologic Renal Disease, 2nd edition* (Neilson, E. G. and Couser, W. G., eds), Lippincott Williams and Willkins, Philadelphia: pp. 1001–1027.
7. Schnaper, H. W. (2003) Idiopathic focal segmental glomerulosclerosis. *Semin. Nephrol.* **23**, 183–193.
8. Wehrmann, M., Bohle, A., Held, H., Schumm, G., Kendziorra, H., and Pressler, H. (1990) Long-term prognosis of focal sclerosing glomerulonephritis. An analysis of 250 cases with particular regard to tubulointerstitial changes. *Clin. Nephrol.* **33**, 115–122.
9. Jones, C. L., Buch, S., Post, M., McCulloch, L., Liu, E., and Eddy, A. A. (1991) Pathogenesis of interstitial fibrosis in chronic purine aminonucleoside nephrosis. *Kidney Int.* **40**, 1020–1031.
10. Mathis, B. J., Kim, S. H., Calabrese, K., Haas, M., Seidman, J. G., Seidman, C. E., and Pollak, M. R. (1998) A locus for inherited focal segmental glomerulosclerosis maps to cromosome 19q13. *Kidney Int.* **53**, 282–286.
11. Coppes, M. J., Liefers, G. J., Higuchi, M., Zinn, A. B., Balfe, J. W., and Williams, B. R. (1992) Inherited WT1 mutation in Denys-Drash syndrome. *Cancer Res.* **52**, 6125–6128.
12. Saylam, K. and Simon, P. (2003) WT1 gene mutation responsible for male sex reversal and renal failure: the Frasier syndrome. *Eur. J. Obstet. Gynecol. Reprod. Biol.* **110**, 111–113.
13. Heathcott, R. W., Morison, I. M., Gubler, M. C., Corbett, R., and Reeve, A. E. (2002) A review of the phenotypic variation due to the Denys-Drash syndrome-associated germline WT1 mutation R362X. *Hum. Mutat.* **19**, 462.
14. Kestila, M., Lenkkeri, U., Mannikko, M., et al. (1998) Positionally cloned gene for a novel glomerular protein—nephrin—is mutated in congenital nephrotic syndrome. *Mol. Cell* **1**, 575–582.
15. Boute, N., Gribouval, O., Roselli, S., et al. (2000) *NPHS2*, encoding the glomerular protein podocin, is mutated in autosomal recessive steroid-resistant nephrotic syndrome. *Nat. Genet.* **24**, 349–354.
16. Caridi, G., Bertelli, R., Di Duca, M., et al. (2003) Broadening the spectrum of diseases related to podocin mutations. *J. Am. Soc. Nephrol.* **14**, 1278.
17. Kaplan, J. M., Kim, S.-H., North, K. N., et al. (2000) Mutations in ACTN4, encoding α-actinin-4, cause familial focal segmental glomerulosclerosis. *Nat. Genet.* **24**, 251–256.
18. Lei, H.-H., Perneger, T. V., Klag, M. J., Whelton, P. K., and Coresh, J. (1998) Familial aggregation of renal disease in a population-based case-control study. *J. Am. Soc. Nephrol.* **9**, 1270–1276.
19. Freedman, B. I., Isakander, S. S., and Appel, R. G. (1995) The link between hypertension and nephrosis. *Am. J. Kidney Dis.* **25**, 207–221.
20. Ingulli, E. and Tejani, A. (1991) Racial differences in the incidence and renal outcome of idiopathic focal segmental glomerulosclerosis in children. *Pediatr. Nephrol.* **5**, 393–397.

21. Pettitt, D. J., Saad, M. F., Bennett, P. H., Nelson, R. G., and Knowler, W. C. (1990) Familial predisposition to renal disease in two generations of Pima Indians with type-2 (non-insulin dependent) diabetes mellitus. *Diabetologia* **33**, 438–443.
22. Roy, L. P., Vernier, R. L., and Michael, A. F. (1972) Effect of protein-load proteinuria on glomerular polyanion. *Proc. Soc. Exp. Biol. Med.* **141**, 870–874.
23. Eddy, A. A., Kim, H., Lopez-Guisa, J., Oda, T., and Soloway, P. D. (2000) Interstitial fibrosis in mice with overload proteinuria: deficiency of TIMP-1 is not protective. *Kidney Int.* **58**, 618–628.
24. Deen, W. M., Maddox, D. A., Robertson, C. R., and Brenner, B. M. (1974) Dynamics of glomerular ultrafiltration in the rat. VII. Response to reduced renal mass. *Am. J. Physiol.* **227**, 556–562.
25. Lan, H. Y., Mu, W., Tomita, N., et al. (2003) Inhibition of renal fibrosis by gene transfer of inducible Smad7 using ultrasound-microbubble system in rat UUO model. *J. Am. Soc. Nephrol.* **14**, 1535–1548.
26. Nakamura, T., Fukui, M., Ebihara, I., Tomino, Y., and Koide, H. (1994) Low protein diet blunts the rise in glomerular gene expression in focal glomerulosclerosis. *Kidney Int.* **45**, 1593–1605.
27. Glasser, R. J., Velosa, J. A., and Michael, A. F. (1977) Experimental model of focal sclerosis. I. Relationship to protein excretion in aminonucleoside nephrosis. *Lab. Invest.* **36**, 519–526.
28. Schulze, M., Pruchno, C. J., Burns, M., Baker, P. J., Johnson, R. J., and Couser, W. G. (1993) Glomerular C3c localization indicates ongoing immune deposit formation and complement activation in experimental glomerulonephritis. *Am. J. Pathol.* **142**, 179–187.
29. Studer, R. K., Craven, P. A., and DeRubertis, F. R. (1993) Role for protein kinase C in the mediation of increased fibronectin accumulation by mesangial cells grown in high-glucose medium. *Diabetes* **42**, 118–126.
30. Tolins, J. P., Stone, B. G., and Raij, L. (1992) Interactions of hypercholesterolemia and hypertension in initiation of glomerular injury. *Kidney Int.* **41**, 1254–1261.
31. Kamanna, V. S. and Kirschenbaum, M. A. (1993) Association between very-low-density lipoprotein and glomerular injury in obese Zucker rats. *Am. J. Nephrol.* **13**, 53–58.
32. Simons, J. L., Provoost, A. P., Anderson, S., et al. (1993) Pathogenesis of glomerular injury in the fawn-hooded rat: early glomerular capillary hypertension predicts glomerular sclerosis. *J. Am. Soc. Nephrol.* **3**, 1775–1782.
33. Esposito, C., He, C. J., Striker, G. E., Zalups, R. K., and Striker, L. J. (1999) Nature and severity of the glomerular response to nephron reduction is strain-dependent in mice. *Am. J. Pathol.* **154**, 891–897.
34. Kos, C. H., Le, T. C., Sinha, S., et al. (2003) Mice deficient in alpha-actinin-4 have severe glomerular disease. *J. Clin. Invest.* **111**, 1683–1690.
35. Rantanen, M., Palmen, T., Patari, A., et al. (2002) Nephrin TRAP mice lack slit diaphragms and show fibrotic glomeruli and cystic tubular lesions. *J. Am. Soc. Nephrol.* **13**, 1586–1594.

36. Shih, N.-Y., Li, J., Karpitskii, V., et al. (1999) Congenital nephrotic syndrome in mice lacking CD2-associated protein. *Science* **286**, 312–315.
37. Schnaper, H. W. and Kopp, J. B. (2003) Renal fibrosis. *Frontiers in Bioscience (online)* **8**, e68–86.
38. Clozel, M., Hess, P., Fischli, W., et al. (1999) Age-dependent hypertension in Mpv17-deficient mice, a transgenic model of glomerulosclerosis and inner ear disease. *Exp. Gerontol.* **34**, 1007–1015.
39. Ljutic, D. and Kes, P. (2003) The role of arterial hypertension in the progression of non-diabetic glomerular diseases. *Nephrol. Dial. Transplant.* **18(Suppl 5)**, v28–30.
40. Velosa, J. A., Torres, V. E., Donadio, J. V., et al. (1985) Treatment of severe nephrotic syndrome with meclofenamate: an uncontrolled pilot study. *Mayo Clin. Proc.* **60**, 586–592.
41. Robson, A. M., Mor, J., Root, E. R., et al. (1979) Mechanism of proteinuria in nonglomerular renal disease. *Kidney Int.* **16**, 416–429.
42. Narkun-Burgess, D. M., Nolan, C. R., Norman, J. E., et al. (1993) Forty-five year follow-up after uninephrectomy. *Kidney Int.* **43**, 1110–1115.
43. Yoshida, Y., Fogo, A., and Ichikawa, I. (1989) Glomerular hemodynamic changes vs. hypertrophy in experimental glomerular sclerosis. *Kidney Int.* **35**, 654–660.
44. Fogo, A., Hawkins, E. P., Berry, P. L., et al. (1990) Glomerular hypertrophy in minimal change disease predicts subsequent progression to focal glomerular sclerosis. *Kidney Int.* **38**, 115–123.
45. Kees-Folts, D., Sadow, J. L., and Schreiner, G. F. (1994) Tubular catabolism of albumin is associated with the release of an inflammatory lipid. *Kidney Int.* **45**, 1697–1709.
46. Kriz, W., Hosser, H., Hahnel, B., Simons, J. L., and Provoost, A. P. (1998) Development of vascular pole-associated glomerulosclerosis in the Fawn-hooded rat. *J. Am. Soc. Nephrol.* **9**, 381–396.
47. Doublier, S., Seurin, D., Fouqueray, B., et al. (2000) Glomerulosclerosis in mice transgenic for human insulin-like growth factor-binding protein-1. *Kidney Int.* **57**, 2299–2307.
48. Border, W. A. and Noble, N. A. (1997) TGF-β in kidney fibrosis: a target for gene therapy. *Kidney Int.* **51**, 1388–1396.
49. Gupta, S., Clarkson, M. R., Duggan, J., and Brady, H. R. (2000) Connective tissue growth factor: potential role in glomerulosclerosis and tubulointerstitial fibross. *Kidney Int.* **58**, 1389–1399.
50. Floege, J., Kriz, W., Schulze, M., et al. (1995) Basic fibroblast growth factor augments podocyte injury and induces glomerulosclerosis in rats with experimental membranous nephropathy. *J. Clin. Invest.* **96**, 2809–2819.
51. Haseley, L. A., Hugo, C., Reidy, M. A., and Johnson, R. J. (1999) Dissociation of mesangial cell migration and proliferation in experimental glomerulonephritis. *Kidney Int.* **56**, 964–972.
52. Uchiyama-Tanaka, Y., Matsubara, H., Mori, Y., et al. (2002) Involvement of HB-EGF and EGF receptor transactivation in TGF-β-mediated fibronectin expression in mesangial cells. *Kidney International* **62**, 799-808.

53. Iida, H., Seifert, R., Alpers, C. E., et al. (1991) Platet-derived growth factor (PDGF) and PDGF receptor are induced in mesangial proliferative nephritis in the rat. *Proc. Natl. Acad. Sci. USA* **88**, 6560–6564.
54. Hocher, B., Thone-Reineke, C., Rohmeiss, P., et al. (1997) Endothelin-1 transgenic mice develop glomerulosclerosis, interstitial fibrosis, and renal cysts but not hypertension. *J. Clin. Invest.* **99**, 1380–1389.
55. Guo, G., Morrissey, J., McCracken, R., Tolley, T., Liapis, H., and Klahr, S. (2001) Contributions of angiotensin II and tumor necrosis factor-alpha to the development of renal fibrosis. *Am. J. Physiol. Renal Fluid Elect.* **280**, F777–F785.
56. Ophascharoensuk, V., Giachelli, C. M., Gordon, K., et al. (1999) Obstructive uropathy in the mouse: role of osteopontin in interstitial fibrosis and apoptosis. *Kidney Int.* **56**, 571–580.
57. Wolf, G., Chen, S., Han, D. C., and Ziyadeh, F. N. (2002) Leptin and renal disease. *Am. J. Kidney Dis.* **39**, 1–11.
58. Yang, J. and Liu, Y. (2002) Dissection of key events in tubular epithelial to myofibroblast transition and its implications in renal interstitial fibrosis. *Am. J. Pathol.* **159**, 1465–1475.
59. Patel, K., Harding, P., Haney, L. B., and Glass, W. F., 2nd. (2003) Regulation of the mesangial cell myofibroblast phenotype by actin polymerization. *J. Cell Physiol.* **195**, 435–445.
60. Hubchak, S. C., Runyan, C. E., Kreisberg, J. I., and Schnaper, H. W. (2003) Cytoskeletal rearrangement and signal transduction in TGF-β1-stimulated mesangial cell collagen accumulation. *J. Am. Soc. Nephrol.* **14**, 1968–1980.
61. Hudson, B. G., Kalluri, R., Gunwar, S., et al. (1992) The pathogenesis of Alport syndrome involves type IV collagen molecules containing the alpha 3(IV) chain: evidence from anti-GBM nephritis after renal transplantation. *Kidney Int.* **42**, 179–187.
62. Hansen, K. M., Berfield, A. K., Spicer, D., and Abrass, C. K. (1998) Rat mesangial cells express two unique isoforms of laminin which modulate mesangial cell phenotype. *Matrix Biol.* **17**, 117–130.
63. Kalluri, R., Shield, C. F., Todd, P., Hudson, B. G., and Neilson, E. G. (1997) Isoform switching of type IV collagen is developmentally arrested in X-linked Alport syndrome leading to increased susceptibility of renal basement membranes to endoproteolysis. *J. Clin. Invest.* **99**, 2470–2478.
64. Kashtan, C. E. (1999) Alport syndrome. An inherited disorder of renal, ocular, and cochlear basement membranes. *Medicine (Baltimore)* **78**, 338–360.
65. Kikkawa, Y., Virtanen, I., and Miner, J. H. (2003) Mesangial cells organize the glomerular capillaries by adhering to the G domain of laminin alpha5 in the glomerular basement membrane. *J. Cell Biol.* **161**, 187–196.
66. Marti, H.-P., McNeil, L., Davies, M., Martin, J., and Lovett, D. H. (1993) Homology cloning of rat 72 kDa type IV collagenase: cytokine and second messenger inducibility in glomerular mesangial cells. *Biochem. J.* **291**, 441–446.
67. Carmago, S., Shah, S. V., and Walker, P. D. (2002) Meprin, a brush-border enzyme, plays an important role in hypoxic/ischemic acute renal tubular injury in rats. *Kidney Int.* **61**, 959–966.

68. Carome, M. A., Striker, L. J., Peten, E. P., et al. (1993) Human glomeruli express TIMP-1 mRNA and TIMP-2 protein and mRNA. *Am. J. Physiol.* **264**, F923–F929.
69. Tomooka, S., Border, W. A., Marshall, B. C., and Noble, N. A. (1992) Glomerular matrix accumulation is linked to inhibition of the plasmin protease system. *Kidney Int.* **42**, 1462–1469.
70. Davies, M., Martin, J., Thomas, G. T., and Lovett, D. H. (1992) Proteinases and glomerular matrix turnover. *Kidney Int.* **41**, 671–678.
71. Eddy, A. A. (2000) Molecular basis of renal fibrosis. *Pediatr Nephrol* **15**, 290–301.
72. Gaedeke, J., Peters, H., Noble, N. A., and Border, W. A. (2001) Angiotensin II, TGF-β and renal fibrosis. *Contrib. Nephrol.* 153–160.
73. Schnaper, H. W., Hayashida, T., Hubchak, S. C., and Poncelet, A.-C. (2003) TGF-β signal transduction and mesangial cell fibrogenesis. *Am. J. Physiol. Renal Physiol.* **284**, F243–F252.
74. Hayashida, T., de Caestecker, M. P., and Schnaper, H. W. (2003) Cross-talk between ERK MAP kinase and Smad-signaling pathways enhances TGF-β-dependent responses in human mesangial cells. *FASEB J.* **17**, 1576–1578.
75. Runyan, C. E., Schnaper, H. W., and Poncelet, A.-C. (2003) Smad3 and PKCδ mediate TGF-β1-induced type I collagen expression in human mesangial cells. *Am. J. Physiol. Renal Physiol.* **285**, F413–F422.
76. Runyan, C. E., Schnaper, H. W., and Poncelet, A.-C. (2004) The phosphatidylinositol 3-kinase Akt pathway enhances Smad3-stimulated mesangial cell collagen I expression in response to TGF-β1. *J. Biol. Chem.* 279, 2632–2639.
77. McGowan, T. A., Madesh, M., Zhu, Y., et al. (2002) TGF-b-induced Ca^{2+} influx involves the type III IP_3 receptor and regulates actin cytskeleton. *Am. J. Physiol. Renal Physiol.* **282**, F910–F920.
78. Poncelet, A.-C. and Schnaper , H. W. (2001) Sp1 and Smad proteins cooperate to mediate TGF-β1-induced α2(I) collagen expression in human glomerular mesangial cells. *J. Biol. Chem.* **276**, 6983–6992.
79. Cheng, J. and Grande, J. P. (2002) Transforming growth factor-β signal transduction and progressive renal disease. *Exp. Biol. Med. (Maywood)* **227**, 943–956.
80. Kawata, Y., Suzuki, H., Higaki, Y., et al. (2002) bcn-1 element-dependent activation of the laminin γ1 chain gene by the cooperative action of transcription factor E2 (TFE3) and Smad proteins. *J. Biol. Chem.* **277**, 11,375–11,384.
81. Higaki, Y., Schullery, D., Kawata, Y., Shnyreva, M., Abrass, C. K., and Bomsztyk, K. (2002) Synergistic activation of the rat laminin γ1 chain promoter by the gut-enriched Kruppel-like factor (GKLF/KLF4) and Sp1. *Nucl. Acids Res.* **30**, 2270–2279.
82. Yang, J., Dai, C., and Liu, Y. (2003) Hepatocyte growth factor suppresses renal interstitial myofibroblast activation and intercepts Smad signal transduction. *Am. J. Pathol.* **163**, 621–632.
83. Yang, J. and Liu, Y. (2002) Blockage of tubular epithelial to myofibroblast tran-

sition by hepatcyte growth factor prevents renal interstitial fibrosis. *J. Am. Soc. Nephrol.* **13**, 96–107.

84. Isono, M., Chen, S., Hong, S. W., Iglesias-de la Cruz, M. C., and Ziyadeh, F. N. (2002) Smad pathway is activated in the diabetic mouse kidney and Smad3 mediates TGF-β-induced fibronectin in mesangial cells. *Biochem. Biophys. Res. Commun.* **296**, 1356–1365.
85. Fujimoto, M., Maezawa, Y., Yokote, K., et al. (2003) Mice lacking Smad3 are protected against streptozotocin-induced diabetic glomerulopathy. *Biochem. Biophys. Res. Commun.* **305**, 1002–1007.
86. Sato, M., Muragaki, Y., Saika, S., Roberts, A. B., and Ooshima, A. (2003) Targeted disruption of TGF-β1/Smad3 signaling protects against renal tubulointerstitial fibrosis induced by unilateral ureteral obstruction. *J. Clin. Invest.* **112**, 1486–1494.
87. Wang, X., Shaw, S., Amiri, F., Eaton, D. C., and Marrero, M. B. (2002) Inhibition of the Jak/STAT signaling pathway prevents the high glucose-induced increase in TGF-β and fibronectin synthesis in mesangial cells. *Diabetes* **51**, 3505–3509.
88. Amiri, F., Shaw, S., Wang, X., Tang, J., Waller, J. L., Eaton, D. C., and Marrero, M. B. (2002) Angiotensin II activation of the JAK/STAT pathway in mesangial cells is altered by high glucose. *Kidney Int.* **61**, 1605–1616.
89. Bhandari, B. K., Feliers, D., Duraisamy, S., et al. (2001) Insulin regulation of protein translation repressor 4E-BP1, and eIF4E-binding protein, in renal epithelial cells. *Kidney Int.* **59**, 866–875.
90. Guan, Y. and Breyer, M. D. (2001) Peroxisome proliferator-activated receptors (PPARs): novel therapeutic targets in renal disease. *Kidney Int.* **60**, 14–30.
91. Routh, R. E., Johnson, J. H., and McCarthy, K. J. (2002) Troglitazone suppresses the secretion of type I collagen by mesangial cells in vitro. *Kidney Int.* **61**, 1365–1376.
92. Ma, L. J., Marcantoni, C., Linton, M. F., Fazio, S., and Fogo, A. B. (2001) Peroxisome proliferator-activated receptor-gamma agonist troglitazone protects against nondiabetic glomerulosclerosis in rats. *Kidney Int.* **59**, 1899–1910.
93. Yorgin, P. D., Krasher, J., and Al-Uzri, A. Y. (2001) Pulse methylprednisolone treatment of idiopathic steroid-resistant nephrotic syndrome. *Pediatr. Nephrol.* **16**, 245–250.
94. Rydel, J. J., Korbet, S. M., Borok, R. Z., and Schwartz, M. M. (1995) Focal segmental glomerulosclerosis in adults: presentation, course and response to treatment. *Am. J. Kid. Dis.* **25**, 534–542.
95. Ingulli, E., Baqi, N., Ahmad, H., Moazami, S., and Tejani, A. (1995) Aggressive, long-term cyclosporine therapy for steroid-resistant focal segmental glomerulosclerosis. *J. Am. Soc. Nephrol.* **5**, 1820–1825.
96. Cattran, D. C. and Rao, P. (1998) Long-term outcome in children and adults with classic focal segmental glomerulosclerosis. *Am. J. Kidney Dis.* **32**, 72–79.
97. Rossing, K., Jacobsen, P., Pietraszek, L., and Parving, H. H. (2003)

Renoprotective effects of adding angiotensin II receptor blocker to maximal recommended doses of ACE inhibitor in diabetic nephropathy: a randomized double-blind crossover trial. *Diabetes Care* **26**, 2268–2274.

98. Levey, A. S., Adler, S., Caggiula, A. W., et al. (1996) Effects of dietary protein restriction on the progression of advanced renal disease in the Modification of Diet in Renal Disease Study. *Am. J. Kidney Dis.* **27**, 652–663.
99. Hansen, H. P., Tauber-Lassen, E., Jensen, B. R., and Parving, H. H. (2002) Effect of dietary protein restriction on prognosis in patients with diabetic nephropathy. *Kidney Int.* **62**, 220–228.
100. Chan, M. K., Kwan, S. Y., Chan, K. W., and Yeung, C. K. (1987) Controlled trial of antiplatelet agents in mesangial IgA glomerulonephritis. *Am. J. Kidney Dis.* **9**, 417–421.
101. Wolf, G., Ziyadeh, F. N., Zahner, G., and Stahl, R. A. (1995) Angiotensin II-stimulated expression of transforming growth factor b in renal proximal tubular cells: attenuation after stable transfection with the c-mas oncogene. *Kidney Int.* **48**, 1818–1827.
102. Iyer, S. N., Gurujeyalakshmi, G., and Giri, S. N. (1999) Effects of pirfenidone on transforming growth factor-b gene expression at the transcriptional level in bleomycin hamster model of lung fibrosis. *J. Pharmacol. Exp. Ther.* **291**, 367–373.
103. Bobadilla, N. A., Tack, I., Tapia, E., et al. (2001) Pentosan polysulfate prevents glomerular hypertension and structural injury despite persisting hypertension in 5/6 nephrectomy rats. *J. Am. Soc. Nephrol.* **12**, 2080–2087.
104. Mishra-Gorur, K., Singer, H. A., and Castellot, J. J., Jr. (2002) Heparin inhibits phosphorylation and autonomous activity of Ca(2+)/calmodulin-dependent protein kinase II in vascular smooth muscle cells. *Am. J. Pathol.* **161**, 1893–1901.
105. Poncelet, A.-C. and Schnaper, H. W. (1998) Regulation of mesangial cell collagen turnover by transforming growth factor-β1. *Am. J. Physiol. Renal Physiol* **275**, F458–F466.
106. Ganta, D. R., McCarthy, M. B., and Gronowicz, G. A. (1997) Ascorbic acid alters collagen integrins in bone culture. *Endocrinology* **138**, 3606–3612.
107. Mott, J. D., Khalifah, R. G., Nagase, H., Shield, C. F., 3rd, Hudson, J. K., and Hudson, B. G. (1997) Nonenzymatic glycation of type IV collagen and matrix metalloproteinase susceptibility. *Kidney Int.* **52**, 1302–1312.
108. Zeisberg, M., Hanai, J., Sugimoto, H., Mammoto, T., Charytan, D., Strutz, F., and Kalluri, R. (2003) BMP-7 counteracts TGF-β1-induced epithelial-to-mesenchymal transition and reverses chronic renal injury. *Nat. Med.* **9**, 964–968.
109. Shi, Y. and Massague, J. (2003) Mechanisms of TGF-β signaling from cell membrane to the nucleus. *Cell* **113**, 685–700.
110. Cochrane, A. L. and Ricardo, S. D. (2003) Oxidant stress and regulation of chemokines in the development of renal interstitial fibrosis. *Contrib. Nephrol.* **139**, 102–119

3

Transforming Growth Factor-β

A Key Mediator of Fibrosis

Alain Mauviel

Abstract

Transforming growth factor (TGF)-β is a prototypic multifunctional cytokine whose broad modulatory mechanisms affect numerous biological functions both at the cell and organism levels. These include, but are not limited to, control of immune functions, embryogenesis, carcinogenesis, tissue responses to injury, cell proliferation, extracellular matrix (ECM) synthesis and degradation, and cell migration. The identification of Smad proteins, TGF-β receptor kinase substrates that translocate into the cell nucleus to act as transcription factors, has increased our understanding of the molecular mechanisms underlying TGF-β action. This introductory chapter will outline the current knowledge on how specific signals initiated by the TGF-β receptors are brought to the nucleus to regulate gene expression, with a specific emphasis on how such signaling relates to connective tissue remodeling, repair, and fibrosis.

Key Words: Growth factors; TGF-β; gene expression; extracellular matrix; pathogenesis of fibrosis; Smad signaling; collagen.

1. Introduction

The transforming growth factor (TGF)-β family is comprised of more than 30 members throughout the animal reign, including TGF-βs *stricto sensu*, activins, and bone morphogenic proteins (BMPs), which are critical in governing cell fate determination and patterning in the developing embryo. They regulate a broad spectrum of biological responses in the adult *(1)*. Deregulation of TGF-β signaling during embryonic development leads to developmental abnormalities and, when occurring after birth, participates in several human diseases, the most prominent ones being cancer, autoimmune disorders, and tissue fibrosis *(2–4)*.

From: *Methods in Molecular Medicine, Vol. 117: Fibrosis Research: Methods and Protocols*
Edited by: J. Varga, D. A. Brenner, and S. H. Phan © Humana Press Inc., Totowa, NJ

2. TGF-β Biosynthesis

The three mammalian TGF-β isoforms, TGF-β1, TGF-β2, and TGF-β3, are encoded by three distinct genes, then secreted as latent precursor molecules (LTGF-β) requiring activation into a mature form for receptor binding and subsequent activation of signal transduction pathways *(5)*. The LTGF-β molecules consist of 390 to 414 amino acids with three specialized regions: an amino-terminal hydrophobic signal peptide region, the latent-associated peptide (LAP) region of 249 residues, and the C-terminal, potentially bioactive region consisting of 112 amino acids per monomer. Each TGF-β molecule is characterized by a cysteine knot composed of six cysteine residues involved in intrachain disulfide bonds that stabilize several β-sheet bands. A seventh cysteine allows an interchain disulfide bond with an identical monomeric TGF-β chain to generate a mature TGF-β dimer. LTGF-β is secreted as a large latent complex (LLC) covalently bound via the LAP region to LTGF-β-binding protein (LTBP), or as a small latent complex (SLC) without LTBP. The LAP confers latency to the complex whereas LTBP binds TGF-β to the extracellular matrix (ECM) and enables its proteolytic activation. Conformational changes of the latent TGF-β complex induced by either cleavage of the LAP by various proteases such as plasmin, thrombin, plasma transglutaminases, or endoglycosylases, or by physical interactions of the LAP with other proteins such as thrombospondin-1, releases bioactive, mature TGF-β (**Fig. 1**).

3. TGF-β Receptors

Following activation, TGF-β transduces its signal across the plasma membrane via specific serine/threonine kinase receptors named type I and type II receptors (TβRI and TβRII) *(6,7)*. Structurally, they both consist in a small cysteine-rich extracellular region and an intracellular portion bearing the kinase domain. TβRII exhibits intrinsic kinase activity whereas TβRI requires activation by TβRII to exert its kinase function. In unstimulated cells, TβRI is stabilized in an inactive conformation by its association with FKBP12 (FK506 binding protein 12) (Fig. 2) *(8)*. Following TGF-β binding to TβRII, recruitment and subsequent activation of TβRI occurs by phosphorylation of serine and threonine residues within the GS domain a region rich in glycine and serine residues preceding the kinase domain of TβRI. Receptors are then rapidly internalized into both caveolin- and EEA1-positive endosome depending on their cell membrane association with either lipid raft or nonraft membrane domains *(9)*.

Of note, a third type of TGF-β receptor, betaglycan, a transmembrane proteoglycan also known as TβRIII, allows high-affinity binding of TGF-β to TβRII but does not transduce signals *(10)*.

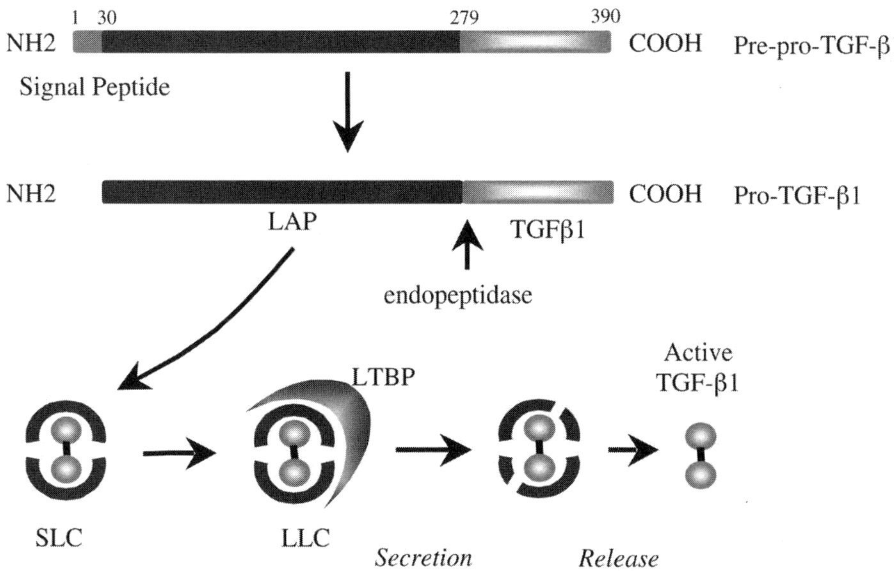

Fig. 1. Transforming growth factor (TGF)-β1 maturation. TGF-β1 is synthesized as pre-pro-TGF-β; that is, cleaved by endopeptidases in the Golgi apparatus to form a small latent complex (SLC) containing a mature 24 kDa TGF-β1 homodimer noncovalently associated with two 80-kDa latency-associated peptides (LAP). It is usually secreted as a large latent complex (LLC), covalently bound with latent TGF-β binding protein (LTBP). Final activation involves the release of mature TGF-β1 from the LLC. From **ref. *57***.

4. From Cell Membrane Receptors to the Nucleus

Specific signal transduction from the TGF-β receptors to the nucleus is mediated by phosphorylation of evolutionarily conserved cytoplasmic proteins of the Smad family ***(6,7)***, divided into three functional groups: receptor-associated Smads (R-Smads), which directly interact with activated TβRI and are ligand-specific; co-Smads, such as Smad4, a common mediator of all TGF-β family members; and inhibitory Smads (I-Smads), including Smad7.

R-Smads are characterized by two highly conserved proline-rich globular domains called Mad-homology (MH) domains, held together by a variable linker region. Mad is the *Drosophila* homolog of Smads. The MH1 domain is located in their N-terminal end and the MH2 domain in their C-terminus. In response to TGF-β, TβRI phosphorylates Smad2 and Smad3 on two serine residues within a conserved, R-Smad-specific, –SSXS motif at the extreme C-terminus of the MH2 domain. Microtubules play an important role in guiding

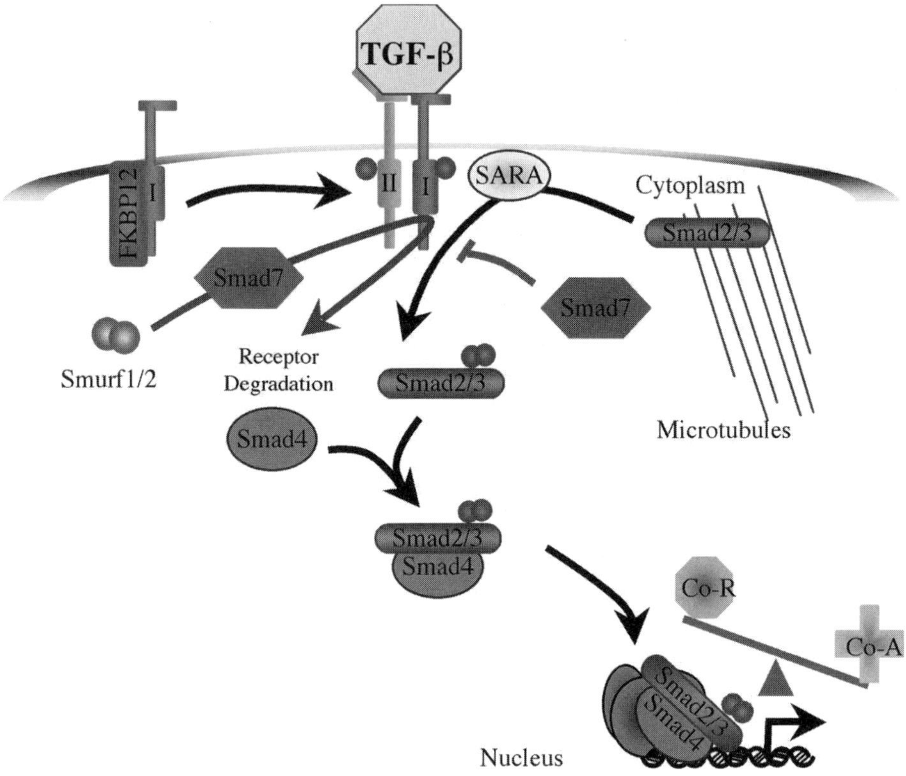

Fig. 2. The Smad pathway. Transforming growth factor (TGF)-β receptor type 1 (TβRI) is stabilized in an inactive conformation by its association with FKBP12. Upon TGF-β ligation to TβRII, the latter phosphorylates TβRI, which in turn phosphorylates Smad2/3. R-Smads are presented to the TβRI by a membrane-bound protein, Smad-anchored for receptor activation (SARA). Activated R-Smads bind Smad4 and translocate to the nucleus to act as transcription factors, controlled by a balance between transcriptional co-activators (co-A) or co-repressors (co-R). Inhibitory Smad7 binds activated TβRI, thereby preventing phosphorylation of R-Smads, or recruits the ubiquitine ligases Smurf1 and Smurf2 to induce proteasomal degradation of the receptor complexes. From **ref. *57***.

R-Smads to the plasma membrane, where a FYVE-domain protein, Smad-anchored for receptor activation (SARA), presents the Smad2 and Smad3 to the receptor ***(11)***. Upon phosphorylation by TβRI, R-Smads partner with Smad4, and translocate into the nucleus where they activate downstream transcriptional responses. Active nuclear import processes regulated by Ran and importins allow for rapid, efficient, and controlled nuclear import of Smad complexes *(12)*. Smad4 only translocates to the nucleus when complexed with R-Smads, whereas ligand-activated Smad2 and Smad3 may translocate into the nucleus in a Smad4-independent fashion *(13)*. In the absence of Smad4, however, neither Smad2 nor Smad3 are capable of transcriptional activity, suggesting that the principal function of Smad4 is to regulate transcription rather than to transmit signals from the cytoplasm to the nucleus.

R-Smad/Smad4 complexes may then function as transcription factors, binding DNA either directly or in association with other DNA binding proteins. Maximal affinity of recombinant Smad3 and Smad4 is observed with the CAGAC nucleotidic sequence, via their MH1 domain *(14)*. The transactivating role of Smad proteins has been ascribed to their MH2 domain. A 30-aa insertion within the Smad2 MH1 domain, as compared with the Smad3 MH1 domain, prevents direct DNA binding of Smad2 *(15)*. The latter requires a nuclear DNA-binding protein of the FAST/FoxH1 family to bind DNA in association with Smad4, to activate transcription in response to TGF-β *(16)*.

Smad7, an inhibitory Smad specific for the TGF-β receptors, binds activated TβRI, thereby preventing phosphorylation of Smad2/3 *(17)*. It also recruits the E3 ubiquitin-ligases Smurf1 and Smurf2 to the activated TβRI, leading to proteasomal degradation of the receptor complexes. Of note, Smad7 may function as a negative feedback loop, as its expression is induced by TGF-β itself in a Smad-dependent manner. Finally, several proteins, such as STRAP or YAP-65, have been shown to stabilize the Smad7–TβRI association, thereby exerting either additive or synergistic activities with Smad7 to prevent R-Smad phosphorylation by TβRI and subsequent intracellular signaling *(18,19)*.

Once in the nucleus, activated Smad complexes may either activate or repress gene expression, depending on the recruitment of transcriptional co-activators or co-repressors into DNA-bound complexes. An essential role for the histone acetyl-transferases CREB binding protein (CBP) and p300 as coactivators of Smad-driven gene expression is well documented *(20–24)*. Inversely, competition for p300/CBP has been suggested to mediate some examples of signal-induced transcriptional repression. For example, p300/CBP squelching by c-Jun or Stat1 may explain, at least in part, the antagonism exerted by tumor necrosis factor (TNF)-α and interferon (IFN)-γ against Smad-driven gene transcription *(25,26)*. Similarly, agents that activate protein kinase A (PKA), e.g., prostaglandin E $(PGE)_2$ and cAMP-elevating agents, antagonize Smad signaling via PKA-dependent, CREB-mediated disruption of Smad-p300/CBP complexes *(27)*.

Smads may also recruit transcriptional corepressors such as TG3-interacting factor (TGIF), Sloan-Kettering Institute proto-oncogene (SKI), Ski-related novel gene N (SnoN), or SNIP1 *(28–31)*. Generally, these proteins bind and recruit chromatin-condensating histone deacetylases, which oppose the histone acetyl-transferase activity associated with p300 and CBP. The level of expression of these co-repressors may thus have important physiological consequences, by either setting a threshold for TGF-β-induced transcriptional activation involving p300/CBP or by helping to terminate TGF-β signal.

5. Role of TGF-β and the Smad Pathway in ECM Gene Expression

A key function for TGF-β in wound healing and fibrosis is to regulate the expression of proteins of the ECM, including fibrillar collagens and fibronectin. TGF-β also represses ECM degradation by inhibiting the expression of metalloproteinases and serine proteases and by enhancing the expression of protease inhibitors such as the tissue inhibitors of metalloproteinases (TIMPs) and plasminogen activator inhibitors (PAIs). TGF-β is therefore considered a potent anabolic factor that enhances connective tissue deposition and repair and whose sustained signaling likely leads to the development of tissue fibrosis *(32)*.

Knockout experiments in mice have revealed that certain functions are specific for one isoform. For example, TGF-β3, which is mostly expressed during embryonic life, exhibits unique antiscarring properties, as exemplified by the fact that anbryonic wound healing in TGF-β3 knockout animals is not scarless, as opposed to embryos expressing TGF-β3 *(33)*. On the other hand, TGF-β1 is also critical for maintenance of proper immune functions, and knockout mice lacking TGF-β1 die a few weeks after birth from aberrant regulation of the immune response, which culminates in lethal cardiopulmonary inflammation. In this context, TGF-β has been shown to play pivotal role in multiple stages of T-cell apoptosis, selection, activation, and clearance *(3)*.

6. Modulation of Collagen Gene Regulation by TGF-β, Antagonistic Activities Exerted by Inflammatory TNF-α and IFN-γ

It is reasonable to hypothesize that a better understanding of the mechanisms of TGF-β-mediated upregulation of ECM gene expression in fibrotic tissue will provide novel approaches to the therapy of these essentially incurable diseases. Accordingly, a better understanding of the mechanisms by which pro-inflammatory cytokines, such as TNF-α, are able to interfere with the TGF-β-induced Smad signaling are of utmost importance. TNF-α have been suggested to block Smad signaling via mechanisms that implicate either c-Jun *(25)* or nuclear factor (NF)-κB *(34)*. The RelA subunit of NF-κB mediates TNF-α-induced expression of the inhibitory Smad, Smad7, which in turn blocks TGF-β signaling. Alternatively, c-Jun and JunB, both activated by TNF-α via the Jun-*N*-terminal kinase (JNK) pathway, are also capable of interrupting Smad3-mediated transcription: Jun/Smad3 complexes promoted by JNK activity may form off-DNA not compatible with Smad3 binding to cognate DNA sequences *(35)*. The outcome of such mechanism in terms of ECM gene expression is best illustrated in *JNK1*$^{-/-}$-*JNK2*$^{-/-}$ (*JNK*$^{-/-}$) fibroblasts, where TNF-α has no effect on TGF-β-induced fibrillar collagen gene transactivation unless ectopic expression of *jnk1* is allowed ***(36)***. In contrast, in NF-κB essential modulator knockout (*NEMO*$^{-}$) fibroblasts, which lack NF-κB activity, TNF-α is able to act as an antagonist of TGF-β, ruling out a possible role for NF-κB in mediating TNF-α effect against TGF-β ***(36)***. With regard to JNK function in the context of ECM turnover, these findings are complementary to a recent study indicating that a synthetic inhibitor of JNK, SP600125, suppresses interleukin (IL)-1-induced phospho-Jun accumulation, Jun–DNA interactions, and interstitial collagenase (matrix metalloproteinase [MMP]-1) gene expression in synovial fibroblasts ***(37)***. Thus, the benefit of JNK targeting in degenerative inflammatory diseases such as rheumatoid arthritis may result not only from the blocking of degradative events induced by IL-1 or TNF-α, but also from preventing cytokines from antagonizing the anabolic functions of TGF-β on ECM deposition. Conversely, means to activate the JNK pathway may be of interest in pathological situations in which interfering with TGF-β signaling and subsequent ECM deposition is critical, such as in fibrosis.

The pleiotropic cytokine IFN-γ exerts opposite effects on diverse cellular functions modulated by TGF-β. First, it has been shown that IFN-γ induces the expression of Smad7 via the activation of the JAK1/STAT1 pathway, Smad7 in turn preventing the interaction of Smad3 with the TβRI ***(38)***. Second, the JAK/STAT pathway may alter Smad-driven transcription because activated STAT1 may compete with Smad3 for limiting amounts of cellular coactivators such as p300/CBP, a mechanism that may explain the antagonistic activity of IFN-γ against TGF-β-induced *COL1A2* gene transcription ***(26)***. Third, IFN-γ may inhibit both basal and TGF-β induced *COL1A2* gene transcription by activating the transcription factor YB-1 ***(39,40)***. The latter not only binds a proximal region of the *COL1A2* promoter identified as a negative IFN-γ-responsive element, but also physically interacts with Smad3 to prevent its binding to the TGF-β-response element of the *COL1A2* promoter.

7. Experimental Targeting of Smad Signaling in Fibrosis

Inactivation of the Smad3 gene in mice has allowed the exploration of the Smad pathway's contribution to tissue repair ***(41)***. In contrast with predictions made on the basis of the ability of exogenous TGF-β to improve wound healing, Smad3-null (Smad3$^{ex8/ex8}$) mice paradoxically show accelerated cutaneous wound healing, characterized by an increased rate of re-epithelialization and significantly reduced local infiltration of monocytes compared with wild-type mice. Interestingly, these Smad3-null mice exhibit resistance to ionizing radiation-induced tissue fibrosis ***(42)***, and are protected from renal fibrosis induced by unilateral ureteral obstruction ***(43)***. Together, these results unequivocally demonstrate the role of the Smad pathway in the pathogenesis of fibrosis.

It has been suggested that defects in SMAD7 may, in certain instances, lead to fibrotic conditions, as reported in the heart and in scleroderma ***(44,45)***. However, ligand-independent constitutive activation of the intracellular TGF-β/Smad signaling axis in scleroderma fibroblasts, without profound differences in Smad7 mRNA levels between control and scleroderma fibroblasts, has also been reported ***(46)***.

The therapeutic potential of targeted delivery of this inhibitory Smad family member to prevent TGF-β-mediated fibrosis in vivo has been investigated in various experimental models of kidney, lung, or liver fibrosis have been developed and confirms this initial hypothesis. Thus, intratracheal injection of a recombinant adenovirus expressing Smad7 prevents bleomycin-induced lung fibrosis in mice ***(47)***. Similar promising results with Smad7 gene transfer have been achieved in in vivo models of liver or renal fibrosis ***(48,49)***. In systemic sclerosis, deficient Smad7 expression is regarded as a putative molecular defect leading to disease development ***(45)***. Furthermore, it was shown in the same study that in vitro adenoviral gene transfer of Smad7 reestablishes normal, not pathologically intensified, TGF-β signaling in SSc fibroblasts.

Most recently, small molecules inhibitors of the TGF-β type I receptor ALK5 are being developed for future clinical use. These molecules, which exhibit high specificity for TbR1, act with an IC50 in the nanomolar range, are able to antagonize TGF-β-induced ECM gene expression in vitro (50). When administered either intravenously or by mouth, they exhibit potent antifibrotic activity in animal models of tissue fibrosis, in the kidney (51), the lung (52), or the liver (53). Whether these new drugs can be used safely in man will be a great challenge, as systemic inhibition of TGF-β may lead to severe secondary effects, given the broad implications of TGF-β in general homeostatsis. To avoid potentially devastating effects such as on the immune system, it may be that therapeutical intervention against fibrosis requires targeted delivery of the inhibitors to the affected organ(s).

8. Conclusions

Several hurdles remain before TGF-β targeting can be considered a therapeutic alternative for the treatment of fibrosis, as significant problems may arise with regard to overall tolerance or biological outcome. For example, transgenic mice expressing a soluble form of TβRII are protected against metastasis without adverse side effects ***(54)***. However, epithelial overexpression of Smad7, or that of a dominant-negative TGF-β type II receptor, results in severe pathological alterations of epithelial tissues in transgenic mice ***(55)***, which could suggest that mesenchyme-specific targeting of the Smad pathway may be required. It gets even more complicated, as it has also been shown that fibroblast-specific expression of a kinase-deficient TβRII in mice leads to paradoxical activation of TGF-β signaling pathways with dermal and pulmonary fibrosis ***(56)***.

References

1. Roberts, A. B. (1998) Molecular and cell biology of TGF-beta. *Miner. Electrolyte Metab.* **24(2–3),** 111–119.
2. de Caestecker, M. P., Piek, E., and Roberts, A. B. (2000) Role of transforming growth factor-beta signaling in cancer. *J. Natl. Cancer Inst.* **92(17),** 1388–1402.
3. Chen, W. and Wahl, S. M. (2002) TGF-beta: receptors, signaling pathways and autoimmunity. *Curr. Dir. Autoimmun.* **5**, 62–91.
4. Varga, J. (2002) Scleroderma and Smads: dysfunctional Smad family dynamics culminating in fibrosis. *Arthritis Rheum.* **46(7),** 1703–1713.
5. Barcellos-Hoff, M. H. (1996) Latency and activation in the control of TGF-beta. *J. Mammary Gland Biol. Neoplasia.* **1(4),** 353–363.
6. Attisano, L. and Wrana, J. L. (2002) Signal transduction by the TGF-beta superfamily. *Science* **296(5573),** 1646–1647.
7. Shi, Y. and Massague, J. (2003) Mechanisms of TGF-beta signaling from cell membrane to the nucleus. *Cell* **113(6),** 685–700.
8. Huse, M., Muir, T. W., Xu, L., Chen, Y. G., Kuriyan, J., and Massague, J. (2001) The TGF beta receptor activation process: an inhibitor- to substrate- binding switch. *Mol. Cell.* **8(3),** 671–682.
9. Di Guglielmo, G. M., LeRoy, C., Goodfellow, A. E., and Wrana, J. L. (2003) Distinct endocytic pathways regulate TGF-beta receptor signalling and turnover. *Nat. Cell Biol.* **5(5),** 410–421.
10. Lopez-Casillas, F., Wrana, J. L., and Massagué, J. (1993) Betaglycan presents ligand to the TGF beta signaling receptor. *Cell* **73(7),** 1435–1444.
11. Tsukazaki, T., Chiang, T. A., Davison, A. F., Attisano, L., and Wrana, J. L. (1998) SARA, a FYVE domain protein that recruits Smad2 to the TGFbeta receptor. *Cell* **95(6),** 779–791.
12. Reguly, T. and Wrana, J. L. (2003) In or out? The dynamics of Smad nucleocytoplasmic shuttling. *Trends Cell Biol.* **13(5),** 216–220.
13. Fink, S. P., Mikkola, D., Wilson, J. K., and Markowitz, S. (2003) TGF-beta-induced nuclear localization of Smad2 and Smad3 in Smad4 null cancer cell lines. *Oncogene* **22(9),** 1317–1323.
14. Zawel, L., Dai, J. L., Buckhaults, P., et al. (1998) Human Smad3 and Smad4 are sequence-specific transcription activators. *Mol. Cell.* **1(4),** 611–617.
15. Dennler, S., Huet, S., and Gauthier, J. M. (1999) A short amino-acid sequence in MH1 domain is responsible for functional differences between Smad2 and Smad3. *Oncogene* **18(8),** 1643–1648.
16. Attisano, L., Silvestri, C., Izzi, L., and Labbe, E. (2001) The transcriptional role of Smads and FAST (FoxH1) in TGFbeta and activin signalling. *Mol. Cell Endocrinol.* **180(1-2),** 3–11.

17. Miyazono, K. (2000) TGF-beta signaling by Smad proteins. *Cytokine Growth Factor Rev.* **11(1-2),** 15–22.
18. Datta, P. K., Chytil, A., Gorska, A. E., and Moses, H. L. (1998) Identification of STRAP, a novel WD domain protein in transforming growth factor-beta signaling. *J. Biol. Chem.* **273(52),** 34,671–34,674.
19. Ferrigno, O., Lallemand, F., Verrecchia, F., et al. Yes-associated protein (YAP65) interacts with Smad7 and potentiates its inhibitory activity against TGF-beta/Smad signaling. *Oncogene* **21(32),** 4879–4884.
20. Janknecht, R., Wells, N. J., and Hunter, T. (1998) TGF-beta-stimulated cooperation of smad proteins with the coactivators CBP/p300. *Genes Dev.* **12(14),** 2114–2119.
21. Feng, X. H., Zhang, Y., Wu, R. Y., and Derynck, R. (1999) The tumor suppressor Smad4/DPC4 and transcriptional adaptor CBP/p300 are coactivators for smad3 in TGF-beta-induced transcriptional activation. *Genes Dev.* **12(14),** 2153–2163.
22. Pouponnot, C., Jayaraman, L., and Massagué, J. (1998) Physical and functional interaction of SMADs and p300/CBP. *J. Biol. Chem.* **273(36),** 22,865–22,968.
23. Shen, X., Hu, P. P., Liberati, N. T., Datto, M. B., Frederick, J. P., and Wang, X. F. (1998) TGF-beta-induced phosphorylation of Smad3 regulates its interaction with coactivator p300/CREB-binding protein. *Mol. Biol. Cell.* **9(12),** 3309–3319.
24. Topper, J. N., Dichiara, M. R., Brown, J. D., et al. (1998) CREB binding protein is a required coactivator for Smad-dependent, transforming growth factor beta transcriptional responses in endothelial cells. *Proc. Natl. Acad. Sci. USA* **95(16),** 9506–9511.
25. Verrecchia, F., Pessah, M., Afti, A., and Mauviel, A. (2000) Tumor necrosis factor-alpha inhibits transforming growth factor-beta /Smad signaling in human dermal fibroblasts via AP-1 activation. *J. Biol. Chem.* **275(39),** 30,226–30,231.
26. Ghosh, A. K., Yuan, W., Mori, Y., Chen, S. J., and Varga, J. (2001) Antagonistic regulation of type I collagen gene expression by interferon-gamma and transforming growth factor-beta. Integration at the level of p300/CBP transcriptional coactivators. *J. Biol. Chem.* **276(14),** 11,041–11,048.
27. Schiller, M., Verrecchia, F., and Mauviel, A. (2003) Cyclic adenosine 3',5'-monophosphate-elevating agents inhibit transforming growth factor-beta-induced SMAD3/4-dependent transcription via a protein kinase A-dependent mechanism. *Oncogene* **22(55),** 8881–8890.
28. Wotton, D., Lo, R. A., Lee, S., and Massague, J. (1999) A Smad transcriptional corepressor. *Cell* **97(1),** 29–39.
29. Luo, K., Stroschein, S. L., Wang, W., et al. (1999) The Ski oncoprotein interacts with the Smad proteins to repress TGFbeta signaling. *Genes Dev.* **13(17),** 2196–2206.
30. Sun, Y., Liu, X., Ng-Eaton, E., Lodish, H. F., and Weinberg, R. A. (1999) SnoN and Ski protooncoproteins are rapidly degraded in response to transforming growth factor beta signaling. *Proc. Natl. Acad. Sci. USA* **96(22),** 12,442–12,447.
31. Kim, R. H., Wang, D., Tsang, M., et al. (2000) A novel smad nuclear interacting protein, SNIP1, suppresses p300- dependent TGF-beta signal transduction. *Genes Dev.* **14(13),** 1605–1616.

32. Verrecchia, F. and Mauviel, A. (2002) Control of connective tissue gene expression by TGF beta: role of Smad proteins in fibrosis. *Curr. Rheumatol. Rep.* **4(2),** 143–149.
33. O'Kane, S. and Ferguson, M. W. (1997) Transforming growth factor beta s and wound healing. *Int. J. Biochem. Cell Biol.* **29(1),** 63–78.
34. Bitzer, M.,von Gersdorff, G., Liang, D., et al. (2000) A mechanism of suppression of TGF-beta/SMAD signaling by NF-kappa B/RelA. *Genes Dev.* **14(2),** 187–197.
35. Verrecchia, F., Tacheau, C., Wagner, E. G., and Mauviel, A. (2003) A central role for the JNK pathway in mediating the antagonistic activity of pro-inflammatory cytokines against transforming growth factor-beta-driven SMAD3/4-specific gene expression. *J. Biol. Chem.* **278(3),** 1585–1593.
36. Verrecchia, F., Wagner, E. F., and Mauviel, A. (2002) Distinct involvement of the Jun-N-terminal kinase and NF-κB pathways in the repression of the human COL1A2 gene by TNF-α. *EMBO Rep.* **3(11),** 1069–1074.
37. Han, Z., Boyle, D. L., Chang, L., et al. (2001) c-Jun N-terminal kinase is required for metalloproteinase expression and joint destruction in inflammatory arthritis. *J. Clin. Invest.* **108(1),** 73–81.
38. Ulloa, L., Doody, J., and Massagué, J. (1999) Inhibition of transforming growth factor-beta/SMAD signalling by the interferon-gamma/STAT pathway. *Nature* **397(6721),** 710–713.
39. Higashi, K., Kouba, D. J., Song, Y. J., Uitto, J., and Mauviel, A. (1998) A proximal element within the human alpha 2(I) collagen (COL1A2) promoter, distinct from the tumor necrosis factor-alpha response element, mediates transcriptional repression by interferon-gamma. *Matrix Biol.* **16(8),** 447–456.
40. Higashi, K., Inagaki, Y., Fujimori, K., Nakao, A., Kaneko, H., and Nakatsuka, I. (2003) Interferon-gamma interferes with transforming growth factor-beta signaling through direct interaction of YB-1 with Smad3. *J. Biol. Chem.* **278(44),** 43,470–43,479.
41. Ashcroft, G. S., Yang, X., Glick, A. B., et al. (1999) Mice lacking Smad3 show accelerated wound healing and an impaired local inflammatory response. *Nat. Cell Biol.* **1(5),** 260–266.
42. Flanders, K. C., Sullivan, C. D., Fujii, M., et al. (2002) Mice lacking Smad3 are protected against cutaneous injury induced by ionizing radiation. *Am. J. Pathol.* **160(3),** 1057–1068.
43. Sato, M., Muragaki, Y., Saika, S., Roberts, A. B., and Ooshmia, A. (2003) Targeted disruption of TGF-β1/Smad3 signaling protects against renal tubulointerstitial fibrosis induced by unilateral ureteral obstruction. *J. Clin. Invest.* **112(10),** 1486–1494.
44. Wang, B., Hao, J., Jones, S. C., Yee, M. S., Roth, J. C., and Dixon, I. M. (2002) Decreased Smad 7 expression contributes to cardiac fibrosis in the infarcted rat heart. *Am. J. Physiol. Heart Circ. Physiol.* **282(5),** H1685–1696.
45. Wang, H., Yang, G. H., Bu, H., Zhou, Q., Gui, L. X., Wang, S. L., and Ye, L. (2003) Systematic analysis of the TGF-beta/Smad signalling pathway in the rhabdomyosarcoma cell line RD. *Int. J. Exp. Pathol.* **84(3),** 153–163.

46. Mori, Y., Chen, S. J., and Varga, J. (2003) Expression and regulation of intracellular SMAD signaling in scleroderma skin fibroblasts. *Arthritis Rheum.* **48(7),** 1964–1978.
47. Nakao, A., Fujii, M., Matsumura, R., et al. (1999) Transient gene transfer and expression of Smad7 prevents bleomycin- induced lung fibrosis in mice. *J. Clin. Invest.* **104(1),** 5–11.
48. Lan, H. Y., Mu, W., Tomita, N., et al. (2003) Inhibition of renal fibrosis by gene transfer of inducible Smad7 using ultrasound-microbubble system in rat UUO model. *J. Am. Soc. Nephrol.* **14(6),** 1535–1548.
49. Dooley, S., Hamzavi, J., Breitkopf, K., et al. (2003) Smad7 prevents activation of hepatic stellate cells and liver fibrosis in rats. *Gastroenterology* **125(1),** 178–191.
50. Laping, N. J., Grygielko, E., Mathur, A., et al. (2002) Inhibition of transforming growth factor (TGF)-beta1-induced extracellular matrix with a novel inhibitor of the TGF-beta type I receptor kinase activity: SB-431542. Mol. Pharmacol. 62(10), 58–64.
51. Grygeiklo, E. T., Martin, W. M., Tweed, C. W., et al. (2005) Inhibition of gene markers of fibrosis with a novel inhibitor of TGF{beta}-type I receptor kinase in puromycin-induced nephritis. J. Pharmacol. Exp. Ther. [Epub ahead of print].
52. Bonniaud, P., Margetts, P. J., Kolb, M., et al. (2005) Progressive transforming growth factor {beta}1-induced lung fibrosis is blocked by an orally active ALK5 kinase inhibitor. Am. J. Resp. Crit. Care Med. 171(8), 889–898.
53. de Gouville, A. C., Boullay, V., Krysa, G., et al. (2005) Inhibition of TGF-beta signaling by an ALK5 inhibitor protects rats from dimethylnitrosamine-induced liver fibrosis. Br. J. Pharmacol. [Epub ahead of print].
54. Yang, Y. A., Dukhanina, O., Tang, B., et al. (2002) Lifetime exposure to a soluble TGF-beta antagonist protects mice against metastasis without adverse side effects. *J. Clin. Invest.* **109(12),** 1607–1615.
55. He, W., Li, A. G., Wang, D., et al. (2002) Overexpression of Smad7 results in severe pathological alterations in multiple epithelial tissues. *EMBO J.* **21(11),** 2580–2590.
56. Denton, C. P., Zheng, B., Evans, L. A., et al. (2003) Fibroblast-specific expression of a kinase-deficient type II transforming growth factor beta (TGFbeta) receptor leads to paradoxical activation of TGFbeta signaling pathways with fibrosis in transgenic mice. *J. Biol. Chem.* **278(27),** 25,109–25,119.
57. Javelaud, D. and Mauviel, A. (2004) Mammalian transforming growth factor-betas: Smad signaling and physio-pathological roles. *Int. J. Biochem. Cell Biol.* **36,** 1161–1165.

II

Regulation of Extracellular Matrix Metabolism: Cultured Cells

4

Isolation and Culture of Skin Fibroblasts

Laure Rittié and Gary J. Fisher

Summary

Dermal fibroblasts synthesize and organize skin connective tissue (dermis). Fibroblast cultures provide a powerful tool for investigating both the molecular mechanisms that regulate skin connective tissue production and the pathophysiology of fibrotic skin diseases. In this chapter, we describe detailed procedures for establishing and maintaining primary cultures of adult human fibroblasts. We also provide protocols for constructing three-dimensional dermal and skin equivalent culture models.

Key Words: Fibrosis; fibroblast; collagen; organ culture; cell culture; organotypic culture; skin equivalent.

1. Introduction

Cultivation of fibroblasts in vitro provides a useful model for studying their functions in normal and pathological states in a controlled environment. Several decades ago, cell culture techniques were considered somewhat esoteric. Today, because of better understanding of cell nutrition, metabolism, and general growth requirements, cell culture has become a routine procedure.

A good cell culture model is one in which the cells faithfully and reproducibly mimic their behavior in their natural in vivo environment. The extent to which these criteria are met is often difficult to access and therefore, caution should always be exercised when extrapolating observations made on cultured fibroblasts to in vivo settings. Nevertheless, fibroblast cultures have proven to be useful tools for understanding molecular mechanisms that regulate fibroblast function. To obtain meaningful data, it is important that culture systems are standardized and maintained in appropriate conditions in order to minimize culture artifacts. In this chapter, we provide detailed protocols for cultivation of primary adult human skin fibroblast used in our laboratory, starting with isolating cells from adult skin. Protocols are given for cultivation of fibroblasts

From: *Methods in Molecular Medicine, Vol. 117: Fibrosis Research: Methods and Protocols*
Edited by: J. Varga, D. A. Brenner, and S. H. Phan © Humana Press Inc., Totowa, NJ

in monolayer on tissue culture dishes, in three-dimensional collagen lattices, and in co-culture with human keratinocytes to form so-called skin reconstructs.

1.1. Fibroblasts in Human Skin

Skin is one of the most suitable tissues that can be used as a source of human fibroblasts. Skin consists of three layers: (1) epidermis, which primarily contains keratinocytes, melanocytes, and Langherans cells; (2) dermis, primarily populated with fibroblasts, blood vessels, and dendritic cells; and (3) subcutaneous tissue. Epidermis is separated from dermis by a basement membrane, which is primarily composed of extracellular matrix proteins (collagens and laminins), synthesized by both fibroblasts and keratinocytes.

Type I collagen is the most abundant protein in the dermis. It is produced by resident fibroblasts, which also synthesize other components of dermal extracellular matrix, including other collagens (III, V, VII), elastin, proteoglycans, and fibronectin. In human skin, the half-life of type I collagen is estimated to be greater than 1 yr *(1)*. Collagen synthesis is increased after a wound, to remodel the injured area *(2,3)*, and in fibrotic diseases such as scleroderma *(4,5)*. Collagen synthesis is decreased after sun exposure and during aging *(6)*. Fibroblasts also produce extracellular matrix-degrading enzymes such as matrix metalloproteinases (MMPs) and plasmin. Homeostasis of extracellular matrix depends on balanced synthesis of all these proteins.

Skin is particularly adaptable to organ cultures. Skin organ cultures have been used for decades to study skin ex vivo *(7)*. Organ cultures allow the use of reagents, which are not approved for human use or not compatible with topical application, to study skin function. However, organ culture is not suitable for the study of individual cell types, as is cell culture.

1.2. Collagen and Fibroblast Culture

In monolayer cultures, numerous reports have shown that proliferation and collagen production of human skin fibroblasts depend on the composition and pH of the medium, the source and concentration of serum, the addition of ascorbate, and the age of the donor. It has also been shown that collagen synthesis per cell decreases with increased cell confluence *(8)*.

1.3. Primary Human Skin Fibroblast Cultures

Normal human dermal fibroblast cultures can be divided into three phases:

1. Primary cultures are established by enzymatic digestion of the dermis, or by outgrowth of fibroblasts from explanted tissue pieces. It is important to note that primary cultures are not derived from a single cell, but rather are a heterogeneous mixture of skin fibroblasts.

2. Secondary cultures are actively proliferating cells, obtained by passage and expansion of primary cultures. After a limited number of cell divisions (30–50 cycles for fibroblasts from skin of young adults), the rate of cell growth gradually decreases.
3. Terminal cultures eventually reach a state of replicative senescence, considered to be aging at the cellular level ***(9,10)***.

One advantage of studying fibroblasts obtained from primary culture is that they contain normal diploid complement of chromosomes, and therefore, in this respect, mimic fibroblasts in vivo. In contrast, fibroblast cell lines typically have numerous chromosomal aberrations and mutations, which are associated with their ability for unlimited growth.

1.4. Culture of Fibroblast in Monolayers

When grown in monolayer culture in their proliferative phase, fibroblast cultures expand, and require subculturing to alleviate overcrowding. If the cell density is not reduced at confluence, cells will detach from their support and die.

Cryogenic preservation of low passage-number fibroblasts is useful for maintaining reserves of cells. In doing so, it is easy for one investigator to rapidly build a bank of fibroblasts from a limited number of skin samples.

1.5. Culture of Fibroblasts With Collagen

In skin, fibroblasts are in contact with type I collagen and other extracellular matrix components. These contacts are critical for normal regulation of fibroblast function. Therefore, culture of fibroblasts on a collagen-coated surface or embedded in collagen gel is commonly done to model in vivo environment.

Culture of skin fibroblasts in collagen gels (also called collagen lattices or dermis equivalents), was first described by Bell et al. ***(11)***. The introduction of fibroblasts into a three-dimensional collagen matrix leads to a reorganization of the matrix by fibroblasts. This reorganization is readily observable as reduction in the size of the gel resulting from fibroblast contraction of the collagen fibrils. Thus the collagen gel serves as a stimulus to modulate fibroblast behavior ***(12)***. When cultured in collagen lattices, fibroblast morphology and many aspects of their behavior differ from those observed in monolayer cultures. Morphologically, fibroblasts in monolayer are flat, spindle-shaped, and organized in parallel arrays. When cultured in a three-dimensional collagen gel, fibroblasts are elongated and have numerous dendrites. Fibroblasts in collagen gels proliferate much slower than in monolayer cultures. Metabolic activities also differ, for example synthesis of collagen is reduced ***(13,14)*** and MMP activities are increased ***(15,16)*** in collagen gels.

Variations of collagen gel models have been developed to assess fibroblast behavior within a three-dimensional matrix. In noncontracting (or attached) collagen lattices, contraction of collagen occurs in the vertical axis but is limited in the other dimensions. Fibroblasts in noncontracting collagen gels spread and elongate but are unable to reorganize the collagen fibers. Downregulation of collagen is less pronounced than in contracted collagen gels. The degree of gel contraction reflects the level of mechanical tension on the cells. Mechanical tension influences a wide array of cellular functions *(17,18)*.

1.6. Skin Equivalents

Skin equivalents consist of fibroblasts embedded in a collagen gel, or dermal equivalent, covered with an epidermis equivalent composed of several layers of differentiated keratinocytes. In contrast with monolayer cultures and collagen gels, skin equivalents include keratinocyte-fibroblast interactions in a physiologically and spatially organized mode. The culture is maintained at the air–liquid interface, allowing formation of a stratified epidermis, which exhibits partial barrier function *(19)*. Skin equivalent models enable the exposure of fibroblasts to topically applied drugs or lights through the epidermis layers, and thereby allow investigation of keratinocyte modulation of fibroblast responses in a collagen gel.

Skin equivalents were originally obtained by growing differentiated keratinocytes on devitalized pigskin dermis *(20)*. Since then, many substrates have been used to support the growth of fibroblasts and keratinocytes, including fibroblast-populated collagen lattices *(21,22)*. Besides type I collagen, artificial dermis may contain additional extracellular matrix proteins including type III or IV collagens and proteoglycans. The degree of complexity of skin equivalents can be further increased by adding other cell types to the culture (e.g., melanocytes, inflammatory cells, cancer cells).

2. Materials

1. Dermal skin fibroblasts are cultured in Dulbecco's modified Eagle medium (DMEM) supplemented with 10% serum (fetal bovine or calf) and antibiotics and antimycotics (optional—*see* **Notes 1–4**). Supplemented culture medium will be called complete medium.
2. Fibroblasts are adherent cells that must be cultured in tissue culture type dishes. For culture maintenance purposes, 75-cm^2 dishes are commonly used (*see* **Note 5**).
3. Volumes stated in the following protocols are for 75-cm^2 dishes; they can be proportionally reduced or increased for culture vessels of other sizes.

2.1. Obtaining Fibroblasts

1. Punch biopsies are obtained from volunteer's non-sun exposed buttock skin. Punch biopsies are 4 to 6 mm in diameter (*see* **Notes 6** and **7**).

2. Skin samples are collected in Hank's balanced salt solution (HBSS), supplemented with penicillin (100 IU/mL), streptomycin (100 µg/mL), and amphotericine B (0.25 µg/mL) (see **Note 8**).

2.2. Skin Organ Cultures

Skin organ cultures are maintained in DMEM-HamF12 1:1 containing 3.75 m*M* glutamine, 1.8 m*M* $CaCl_2$, and 2% serum.

2.3. Primary Culture of Fibroblasts

2.3.1. Enzymatic Digestion of Dermis

1. 0.25% Trypsin (w/v) in phosphate-buffered saline (PBS).
2. Sterile forceps.
3. Ethanol sterilized nylon mesh.
4. Enzyme solution: *N*-2-hydroxyethylpiperazine-*N*'-2-ethanesulfonic acid [HEPES] containing Richter's improved MEM insulin medium [RPMI], supplemented with 1 m*M* sodium pyruvate, 2.75 mg/mL bacterial collagenase, 1.25 mg/mL hyaluronidase, and 0.1 mg/mL DNase I.

2.3.2. Outgrowth of Fibroblasts From Explants

1. 150-mm sterile dish (type Pyrex®).
2. Storage medium: HBSS supplemented with antibiotics and antimycotics.
3. Sterile scalpel and forceps.
4. Explantation medium: DMEM containing 20% serum, antibiotic/antimycotic supplement.

2.4. Subculture of Fibroblasts

1. Trypsin-ethylenediamine tetraacetic acid (EDTA) solution: 0.05% (w/v) trypsin in PBS containing 1 m*M* EDTA (*see* **Note 9**).

2.5. Freezing Fibroblasts

1. Freezing medium: DMEM containing 20% serum and 10% dimethylsulfoxide (DMSO).
2. Cryogenic vials.
3. Slow cooling rate device: programmable electronic freezer unit (–1 to –3°C per minute) or mechanical freezer unit (Mr. Frosty™ from Nalge Nunc International, Rochester, NY; StrataCooler™ from Stratagene, La Jolla, CA).
4. Liquid nitrogen freezer and protective gloves and glasses.

2.6. Culture of Fibroblasts With Collagen

Important: *see* **Note 10** for handling collagen solutions.

2.6.1. Collagen Coating

1. Type I collagen solution (BD Biosciences, San Jose, CA) diluted to 250 μg/mL with 18 m*M* acetic acid.
2. 24-Well plates.
3. 2% (w/v) serum albumin solution in PBS, sterilized by filtration.
4. Sterile PBS.

2.6.2. Collagen Lattice Cultures

1. "Bacterial type" Petri dishes. The method is described for 35-mm diameter dishes. Stated volumes can be proportionally increased for culture dishes of bigger sizes.
2. Stock solution of 2.5X DMEM: DMEM prepared from powder, sterilized by filtration, and stored at 4°C up to 1 mo. This stock solution is used to counteract dilution of medium obtained by addition of collagen (solubilized in acetic acid) and sodium hydroxide (used to neutralize acetic acid).
3. Lattice medium: for 1.25 mL per 35-mm diameter dish, mix 0.70 mL 2.5X DMEM, 0.26 mL distilled H_2O, 0.09 mL 0.1 *M* NaOH, and 0.20 mL serum.
4. Type I collagen solution (BD Biosciences) diluted to 2 mg/mL with 18 m*M* acetic acid.
5. 18-Gage needles and 1-mL syringes for collagen and cell suspension pipetting make the manipulation easier (they can easily be placed back in the tube between two samples).

2.6.3. Collagenase Digestion for Isolation of Cells

1. Bacterial collagenase solution: dilute bacterial collagenase from *Clostridium histolyticum* (Sigma, St. Louis, MO) to 1 mg/mL in collagenase buffer (50 m*M* Tris, 0.15 *M* NaCl, 4 m*M* $CaCl_2$, pH = 7.4) before each use. Prepare 1 mL per lattice in microtubes (*see* **Note 11**).

2.7. Skin Equivalents

1. 24-mm diameter culture inserts with a 0.4-μm pore sized polyester membrane, and placed in individual wells of 6-well plates (Costar, Corning Inc, Acton, MA). The clear membrane allows observation of the culture with an inverted microscope.
2. Type I collagen solution (BD Biosciences) diluted to 3 mg/mL in 0.18 m*M* acetic acid.
3. 2.5X DMEM, 0.1 *M* NaOH (*see* collagen lattice protocol).
4. Human adult keratinocytes needed for establishing skin equivalents can be obtained from primary cultures of skin samples *(23)*. Human adult keratinocytes are also commercially available either as cryopreserved vials or proliferating cultures (Cascade Biologics, Portland, OR; BD Bioscience-Clontech, Palo Alto, CA). Keratinocytes are handled according to the protocol provided with the cells.
5. Compositions of the different culture media used for skin equivalents are detailed in **Table 1**. Stock solutions for making media can be stored up to 3 mo at indicated temperatures. Once prepared, skin equivalent media must be sterilized by filtration and can be stored up to 2 wk at 4°C.

Table 1
Composition of Skin Equivalent (SE) Media

	Stock (X)	Storage temp.	SE1	SE2	SE3
Ca^{2+}-free DMEM		4°C	725 mL/L	725 mL/L	474 mL/L
Ham-F12		4°C	240 mL/L	240 mL/L	474 mL/L
Antibiotics supplement	100	–20°C	10 mL	10 mL	10 mL
L-Glutamine	50	–20°C	4 m*M*	4 m*M*	4 m*M*
Hydrocortisone	100	–20°C	1.4 µ*M*	1.4 µ*M*	1.4 µ*M*
ITS-G supplement[a]	100	4°C	10 mL	10 mL	10 mL
Adenine	250	R.T.	0.18 m*M*	0.18 m*M*	0.18 m*M*
o-Phosphorylethanolamine	500	–20°C	0.1 m*M*	0.1 m*M*	0.1 m*M*
$CaCl_2$	500	R.T.	—	1.8 m*M*	1.8 m*M*
Progesterone	500	–20°C	4 p*M*	4 p*M*	4 p*M*
Tri-iodo-thyronine	1000	4°C	20 p*M*	20 p*M*	20 p*M*
Ethanolamine	5000	–20°C	10 m*M*	10 m*M*	10 m*M*
Chelated serum[b]		4°C	0.1%	—	—
Serum		4°C	—	0.1%	2%

R.T., room temperature.

[a] ITS-G = 1 g/L insulin, 0.67 mg/mL sodium selenite, 0.55 g/L transferrin (Invitrogen, San Diego, CA).

[b] Mix 4 g Chelex-100 (Sigma) with 40 mL serum. Stir 3 h at 4°C. Centrifuge 10 min at 400 *g* at 4°C. Sterilize supernatant by filtration.

3. Methods

3.1. Obtaining Fibroblasts

1. Thoroughly wash the biopsy site with an antiseptic soap and swab with 70% ethanol. Ethanol should be allowed to completely air-dry before the biopsy is taken. A local anesthetic (e.g., 1% lidocaine) is administered prior to biopsy. The anesthetic should be injected adjacent to the biopsy site rather than directly into it.
2. Stabilize the skin with the thumb and forefinger, stretching it slightly perpendicular to the normal skin tension lines.
3. Place the punch instrument perpendicular to the skin and apply firm and constant downward pressure with a circular motion, avoiding back-and-forth twisting motions. A definite "give" occurs when the punch instrument reaches the subcutaneous fat, indicating that a full thickness cut has been made.
4. Remove the punch instrument and apply downward pressure at the sides of the wound. Gently elevate the core, using aseptic forceps, and excise it at its base using small scissors. While applying pressure on the wound in preparation for closure, store the biopsy into a sterile vial containing storage medium.
5. Wounds 3 mm or less can be treated with a hemostatic agent and allowed to heal freely, whereas larger wounds require one or two sutures (in this case, no hemostatic agent is needed).

After removal, skin is able to withstand prolonged storage in the cold, simplifying the time schedule for culture preparations. Successful cultures can be made from material stored up to 48 h at 4°C.

3.2. Skin Organ Cultures

Skin is particularly adaptable to organ culture methods. However, small biopsies (2 mm) should be used to allow sufficient penetration of nutriments and oxygen through the entire specimen.

Skin biopsies are placed into organ culture medium immediately after removal. The culture should be started as soon as possible after biopsies are obtained.

1. Transfer each skin sample into a culture plate (e.g., 6-well plate) using sterile forceps, orientating the tissue so that the dermis is in contact with the bottom of the dish.
2. Incubate the plate 15 min at room temperature to allow good adhesion of the dermis onto the culture dish.
3. Gently add a small amount of medium on the side of the biopsy, making sure that the epidermis is exposed to the air. Culture up to 48 h in the 5% CO_2 incubator at 37°C.

3.3. Primary Culture of Fibroblasts

3.3.1. Enzymatic Digestion vs Outgrowth Procedures

Fibroblast primary cultures can be obtained by two methods: enzymatic digestion of dermis, or outgrowth of cells from explanted tissue pieces. The first method is faster, and yields higher recovery of cells from the skin sample. Enzymatic digestion should be utilized when fibroblast motility may be impaired (e.g., skin sample from elderly people). Although the cultures initially contain a variety of cell types, culture conditions select for fibroblast growth.

The outgrowth method relies on the capacity of fibroblasts to migrate out of the skin and adhere to the surface of the culture vessel. This method has the advantage that the migrating cells are highly enriched in fibroblasts. However, this method may also select for fibroblasts with higher rates of motility.

3.3.2. Enzymatic Digestion of Dermis

1. Transfer the biopsy and medium into a sterile plastic dish.
2. Add 10 mL of 0.25% trypsin. Incubate 30 min at room temperature.
3. After incubation, isolate the dermis from epidermis using sterile forceps. Cut the dermis into small pieces. Add 10 mL of enzyme solution and incubate at room temperature for 3 h.
4. After incubation, mechanically dissociate the tissue by pipetting up and down 10 times.
5. Filter the cell suspension through a sterile nylon mesh to remove tissue fragments.
6. Centrifuge at 400*g* for 10 min at room temperature.

7. Discard the supernatant, resuspend the cell pellet in 10 mL of complete medium and transfer cell suspension into a 75-cm^2 culture dish. Place cultures in the 5% CO_2 incubator at 37°C.
8. Change the medium 24 h later to remove nonadherent material.

3.3.3. Outgrowth of Fibroblasts From Explants

1. Transfer the skin sample into a 150-mm sterile dish containing 25 mL of storage medium.
2. Dissect the dermis from the rest of the skin (epidermis, subcutaneous tissue, vascular structures) using scalpel and forceps. The dermis can be distinguished from other structures in that it sticks to dissection instruments.
3. Mince the dermis into small pieces (about 1 mm^3) and place about eight fragments on the bottom of a 75-cm^2 culture dish, separated from one another.
4. Allow explants to air-dry for 15 min to increase attachment to the bottom of the dish.
5. Gently add 8 mL of explant medium, to cover each tissue piece. Place cultures back in the 5% CO_2 incubator at 37°C.
6. Change the medium 24 h later and discard nonadherent material. Change the medium once per week, until substantial number of fibroblasts is observed.

Fibroblast migration out of tissue fragments should be regularly monitored using an inverted microscope. Fibroblasts should be subcultured when they occupy most of the dish surface between explants (approx 2–3 wk after start of the culture—*see* subculturing protocol below). After detaching cells from the dish, the explantation process can be repeated up to three times feeding the explant with 10 mL of explantation medium.

3.4. Subculture of Fibroblasts

1. Remove and discard culture medium.
2. Rinse cell layer with 2 mL of trypsin–EDTA solution to remove residual cellular debris and serum-containing medium, which contains trypsin inhibitors.
3. Add 3 mL of trypsin–EDTA to the cell layer and incubate at 37°C.
4. Observe regularly under an inverted microscope until cells are detached and float in the solution. This should occur after 2 to 5 min (if cells are difficult to detach, the incubation can be prolonged up to 10 min).
5. Add 5 mL of complete medium (to inactivate trypsin), gently aspirate cell suspension, and transfer it to a centrifugation tube.
6. Centrifuge at 400*g* for 10 min at room temperature (*see* **Note 12**).
7. Discard the supernatant, resuspend the pellet in 1 mL of complete medium, and transfer the cell suspension into a new dish containing 10 mL of complete medium.

One confluent 75-cm^2 dish contains approx 3×10^6 cells. New dishes can be seeded at $0.75–1 \times 10^6$ cells/dish.

3.5. Freezing and Thawing Fibroblasts

3.5.1. Freezing Fibroblasts

1. Prior to freezing, the culture should be in actively growing phase, and free from any fungal, bacterial or mycoplasma contamination.
2. Use previously described protocol for subculturing fibroblasts to detach and isolate the cells.
3. After centrifugation, remove and discard the supernatant and slowly resuspend the cell pellet with freezing medium using approx 1 mL per 75-cm^2 dish.
4. Label cryogenic vials (cell source, passage number, and date) with low temperature resistant ink.
5. Add 1 mL of cell suspension per vial and seal.
6. Place in a slow cooling rate device overnight at –80°C.
7. Transfer the vials to a liquid nitrogen freezer. Make sure that the location and labeling recording system is suitable for long-term cryogenic storage (*see* **Note 13**).

3.5.2. Thawing Fibroblasts

1. Using protective gloves and clothing, remove vials from the liquid nitrogen freezer. Update the freezer log appropriately.
2. Loosen the cap on each vial one-quarter turn to release liquid nitrogen from the threads, and re-tighten on the caps.
3. Thaw the vials by gentle agitation in a 37°C water bath, making sure to keep the cap out of the water to avoid contamination.
4. As soon as the content is thawed, remove vial from the water and disinfect the vial with 70% ethanol.
5. Transfer the vial content to a 75-cm^2 culture dish containing 10 mL complete medium.
6. Place the cultures in the incubator. Change the medium 24 h later to remove nonadherent cells.

3.6. Culture of Fibroblasts With Collagen

3.6.1. Collagen Coating

Stated volumes are for coating a 24-well plate. They can be proportionally increased or decreased for culture dishes of different sizes.

1. Spread 500 μL of type I collagen solution per well over the surface of a sterile 24-well plate.
2. Air-dry overnight in a tissue culture hood to allow complete evaporation of solution and fixation of collagen.
3. Incubate 1 h with 500 μL of a 2% serum albumin solution to saturate free binding sites.
4. Rinse three times with 500 μL of PBS before seeding fibroblasts (*see* **Note 14**).

3.6.2. Collagen Lattice Cultures

3.6.2.1. Contracting Collagen Gels

1. Dispense 1.25 mL of lattice medium into a 35-mm diameter dish. Incubate at 37°C until needed (**step 3**).
2. Prepare fibroblast suspension from monolayer cultures, according to subculturing protocol (**Subheading 3.4.**). Resuspend the resulting cell pellet in 1X DMEM. Adjust the cell density to 0.4×10^6 cells/mL.
3. For each lattice:
   a. Add 0.5 mL of collagen solution to the lattice medium.
   b. Agitate the dish in a circular motion, to allow an even neutralization of collagen by NaOH (homogeneous color).
   c. Gently mix the cell suspension and add 0.25 mL to the dish. Repeat the agitation procedure.
   d. After cell suspension is well mixed, allow collagen to gel without disturbing, i.e., at room temperature for 15 min.
4. The gel should be detached from the side of the dish. If not, gently agitate the dish to detach the lattice. Place dish in the 5% CO_2 incubator at 37°C.

Culture medium should be replaced at least every week with fresh complete medium (*see* **Note 15**).

3.6.2.2. Noncontracting Collagen Gels

Prior to making noncontracting collagen gels, place an ethanol-sterilized nylon mesh, of the same diameter as the Petri dish, onto the bottom of the dish. Then, follow the same protocol as for contracting gels.

3.6.3. Collagenase Digestion of Collagen Gels for Recovery of Cultured Fibroblasts

1. Pre-warm bacterial collagenase solution at 37°C (1 mL/lattice in microtubes).
2. Transfer each lattice into the bacterial collagenase solution using forceps, and incubate in a water bath at 37°C for 10 min. Agitate the tubes after 5 min by inverting them.
3. When lattices are completely digested, stop the digestion by addition of 1 m*M* EDTA and centrifuge for 10 min at 400*g* at room temperature to pellet the cells.

3.7. Skin Equivalents

3.7.1. General Design

Table 2 summarizes the different steps for generating skin equivalents.

3.7.2. Skin Equivalent

The following protocol is described for six wells. Volumes can be proportionally changed for different quantities.

Table 2
Different Steps for Building Skin Equivalents

Time	Description	Medium	mL (insert)	mL (well)
D 1	Collagen gel, without cells, is formed on surface of the insert.	Lattice	1.3	0
D 2	Collagen gel, with fibroblasts, is formed on top of the acellular gel.	Lattice	3	0
D 8	Keratinocytes are seeded on top of the dermis equivalent.	SE1	2	3
D 11	Calcium-containing medium is added to support viability of fibroblasts and differentiation of keratinocytes.	SE2	2	3
D 13	Medium is removed from the insert to allow keratinocytes contact with the air. Cultures are fed from the bottom, through the membrane.	SE3	0	1
D 13–21	Medium is changed every other day until total differentiation of the epidermis is achieved.	SE3	0	1

A. D 1: Collagen gel without cells.
   1. Using sterile and prechilled reagents, mix on ice and in the order indicated 3.2 mL of 2.5X DMEM, 0.8 mL of serum, 0.85 mL of distilled water, 0.48 mL of 0.1 *M* NaOH, and 2.67 mL of 3 mg/mL type I collagen.
   2. Immediately mix, by gently pipetting up and down, until color is homogeneous, and immediately dispense 1.3 mL of solution per insert.
   3. Incubate 15 min at room temperature without disturbing to allow collagen to gel, and place the plate in the 5% CO_2 incubator at 37°C.

B. D 2: Dermis equivalent.
   1. Prepare a cell suspension of fibroblasts at 245,000 cells/ml in 1X DMEM, according to subculturing fibroblast protocol (**Subheading 3.4.**).
   2. Using prechilled reagents, mix on ice and in order 7.8 mL of 2.5X DMEM, 1.95 mL of serum, 1.17 mL of 0.1 *M* NaOH, and 6.5 mL of 3 mg/mL type I collagen.
   3. Gently mix, by pipetting up and down, until color is homogeneous, and add 2 mL of the cell suspension prepared in **step 1**.
   4. Mix by pipetting up and down, and dispense 3 mL of cell suspension into each insert, on top of acellular gels.

   5. Incubate 15 min at room temperature without disturbing to allow collagen to gel, and place the plate in the 5% CO_2 incubator at 37°C for 7 d.

C. D 9: Seeding keratinocytes. After 7 d, the dermal equivalent is partially contracted, to form a concave upper surface.
   1. Remove and discard culture medium without disturbing collagen gels, and rinse three times (5 min between rinses) with SE1 medium: 2 mL in the insert and 3 mL in the well.
   2. After the third rinse, remove and discard medium. Place in sterile hood during preparation of keratinocytes (approx 20 min).
   3. Prepare a suspension of keratinocytes at 3×10^6 cells/mL in SE1 medium.
   4. Dispense drop-wise 100 µL of keratinocyte suspension on top of each dermal equivalent. During this step, maintain pipet as vertical as possible and tip as close as possible to the dermis equivalent. Do not try to spread the cell suspension, but rather target each drop to the center of the gel.
   5. Carefully place the plate back in the incubator, keeping it as horizontal as possible. Incubate for 2 h without medium to promote keratinocyte attachment to the collagen gel.
   6. Gently add 2 mL of SE1 medium to the insert on top of the gel, and 3 mL of SE1 medium to the well.
   7. Place the plate back in the 5% CO_2 incubator at 37°C.

D. D 13: Replace SE1 by SE2 medium.
   1. Remove and discard medium as completely as possible without disturbing the reconstructs.
   2. Gently add 2 mL of SE2 medium in each insert and 3 mL of SE2 medium in each well.
   3. Place the plate back in the 5% CO_2 incubator at 37°C.

E. D 15: Exposing keratinocytes to air.
   1. Remove and discard medium from the insert and the well.
   2. Add 1 mL of SE3 medium in the well; no medium is added to the insert. Placing medium only in the well allows keratinocytes to be in contact with the air, which promotes stratification and differentiation.
   3. Exchange medium in the well three times a week until d 21, when reconstructs are ready for experiments.

Once ready for experiments, skin equivalents can be maintained in SE3 medium for up to 1 wk. After this time, keratinocytes proliferation diminishes.

4. Notes

1. All techniques described must be performed in sterile conditions and proper disposal and decontamination practices should be followed. Moreover, all human samples should be considered as possible sources of infectious agents and should be handled appropriately.
2. Culture media are supplemented with antibiotics and antimycotics. However, antibiotics do not eliminate problems of contamination resulting from poor sterilization techniques or antibiotic-resistant micro-organisms.

3. In order to avoid exposure of cultures to temperature fluctuations, reagents used for cell culture should be prewarmed to 37°C, in water bath, and the container outsides should be rinsed with 70% ethanol before use, in order to prevent contamination.
4. It is good practice to routinely and carefully examine cultures to determine their status and health.
5. Adherent cells like fibroblasts must be cultured in specially treated vessels (dishes or flasks) commonly called "tissue culture" type. The bottom surface of these vessels is specially treated to enhance cell attachment and cell survival. Several vessel sizes are commercially available.
6. Before any material can be collected from a human volunteer, ethical approval for the research must be obtained from the local Institutional Review Board. Only trained and authorized personnel should perform skin biopsies, and every subject from whom skin is taken must give written informed consent. Furthermore, it is essential that the designation of the cell strain is unambiguous. It should be unique and maintain donor anonymity.
7. Using cells derived from laboratory staff for research purposes is not recommended. The use of tissue from laboratory staff for the development of transformed cell lines is prohibited, as the person concerned would have no immunity to the transformed cells.
8. Adult skin is invariably contaminated with micro-organisms, mainly nonpathogenic bacteria or molds. In order to insure good sterility of the tissue for cell culture, these micro-organisms must be removed as much as possible prior to skin biopsy.
9. Cells can also be detached using nonproteolytic methods. These methods should be used especially when use of cells with intact plasma membrane is required (adhesion studies, membrane protein extraction). To detach cells without proteolysis, use Versene buffer (0.8 m*M* EDTA, 0.15 *M* NaCl, 2.7 m*M* KCl, 8 m*M* Na_2HPO_4, 1.6 m*M* KH_2PO_4, pH 7.2.; 20 min at 37°C) or EDTA (1–5 m*M* at 4°C, 20–30 min).
10. Type I collagen is soluble only at low temperature and low pH. It will start to gel and become insoluble if either the temperature or the pH is raised. For this reason, the stock collagen solution should be kept at 4°C until it is needed. During handling, it should be maintained at 4°C. Keep in mind that collagen will start to gel as soon as it is mixed with sodium hydroxide. Therefore, as soon as the collagen is added to the solution, the following steps should be performed as quickly as possible.
11. Unlike human collagenase, bacterial collagenase is able to digest mature collagen into small fragments. The main source of bacterial collagenase is *Clostridium histolyticum*. Collagenase preparations are rarely pure and contain other proteases, including trypsin- and chymotrypsin-like activities. Thus, to avoid cellular damage resulting from proteolysis, incubations with bacterial collagenase should be kept to the minimum time necessary to release cells from the collagen gel.

12. Centrifugation following trypsin detachment of cells removes trypsin and cell debris. This removal helps to maintain viability and longevity of cultures.
13. It is recommended to record the details concerning cell cultures, including the type, sources, and batch numbers of all media and additives, and the methods by which the cultures were established. It is helpful to record the subculture ratios and the passage number.
14. Collagen coatings tend to detach in long-term cultures. Alternatively, a double-layered collagen coating can provide a stable substrate. The second layer is dispensed after the first one is completely dry.
15. Collagen reorganization is observed as a reduction in size of the collagen gel. Under the conditions described, contraction of the gel can be observed 2 to 6 h after seeding cells, is half complete after 24 h, and complete after 4 d. To quantify gel contraction, the diameter of the gel can be measured using a ruler on top of the dish placed on a dark background.

References

1. Verzijl, N., DeGroot, J., Thorpe, S., et al. (2000) Effect of collagen turnover on the accumulation of advanced glycation end products. *J. Biol. Chem.* **275,** 39,027–39,031.
2. Heughan, C. and Hunt, T. (1975) Some aspects of wound healing research: a review. *Can. J. Surg.* **18,** 118–126.
3. Gabbiani, G. (2003) The myofibroblast in wound healing and fibrocontractive diseases. *J. Pathol.* **200,** 500–503.
4. LeRoy, E. (1974) Increased collagen synthesis by scleroderma skin fibroblasts *in vitro*: a possible defect in the regulation or activation of the scleroderma fibroblast. *J. Clin. Invest.* **54,** 880–889.
5. Jimenez, S. and Saitta, B. (2000) Alternations in the regulation of expression of the α1(I) collagen gene (COL1A1) in systemic sclerosis (scleroderma). *Springer Semin. Immunopathol.* **21,** 397–414.
6. Rittié, L. and Fisher, G. (2002) UV-light-induced signal cascades and skin aging. *Ageing Res. Rev.* **1,** 705–720.
7. Hiebert, C. (1959) The carcinogenic action of methylcholanthrene on mouse skin in organ culture. *Cancer* 12, 663-672.
8. Aumailley, M., Krieg, T., Razaka, G., Müller, P., and Bricaud, H. (1982) Influence of cell density on collagen biosynthesis in fibroblast cultures. *Biochem. J.* **206,** 505–510.
9. Hayflick, L. and Moorhead, P. (1961) The serial cultivation of human diploid cell strains. *Exp. Cell Res.* **25,** 585–621.
10. Cristofalo, V. and Pignolo, R. (1993) Replicative senescence of human fibroblast-like cells in culture. *Physiol. Rev.* **73,** 617–638.
11. Bell, E., Ivarsson, B., and Merrill, C. (1979) Production of a tissue-like structure by contraction of collagen lattices by human fibroblasts of different proliferative potential *in vitro*. *Proc. Natl. Acad. Sci. USA* **76,** 1274–1278.
12. Grinnell, F. (2003) Fibroblast biology in three-dimensional collagen matrices. *Trends Cell Biol.* **13,** 264–269.

13. Eckes, B., Mauch, C., Hüppe, G., and Krieg, T. (1993) Downregulation of collagen synthesis in fibroblasts within three-dimensional collagen lattices involves transcriptional and posttranscriptional mechanisms. *FEBS* **318,** 129–133.
14. Mauch, C., Hatamochi, A., Scharffetter, K., and Krieg, T. (1988) Regulation of collagen synthesis in fibroblasts within a three-dimensional collagen gel. *Exp. Cell Res.* **178,** 493–503.
15. Mauch, C., Adelmann-Grill, B., Hatamochi, A., and Krieg, T. (1989) Collagenase gene expression in fibroblasts is regulated by a three-dimensional contact with collagen. *FEBS* **250,** 301–305.
16. Seltzer, J., Lee, A.-Y., Akers, K., et al. (1994) Activation of 72-kDa type IV collagenase/gelatinase by normal fibroblasts in collagen lattices is mediated by integrin receptors but is not related to lattice contraction. *Exp. Cell Res.* **213,** 365–374.
17. Arora, P., Narani, N., and McCulloch, C. (1999) The compliance of collagen gels regulates transforming growth factor-ß induction of a-smooth muscle actin in fibroblasts. *Am. J. Pathol.* **154,** 871–882.
18. Kessler, D., Dethlefsen, S., Haase, I., et al. (2001) Fibroblasts in mechanically stressed collagen lattices assume a "synthetic" phenotype. *J. Biol. Chem.* **276,** 36,575–36,585.
19. Roguet, R., Cohen, C., Dossou, K., and Rougier, A. (1994) Episkin, a constituted human epidermis for assessing *in vitro* the irritancy of topically applied compounds. *Toxicol. Vitro* **8,** 283–291.
20. Freeman, A., Igel, H., Herrman, B., and Kleinfeld, K. (1976) Growth and characterization of human skin epithelial cell cultures. *In Vitro* **12,** 352–362.
21. Bell, E., Ehrlich, H., Buttle, D., and Nakatsuji, T. (1981) Living tissue formed *in vitro* and accepted as skin-equivalent tissue of full thickness. *Science* **211,** 1052–1054.
22. Pouliot, R., Germain, L., Auger, F., Tremblay, N., and Juhasz, J. (1999) Physical characterization of the stratum corneum of an *in vitro* human skin equivalent produced by tissue engineering and its comparision with normal human skin by ATR-FTIR spectroscopy and thermal analysis (DSC). *Biochim. Biophys. Acta* **1439,** 341–352.
23. Nickoloff, B., Mitra, R., Fisher, G., and Voorhees, J. (1989) Decreased growth inhibition by recombinant gamma interferon is associated with increased transforming growth factor-α production in keratinocytes cultured from psoriatic lesions. *Brit. J. Dermatol.* **121,** 161–174.

5

Isolation and Culture of Hepatic Stellate Cells

Ralf Weiskirchen and Axel M. Gressner

Summary

Hepatic stellate cells (HSCs) are routinely prepared by collagenase/pronase digestion of liver using a perfusion system and subsequent fractionation of the heterogenous cell suspension on continuous density gradients made out of Nycodenz, metrizamide, stractan, or percoll. Because of their lipid content, stellate cells are the least dense fraction of the nonparenchymal cells, and during centrifugation they float effectively away from other hepatic cells resulting in preparations containing almost 80% stellate cells. The degree of purity can be increased by further enrichment of cells by methods like centrifugal elutriation or Scatter-activated cell sorting. We present a detailed protocol from our laboratory to obtain a high number of pure, viable, freshly isolated hepatic stellate cells from rat liver. This two-step protocol (collagenase/pronase digestion and Nycodenz gradient) yields a preparation of approx 4–5 × 10^7 cells enriched in 74% HSC having a viability of at least 76% as estimated by Trypan blue exclusion test. Further purification by centrifugal elutriation results in virtually pure HSC preparations (>98%).

Key Words: Centrifugal elutriation; density-gradient; fibrosis; hepatic stellate cells; liver; Metrizamide; Nycodenz; myofibroblasts; Percoll; perfusion; stractan; transdifferentiation.

1. Introduction

The liver consists mainly of five cell types: the parenchymal cells (hepatocytes, PC), Kupffer cells (KC), endothelial cells (EC), and hepatic stellate cells (HSC), also referred to as vitamin A-storing cells, fat storing cells, lipocytes, interstitial cells, or Ito cells and pit cells (liver-specific natural killer [NK] cells). In the rat, HSC represent approx 10% of the total resident liver cells *(1)*, which play a central role in the uptake and storage of vitamin A. During liver injury of any etiology, HSC undergo a response known as activation, which is the transition of quiescent cells into proliferative, fibrogenic, and contractile MFB (reviewed in **ref.** ***2***). Many of the characteristic changes are also observed when primary HSC are cultured on uncoated plastic surfaces. Therefore, isolation and culturing of HSC is a common in vitro model for the investigation of processes involved in molecular regulation of hepatic fibrosis. HSC were origi-

From: *Methods in Molecular Medicine, Vol. 117: Fibrosis Research: Methods and Protocols*
Edited by: J. Varga, D. A. Brenner, and S. H. Phan © Humana Press Inc., Totowa, NJ

nally identified in 1876 by Carl von Kupffer as intralobular star-shaped cells that appeared dark with a selective gold chloride staining method (for review, *see* **ref. *3***). Since then, these cells have attracted attention of many investigators because of their exceptional pathophysiological importance indicated by their ability to transdifferentiate phenotypically into myofibroblasts (MFB). However, the usage of different names for this hepatic cell population has contributed to confusion. Accordingly, in 1996 the scientific community decided to denote this cell population as HSC ***(4)***.

HSC are located in the subendothelial space of Disse in the recess of neighboring hepatocytes, their star-shaped branches encompass the sinusoidal endothelial cell tube, and they exhibit intralobular and local heterogeneity in regard to phenotypical markers ***(5,6)***. Quantitative analysis has demonstrated that the number of HSC per thousand PC (Ito cell index) is 63.45 ± 19.18 in normal human liver ***(7)***. Typical features of these cells are the presence of cytoplasmic triacylglycerol-rich droplets, a distinct rough endoplasmic reticulum, small numbers of mitochondria, existence of interstitial collagen bundles in close apposition to the cell body, and a near absence of cytosolic vesicles and vacuoles (for further details, *see* **ref. *3***).

The histological visualization of HSC in liver tissue by light microscopy is difficult. Therefore, specialized methods for selective staining of these nonparenchymal cells were developed. In most protocols, the reduction of gold chloride by the retinoids results in dark staining of HSC. Alternatively, the vitamin A-autofluorescence or unspecific lipid stains (e.g., oil red O staining) are applied for the identification of HSC in tissue. In rat liver, HSC are the only sinusoidal cell type to express desmin and glial fibrilliary acidic protein (GFAP). Therefore, specific detection of HSC in liver sections by immunohistochemistry is another potential method to visualize this cell type. However, it should be noted that the expression of desmin appears to be (in part) dependent on the location of the cells within the liver ***(5)*** and that, undoubtedly, identification of HSC is only possible by use of transmission electron microscopy.

The available stellate cell isolation and purification methods are commonly based on enzymatic digestion of the liver by collagenase, pronase, and DNase, followed by centrifugation of the crude cell suspension through a density gradient (Nycodenz, Metrizamide, Stractan, or Percoll). Further enrichment of the resulting preparations can be obtained by centrifugal elutriation or by side-scatter activated cell sorting.

We here describe a detailed protocol for isolation and culturing of rat HSC. The protocol includes the steps necessary to release HSC from liver tissue (pronase/collagenase step), their enrichment by centrifugal elutriation, and a procedure for determination of cellular integrity (Trypan exclusion stain).

2. Materials

2.1. Animals/Anesthetics

1. Male Sprague-Dawley rats, weighing 550 to 800 g. In order to improve the yield of HSC isolations, heavy (older) animals should be used, as lipid content has been found to be higher within cells of aged animals.
2. 10% Ketamin (CEVA Tiergesundheit GmbH, Düsseldorf, Germany)
3. Xylazin (2% Xylazinhydrochlorid, 0.7% Methyl-4-hydroxybenzoat) (Medistar, Holzwickede, Germany).

2.2. Solutions, Culture Media

1. Hank's balanced salt solution (HBSS) (with Ca^{2+}/Mg^{2+}): 0.185 g $CaCl_2 \cdot H_2O$, 0.4 g KCl, 0.06 g KH_2PO_4, 0.1 g $MgSO_4 \cdot 7\ H_2O$, 8 g NaCl, 0.35 g $NaHCO_3$, 0.048 g Na_2HPO_4, and 1 g D-glucose per liter water. The solution must be sterile filtered, when not obtained in ready-to-use form. We obtain the solution from PAA Laboratories GmbH (Linz, Austria, PN # H15-008).
2. HBSS (with Ca^{2+}/Mg^{2+}) + bovine serum albumin (BSA), contains 0.25% (w/v) BSA (Sigma, Taufkirchen, Germany, PN #A-7030) in HBSS (with Ca^{2+}/Mg^{2+}).
3. HBSS (without Ca^{2+}/Mg^{2+}): 0.4 g KCl, 0.06 g KH_2PO_4, 8 g NaCl, 0.35 g $NaHCO_3$, 0.048 g Na_2HPO_4, and 1 g D-glucose per liter water. The solution must be sterile filtered when not obtained in ready to use form. We obtain the solution from PAA Laboratories GmbH (PN# H15-009).
4. Dulbecco's modified Eagle medium, *N*-2-hydroxyethylpiperazine-*N*'-2-ethansulfonic acid (HEPES) buffered (DMEM): 200 mg $CaCl_2$ (anhydrous), 0.10 mg $Fe(NO_3)_3 \cdot 9\ H_2O$, 400 mg KCl, 200 mg $MgSO_4 \cdot 7\ H_2O$, 6400 mg NaCl, 3700 mg $NaHCO_3$, 141 mg $NaH_2PO_4 \cdot 2H_2O$, 4500 mg D-glucose, 110 mg Na-pyruvate, 84 mg L-arginine · HCl, 48 mg L-cystin, 30 mg glycine, 42 mg L-histidine · HCl · H_2O, 105 mg L-isoleucine, 105 mg L-leucine, 146 mg L-lysine · HCl, 30 mg L-methionine, 66 mg phenylalanine, 42 mg L-serine, 95 mg L-threonine, 16 mg tryptophane, 72 mg L-tyrosine, 94 mg L-valine, 4 mg D-calcium pantothenat, 4 mg choline chloride, 4 mg folic acid, 7.2 mg i-inositol, 4 mg nicotinamide, 4 mg pyrridoxine · HCl, 0.4 mg riboflavine, 4 mg thiamine · HCl, 15 mg/mL phenol red, and 25 m*M* HEPES. The solution must be sterile filtered when not obtained in ready to use form. We obtain the solution from BioWhittaker/Cambrex, Verviers, Belgium (PN # BE12-709F).
5. L-Glutamine (200 m*M*): 29.23 mg/mL L-glutamine in 0.85% (w/v) NaCl solution (BioWhitaker/Cambrex, PN # BE17-605E).
6. Penicillin/Streptomycin (X100) solution: per mL 10.000 IU penicillin and 10 mg streptomycin (BioWhitaker/Cambrex, PN # DE17-602E).

2.3. Proteases/DNase

1. Pronase E-solution: Pronase E (EC 3.4.24.4, 4.000.000 U/g) from *Streptomyces griseus* (Merck, Darmstadt, Germany) is dissolved to 3.5 mg/mL in HBSS (with Ca^{2+}/Mg^{2+}) and sterile filtered (0.22 μ*M*).

2. Collagenase H-solution: Collagenase H (0.23 U/mg) from *Chlostridium histolyticum* (Roche, Mannheim, Germany, PN #1074049) is dissolved to 0.25 mg/mL in HBSS (with Ca^{2+}/Mg^{2+}) and sterile filtered (0.22 μ*M*).
3. DNaseI-solution: desoxyribonuclease I (grade II) from bovine pancreas (Roche, PN #70014820) is dissolved to 0.1 mg/mL in HBSS (with Ca^{2+}/Mg^{2+}) and sterile filtered (0.22 μ*M*).

2.4. Miscellaneous

1. Nycodenz solution contains 28.7% (w/v) Nycodenz (Axis-Shield PoC AS, Oslo, Norway, PN #1002424) in modified HBSS (with Ca^{2+}/Mg^{2+}, without NaCl). Nycodenz is also referred to as Iohexol.
2. Trypan blue solution contains 0.4% (w/v) Trypan blue (Sigma, PN #T-8154) dissolved in 0.81% sodium chloride and 0.06% potassium phosphate.
3. Braunüle MT® (luer lock) allows easy cannulation of vena porta. They can be obtained by B. Braun Melsungen AG, Melsungen, Germany (PN#4206274).
4. Centrifugation tubes (25 mL, canonical tip, made out of glass), can be obtained by Roth, Karlsruhe, Germany (PN#K212.1).

3. Methods

3.1. Isolation of HSC

Current protocols for HSC isolation and purification are based on enzymatic digestion of the liver by collagenase, pronase, and DNase, followed by centrifugation of the crude cell suspension through a density gradient of Nycodenz. These basic procedures result in cell suspensions enriched in stellate cells (70–85%). An important prerequisite for successful isolation is that the cells contain sufficient lipid droplets. This mandatory can be more easily achieved by using "old" rats (6–12 mo of age) or animals that received supplementary vitamin A. In our laboratory, we use male rats of the Sprague-Dawley strain.

3.2. Perfusion Apparatus

A schematic representation of the perfusion apparatus is shown in **Fig. 1A**. All solutions are pre-equilibrated at 37°C (99°F), and an adjustable peristaltic pump is set into flow to allow recirculating liver perfusion with HBSS, pronase, and collagenase. The possibility of changing between individual solutions used for perfusion is allowed by clips. A bubble trap prevents air bubbles entering into the system and an ordinary hair dryer allows setting of the appropriate temperature. We use lockable cupboards with doors made of glass allowing permanent view to the perfused liver (*see* **Fig. 1B**).

3.3. Anesthesia and Withdrawal of Liver

For anesthesia, animals receive 1 mL Ketamin (10%) and 50 μL Xylazin (2%) per kg body weight. The rat is entirely shaved at the abdomen and fixed

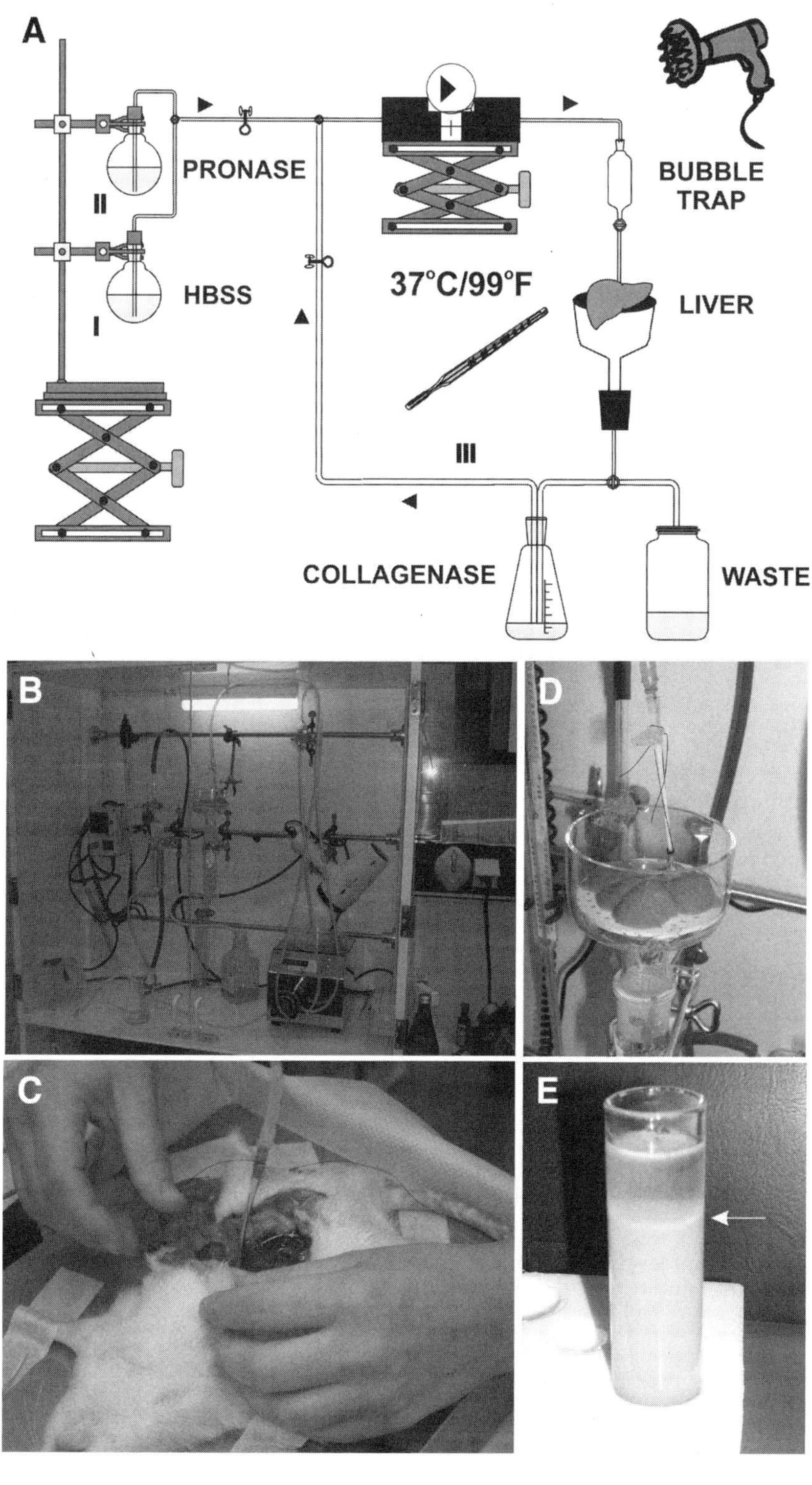
A
PRONASE
HBSS
II
I
37°C/99°F
BUBBLE
TRAP
LIVER
III
COLLAGENASE
WASTE
B
C
D
E

upside-down with tape (*see* **Fig. 1C**). The abdominal wall is cut with a scalpel through a longitudinal line and with a transverse cut up to the sternum. Thereafter, to expose the vena cava and the vena porta, the gut is gently moved to the side. After setting of a ligature around the vena porta (use a thread or a clip made out steel), this vessel is cut and a fine cannula (Braunüle MT) is inserted. When the cannula is properly in place, the ligature is strengthened and cannula is adjusted to allow perfusion of liver.

3.3.1. Liver Perfusion

After the first drops of blood out the cannula, the aorta abdominalis is cut and the cannula is connected (avoid bubbles) with the tube of perfusion apparatus and liver is *in situ* rinsed with HBSS (without Ca^{2+}/Mg^{2+}) at a flow rate of 10 mL/min until liver is free of blood (the reddish-brown color changes to loam-color). Then, the liver is gently removed (take care not to damage the liver capsule) from the body cavity. The peristaltic pump is turned off and liver is transferred to the perfusion dish in the lockable cupboard. Subsequently, the liver is perfused with 100 mL pronase-E solution (flow rate 10 mL/min). In the following, recirculating liver perfusion is performed with 60 mL collagenase solution until liver architecture is massively destroyed (approx 30 min, *see* **Fig. 1D**). The liver is then removed from the perfusion dish, cleaned from attachments, and placed into a sterile plastic culture dish. The soaked liver is poured with approx 30 mL DNaseI solution and the liver capsule is opened and tissue is torn into small pieces. Another 70 mL of DNaseI solution is added and the tissue pieces are further dissected by rotating on a magnetic stirrer (200

Fig. 1. *(previous page)* Recirculating liver perfusion. **(A)** Schematic representation of apparatus used for recirculating liver perfusion. Liver is subsequently perfused with Hank's balance salt solution (HBSS) (I), pronase E-solution (II), and collagenase-solution (III) at a flow rate of 10 mL/min. All solutions are pre-equilibrated at 37°C/99°F. The possibility of changing between individual solutions used for perfusion is permitted by clips. A bubble trap prevents air bubbles entering into the system. In the figure, the direction of flow is marked by triangles. **(B)** Photograph of a working liver perfusion apparatus. **(C)** For withdrawal of liver, the extremities of a deeply anesthetized rat are fixed with silk and the entire abdomen is opened by a transverse cut across the lower abdomen and a longitudinal cut up to the sternum. To expose the vena cava and the vena porta, the gut is gently moved to the side. After ligation and cutting through the vena porta, a fine cannula is inserted to allow perfusion of liver. **(D)** Photograph of perfusion dish after recirculation perfusion. Note that the liver is swelled. **(E)** Nycodenz gradient after centrifugation of total liver cell suspension. Hepatic stellate cell layering at the top of the Nycodenz gradient appear as a white condensed band (marked by a white arrow).

rpm) at 37°C for several minutes (the pH should be approx 7.3). The obtained cell suspension is subsequently filtered through nylon meshes (250 μm and 100 μm), which were sterilized by dipping in 70% ethanol. All further steps are then performed at 4°C. The suspension is centrifuged for 7 min at 450*g* and the resulting pellet is resuspended in ice-cold HBSS (with Ca^{2+}/Mg^{2+}) + BSA (final volume is adjusted to 15–55 mL).

3.3.2. Nycodenz Density Gradient Centrifugation

There are several nontoxic, chemically near-inert components commonly used for differential centrifugation of HSC (*see* **Fig. 2**). These substances allow separation of this nonparenchymal liver cell population from parenchymal cells. All protocols are simply based on the circumstance that the average volume of parenchymal cells is an order of magnitude higher than from HSC. Further, the retinoid content of HSC results in a low cell density allowing flotation on the gradient. In the protocol originally described by Schafer et al. *(8)*, the resuspended cell pellet (previously described) is mixed with 0.4 vol of Nycodenz-solution (precooled to 4°C). Twenty-milliliter portions of this solution are then transferred under a cushion of 6 mL HBSS (with Ca^{2+}/Mg^{2+}) + BSA (use 25-mL centrifugation tubes made out of glass, previously described). Tubes are centrifuged at 1400*g* for 22 min (low acceleration) and the resulting upper top layer (**Fig. 1E**) of the gradient is removed with a fine tip. This step is critical because the white band (containing HSC) is bordered on other cell types (mainly KC). The removed cells are washed in 50 mL HBSS (with Ca^{2+}/Mg^{2+}) and centrifuged at 450*g* for 7 min. Subsequently, the cell pellet is washed in HBSS (with Ca^{2+}/Mg^{2+}) including 1% fetal calf serum (FCS) and cells are counted in a Neubauer chamber. At this point, fairly pure HSC preparations (>85%) with high rates of viability, as estimated by Trypan blue exclusion test (*see* **Subheading 3.3.4.**), are obtained. The cells can be plated in DMEM including 10% FCS, 4 m*M* L-glutamin, and 1X penicillin/streptomycin.

Note that other investigators use gradients made out of stractan, metrizamide, or percoll. The characteristics of these components are briefly described in **Note 9**.

3.3.3. Centrifugal Elutriation

The cell preparations obtained by pronase/collagenase digestion followed by density gradient centrifugation contain contaminations of other liver cells. During cultivation, some of these cells are removed, but additional purification following density gradient centrifugation is necessary to obtain virtually pure HSC. We use a JE-5.0 elutriation system for use with J6 series centrifuges (Beckman instruments, Palo Alto, CA), which combines the process of sedimentation under the influence of a centrifugal force and counterflow elutriation.

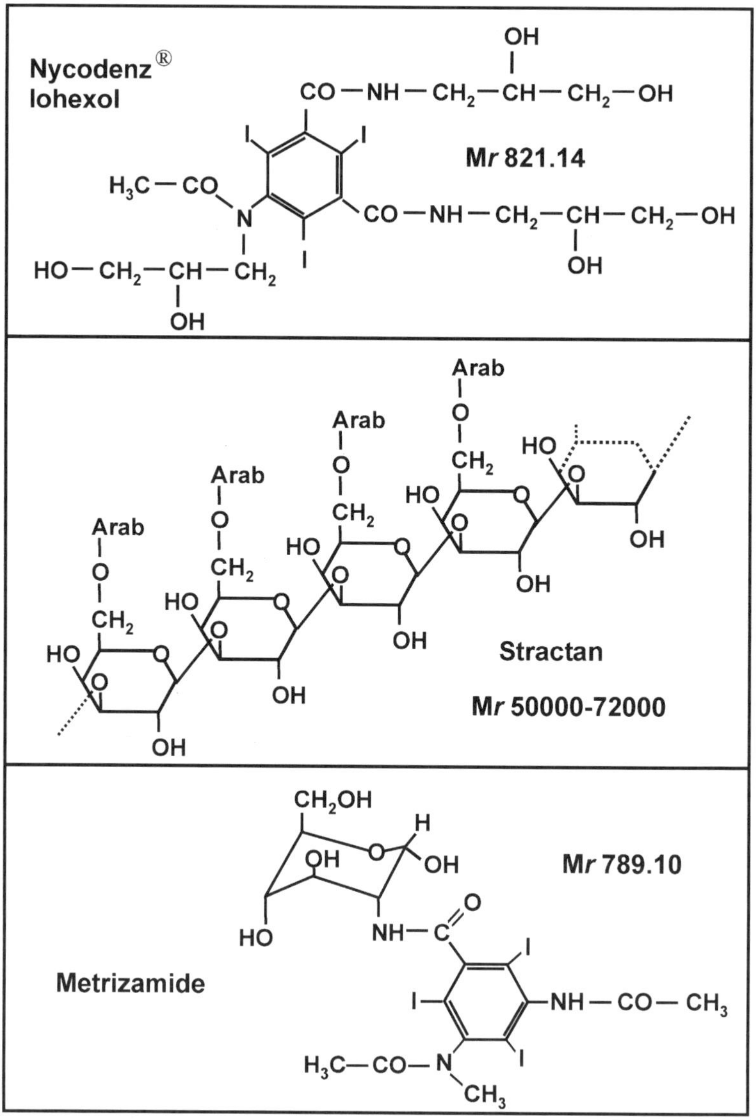

Fig. 2. Components used for purification of hepatic stellate cells by differential density centrifugation. Nycodenz 5-(*N*-2,3-dihydroxypropylacetamido)-2,4,6-triiodo-*N*,*N*'-*bis*(2,3-dihydroxypropyl)isophthalamide) **(top)**, Stractan **(middle)**, Metrizamide (2-[3-acetamido-2, 4, 6-triiodo-5(*N*-methylacetamido-benzamido]-2-deoxy-D-glucose) **(bottom)** are commonly used for preparing density gradients for differential centrifugation. Molecular weights of components (M*r*) are given. These components are nontoxic, almost chemically inert, and are not adhering to membranes. Usually they are used as iso-osmotic solutions.

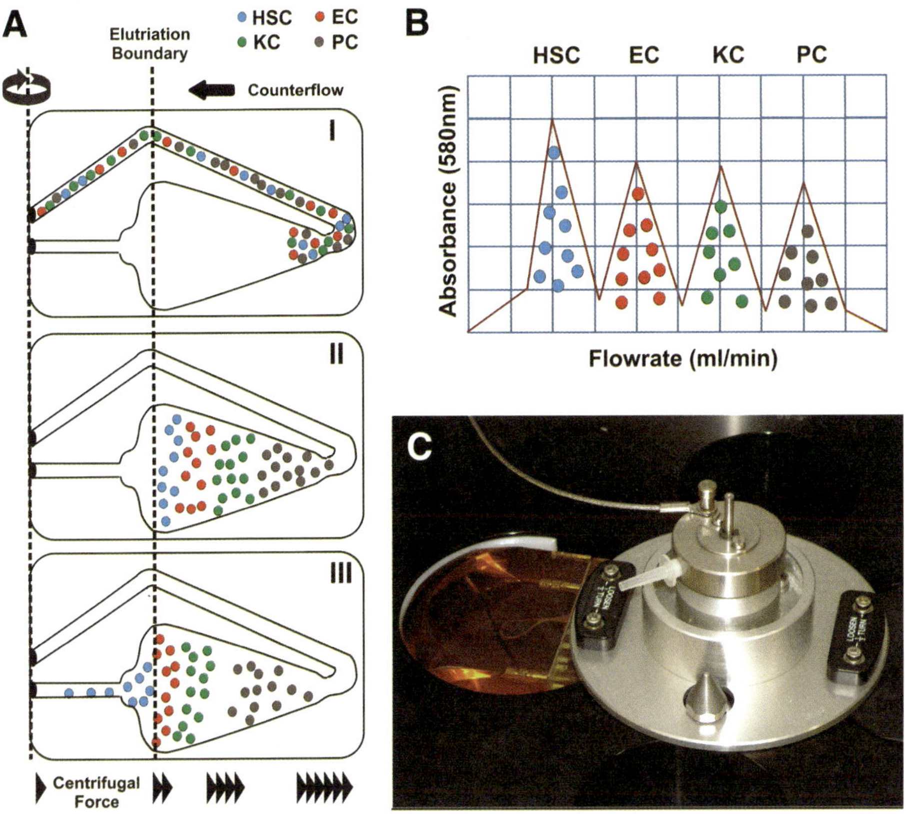

Fig. 3. Centrifugal elutriation for separation of various liver cells. **(A)** Principle of centrifugal elutriation. Driven by the centrifugal force cells suspended in medium enter the elutriation chamber (I). In the chamber the sedimentation tendency of different cell populations is balanced by the counterflow (II). Subsequent increase of the counterflow results in differential elutriation of cells (hepatic stellate cells [HSC], endothelial cells [EC], Kupffer cells [KC], parenchymal cells [PC]) from the elutriation chamber (III). **(B)** Based on their cell sizes, different liver cell subpopulations are separated at different flow rates. Increase of the counterflow rate results in differential elutriation of HSC, EC, KC, and PC as assessed by absorbance at 580 nm. **(C)** Overview of the JE-5.0 separation chamber (Beckman Instruments) most commonly used for differential elutriation.

The principle of centrifugal elutriation is given in **Fig. 3A** and more details about the principles of centrifugal elutriation of living cells are outlined in **Note 2**. For elutriation, cells are rotated at 2500 rpm in HBSS (+1% FCS) at 4°C. Under these conditions, liver cells are obtained in the following order:

HSC (flow rate approx 13.5 mL/min), SEC (approx 18–22 mL/min), KC (35–41 mL/min), and contaminating PC (>41 mL/min), respectively (*see* **Fig. 3B**). Beckman's elutriation chambers are made of Novolac, a clear phenolic resin (*see* **Fig. 3C**). During the run, the processes taking place in the chamber can be viewed through the port in the centrifuge door. In general, this equipment is robust, but intensive purification of elutriation chambers, tubes, and seals after each run are necessary to allow separation of vital cells.

3.3.4. Cell Viability

Following centrifugal elutriation, the viability of cell preparations can be estimated by Trypan blue stain, a dye staining dead or dying cells. In contrast, living cells repel the dye and do not stain. This exclusion test is simple, fast, and allows determination of the number of living cells for plating. For staining, an equal volume HSC (suspended in HBSS) is mixed with 0.4% Trypan blue solution. After 5 min, an aliqout is analyzed in a Neubauer chamber, and viable and nonviable cells are counted. The cell viability (in %) is calculated as follows:

[total viable cells (unstained)/total cells (stained and unstained)] ·100.

3.4. Cell Purity

In our hands, the purity of HSC preparations obtained after density centrifugation range from 75 to 85% as estimated by analysis of the vitamin A-autofluorescence (*see* **Note 5**). After seeding and culturing, the purity grades increase to values higher than 95%. Based on the high difference in sedimentation rates of HSC compared with other liver cells, elutriation results in virtually pure HSC cultures. However, although recoveries close to 100% have been reported for other cell systems ***(9)***, elutriation results in a loss of approx 25% of HSC.

3.5. Cell Recovery

If cells are purified on Nycodenz density gradient, the preparation of one rat liver leads to high yield of HSC (typically about 4–5 × 10^7 cells). It has been reported that the yield is strongly dependent on age and nutrition of the rats. Therefore, it should be noted that during establish most of these protocols, animals from different suppliers should be tested.

3.6. Culturing of HSC and Transdifferentiation Into Myofibroblasts

Freshly prepared, we seed rat HSC in DMEM supplemented with 10% FCS, 4 m*M* L-glutamine and 1X penicillin/streptomycin at a density of 2.5 × 10^6 cells per 10-cm Petri dish. During the contact with uncoated plastic, the cells become spontaneously activated and develop features of fibrogenically activated HSC (*see* **Fig. 4**). After 7 d in culture, we subcultivate HSC by trypsinization. Therefore, the culture medium is aspirated, and cells are washed with HBSS (–Ca^{2+}/–Mg^{2+}). Subsequently, the cells are overlaid with 1X trypsin and incubated at 37°C. After the cells are detached (this takes approx 5–10 min), they are carefully suspended in DMEM (+10% FCS, + 4 m*M* L-glutamine, + 1X penicillin/streptomycin) and replated. After subcultivation, these cells are referred to as myofibroblasts.

4. Notes

1. Generally, the separation of HSC from human or murine livers should follow the same protocol. However, obtaining human livers is difficult and is ethically problematic. Therefore, most investigators have established protocols for the use of explant cells from human liver biopsy samples (e.g., **ref. *10***; *see* also **Note 8**). The isolation of murine HSC is more complex in regard to handling. The separation by density gradient of (pooled) murine HSC needs strain-specific adaptation in regard to their different size and lipid content.
2. In centrifugal elutriation, cells are subjected to two opposing forces within the separation chamber; the centrifugal field generated by the spinner rotor, and the viscous drag of the fluid flowing in the opposite (centripetal) direction. Each cell tends to migrate to a zone where its sedimentation rate is balanced by the flow rate of the fluid through the separation chamber. Because the chamber's geometry produces a gradient of flow rates from one end to the other, cells with a wide range of different sedimentations rates can be held in suspension. By increasing the flow rate of the elutriating fluid in steps, or by decreasing the rotor speed, successive populations of relatively homogeneous cell sizes can be washed from the chamber (for details, *see* **ref. *11***). Each population contains larger (or more dense) cells (i.e., faster-sedimenting) than those of the previous fraction. Note: details for developing elutriation protocols are available on-line (at http://www.beckmancoulter.com).
3. The purification of rat hepatic stellate cells by side scatter-activated cell sorting offers another possibility for preparation of very pure HSC ***(12)***.
4. A characteristic feature of HSC is the appearance of intracellular lipid droplets, which resemble a bunch of grapes. The lipid droplets can be easily detected in light microscopy, or alternatively, by transmission electron microscopy ***(13)***.
5. HSC contain considerable amounts of vitamin A, allowing their identification in a fluorescence microscope ***(14)***. Retinol and its esters show an intense but rapidly fading vitamin A autofluorescence after excitation at 330 nm.
6. Typical markers of HSC, e.g., desmin, vimentin, N-CAM, or GFAP, can be visualized by immunostaining. To rule out contaminations with endothelial cells, preparations can be stained with 1,1'-dioctadecyl-3,3,3',3'-tetramethylindocarbocyanine perchlorate (Dil-Ac-LDL). When EC are incubated with Dil-Ac-LDL for 4 h at 37°C and subsequently examined by fluorescence microscopy, they appear brilliantly fluorescent under ultraviolet light.

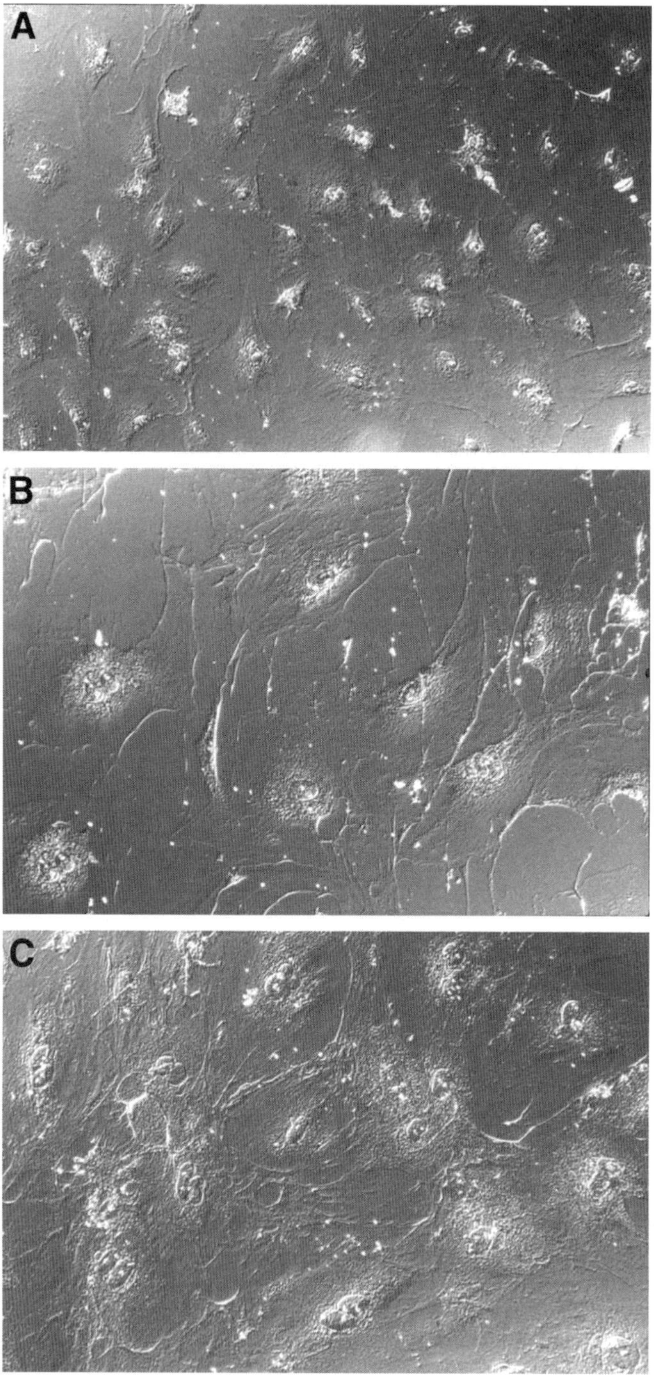

Fig. 4. Morphology of hepatic stellate cells (HSC)/myofibroblasts. Light micrograph of HSC at day 2 (**A**), 5 (**B**), and 7 (**C**) of primary culture. Note that the phenotypic changes on culturing on uncoated plastic.

7. Studies of biologically relevant changes during the transition from quiescent to activated myofibroblastic phenotype are most convincing when performed with primary cultures of HSC. However, several groups reported about the establishment of different stellate cell lines of murine (GRX, SV68c-IS), rat (NFSC, CFSC, CFSC-2G, HSC-T6, PAV-1) or human (LI90, GREF-X, LX-1, LX-2) origin ***(15–23)***. Some of these immortalized cell lines were shown to take up and esterify retinal, express some characteristic HSC markers, and respond to transforming growth factor-β1, suggesting that they actually derive from HSC. However, differences in morphology, growth characteristics, and several anomalies of chromosome number and structure in some of these cell lines were reported. Therefore, these cell lines are potentially useful for exploring some specialized questions on the biology of HSC, but confirmation of the observation in primary cell culture is strongly recommended.
8. Another possibility for obtaining human HSC in their myofibroblastic phenotype is the outgrowth from explants of normal liver isolated after surgery of benign of malignant liver tumors. Typically, these cells are cultured in DMEM containing 10% serum (5% FCS, 5% pooled human serum). The cells were reported to show typical features of myofibroblast-like cells, such as abundant rough endoplasmic reticulum and large bundles of microfilaments ***(24,25)***. Additionally, immunocytochemical studies indicate that these cells are positive for smooth muscle α-actin and desmin, two markers of human HSC in their myofibroblastic phenotype. Note, that the isolation of cells from human livers must be in accordance with ethical regulations imposed by the national legislation.
9. Other reagents used for density gradient centrifugation:
   a. Metrizamide (2-[3-acetamido-2,4,6-triiodo5(*N*-methylacetamido-benzamido]-2-deoxy-D-glucose) is a water-soluble component commonly used in radiology or in preparing gradients for ultracentrifugation. A detailed protocol for HSC peparation using metrizamide is given in **ref. *14***.
   b. Stractan is an arabinogalactan consisting mainly of polymeric galactose linked to arabinose side chains. HSC are separated efficiently from other nonparenchymal cells from the top of a discontinuous gradient made out of 6, 8, 12, and 20% stractan ***(26,27)***.
   c. Percoll is adjustable to physiological ionic strength and pH. Gradients can either be preformed or spontaneously generated by centrifugation at moderate speeds in an angle-head rotor. Gradients are iso-osmotic throughout and cover a range of densities up to 1.3 g/mL. Percoll's low viscosity means that cell separations on preformed gradients can be completed in only a few minutes using low centrifugal forces. Typically, HSC can be enriched at densities in the range of 1.025 to 1.035 g/mL ***(28)***.
10. We have recently developed protocols for cryopreservation of rat HSC ***(29)***.

Acknowledgments

The author's work is supported by grants from the Deutsche Forschungsgemeinschaft (DFG) and from the Federal Ministry of Education and Research of Germany (BMBF), e.g., IZKF Biomat and Hep-Net.

References

1. Hendriks, H. F., Verhoofstad, W. A., Brouwer, A., de Leeuw, A. M., and Knook, D. L. (1985) Perisinusoidal fat-storing cells are the main vitamin A storage sites in rat liver. *Exp. Cell Res.* **160,** 138–149.
2. Friedman, S. L. (2000) Molecular regulation of hepatic fibrosis, an integrated cellular response to tissue injury. *J. Biol. Chem.* **275,** 2247–2250.
3. Geerts, A. (2001) History, heterogeneity, developmental biology, and functions of quiescent hepatic stellate cells. *Sem. Liv. Dis.* **21,** 311–335.
4. Hepatic stellate cell nomenclature (1996) [Letter] *Hepatology* **23,** 193.
5. Ballardini, G., Groff, P., Badiali de Giorgi, L., Schuppan, D., and Bianchi, F. B. (1994) Ito cell heterogeneity: desmin-negative Ito cells in normal rat liver. *Hepatology* **19,** 440–446.
6. Zhou, Z., Ekataksin, W., and Wake, K. (1998) Zonal and regional differences identified from precision mapping of vitamin A-storing lipid droplets of the hepatic stellate cells in pig liver: a novel concept of addressing the intralobular area of heterogeneity. *Hepatology* **27,** 1098–1108.
7. Giampieri, M. P., Jezequel, A. M., and Orlandi, F. (1981) The lipocytes in normal human liver. A quantitative study. *Digestion* **22,** 165–169.
8. Schafer, S., Zerbe, O., and Gressner, A. M. (1987) The synthesis of proteoglycans in fat-storing cells of rat liver. *Hepatology* **7,** 680–687.
9. Grabske, R. J., Lake, S., Gledhill, B.L., and Meistrich, M. L. (1975) Centrifugal elutriation: separation of spermatogenic cells on the basis of sedimentation velocity. *J. Cell Physiol.* **86,** 177–189.
10. Galambos, J. T., Hollingsworth, M. A. Jr, Falek, A., Warren, W. D., and McCain, J. R. (1977) The rate of synthesis of glycosaminoglycans and collagen by fibroblasts cultured from adult human liver biopsies. *J. Clin. Invest.* **60,** 107–114.
11. Beckman Instruments: The JE-5.0 elutriation system for use with J6 series centrifuges. Instruction manual JE5-IM-7 (Beckman Coulter, Palo Alto, CA).
12. Geerts, A., Niki, T., Hellemans, K., et al. (1998) Purification of rat hepatic stellate cells by side scatter-activated cell sorting. *Hepatology* **27,** 590–598.
13. Wake, K. (1980) Perisinusoidal stellate cells (fat-storing cells, interstitial cells, lipocytes), their related structure in and around the liver sinusoids, and vitamin A-storing cells in extrahepatic organs. *Int. Rev. Cytol.* **66,** 303–353.
14. de Leeuw, A. M., McCarthy, S. P., Geerts, A., and Knook D. L. (1984) Purified rat liver fat-storing cells in culture divide and contain collagen. *Hepatology* **4,** 392–403.
15. Borojevic, R., Monteiro, A. N., Vinhas, S. A., et al. (1985) Establishment of a continuous cell line from fibrotic schistosomal granulomas in mice livers. *In Vitro Cell. Dev. Biol.* **21,** 382–390.
16. Horie, S., Kitamura, Y., Kawasaki, H., and Terada, T. (2000) Inhibitory effects of antisense oligonucleotides on the expression of procollagen type III gene in mouse hepatic stellate cells transformed by simian virus 40. *Pathol. Int.* **50,** 937–944.
17. Greenwel, P., Rubin, J., Schwartz, M., Hertzberg, E. L., and Rojkind, M. (1993) Liver fat-storing cell clones obtained from a CCl4-cirrhotic rat are heterogeneous

with regard to proliferation, expression of extracellular matrix components, interleukin-6, and connexin 43. *Lab. Invest.* **69,** 210–216.

18. Greenwel, P., Schwartz, M., Rosas, M., Peyrol, S., Grimaud, J. A., and Rojkind, M. (1991) Characterization of fat-storing cell lines derived from normal and CCl4-cirrhotic livers. Differences in the production of interleukin-6. *Lab. Invest.* **65,** 644–653.
19. Kim, Y., Ratziu, V., Choi, S. G., et al. (1998) Transcriptional activation of transforming growth factor beta1 and its receptors by the Kruppel-like factor Zf9/core promoter-binding protein and Sp1. Potential mechanisms for autocrine fibrogenesis in response to injury. *J. Biol. Chem.* **273,** 33,750–33,758.
20. Sauvant, P., Sapin, V., Abergel, A., et al. (2002) PAV-1, a new rat hepatic stellate cell line converts retinol into retinoic acid, a process altered by ethanol. *Int. J. Biochem. Cell. Biol.* **34,** 1017–1029.
21. Murakami, K., Abe, T., Miyazawa, M., et al. (1995) Establishment of a new human cell line, LI90, exhibiting characteristics of hepatic Ito (fat-storing) cells. *Lab. Invest.* **72,** 731–739.
22. Weill, F. X., Blazejewski, S., Blanc, J. F., et al. (1997) Characterization of a new human liver myofibroblast cell line: transcriptional regulation of plasminogen activator inhibitor type I by transforming growth factor beta 1. *Lab. Invest.* **77,** 63–70.
23. Xu, L., Hui, A. Y., Albanis, E., et al. (2005) Human hepatic stellate cell lines, LX-1 and LX-2: new tools for analysis of hepatic fibrosis. *Gut* **54,** 142–151.
24. Friedman, S. L., Rockey, D. C., McGuire, R. F., Maher, J. J., Boyles, J. K., and Yamasaki, G. (1992) Isolated hepatic lipocytes and Kupffer cells from normal human liver: morphological and functional characteristics in primary culture. *Hepatology* **15,** 234–243.
25. Blazejewski, S., Preaux, A. M., Mallat, A., et al. (1995) Human myofibroblastlike cells obtained by outgrowth are representative of the fibrogenic cells in the liver. *Hepatology* **22,** 788–797.
26. Friedman, S. L. and Roll, F. J. (1987) Isolation and culture of hepatic lipocytes, Kupffer cells, and sinusoidal endothelial cells by density gradient centrifugation with Stractan. *Anal. Biochem.* **161,** 207–218.
27. Pinzani, M., Gesualdo, L., Sabbah, G. M., and Abboud, H. E. (1989) Effects of platelet-derived growth factor and other polypeptide mitogens on DNA synthesis and growth of cultured rat liver fat-storing cells. *J. Clin. Invest.* **84,** 1786–1793.
28. Blomhoff, R. and Berg, T. (1990) Isolation and cultivation of rat liver stellate cells. *Meth. Enzymol.* **190,** 58–71.
29. Neyzen, S., Van de Leur, E., Hollweg, G., Gressnerm, A. M., and Weiskirchen, R. (2005) Cryopreservation of hepatic stellate cells: methodology to conserve fibrogenic progenitor cells. Submitted.

6

Isolation and Phenotypic Characterization of Lung Fibroblasts

Carolyn J. Baglole, Sireesha Y. Reddy, Stephen J. Pollock, Steven E. Feldon, Patricia J. Sime, Terry J. Smith, and Richard P. Phipps

Summary

Primary fibroblasts represent a heterogeneous population of cells that can be separated into subsets on the basis of cell surface markers such as Thy-1. Deriving fibroblasts initially involves obtaining tissue explants from tissues such as the lung, heart, cornea, skin, and orbit. The tissue is mechanically dissociated and cells are allowed to proliferate from the fragments. Following establishment of a primary culture of fibroblasts, it is necessary to characterize the new strain of cells to ensure their purity and fibroblastic phenotype using immunofluorescence and immunohistochemistry to detect the presence or absence of cell-specific surface markers. Characterizing the cells as expressing or lacking Thy-1 can also be performed by immunofluorescence in concert with microscopy or by flow cytometry using an anti-human Thy-1 antibody. In addition, fibroblasts may be sorted according to their expression of Thy-1 by fluorescence-activated cell sorting and/or magnetic beading; use of these techniques can yield greater than 99% purity. Once separated, the pure Thy-1 expressing or lacking fibroblast subsets can be propagated. These subsets can then be used for experimentation to determine functional differences between fibroblasts derived from normal and pathological tissue such as scarred lung.

Key Words: Fibroblasts; flow cytometry; fibrosis; lung; Thy-1; magnetic beading; heterogeneity; fluorescence-activated cell sorting.

1. Introduction

Fibroblasts are a heterogeneous population of cells that play a vital role in maintaining the structural integrity of organs such as the lung, integument, heart, sclera, and orbit under conditions of health and disease. This includes healing and reparative processes, and in the pathogenesis of scarring (fibrosis) disorders *(1)*. Fibrosis results from abnormal or altered production of extracellular matrix and from fibroblast hyperplasia *(2,3)*. Such responses are also associated with the activation of fibroblasts *(4)*. Recent evidence indicates that subpopulations of fibroblasts have differing roles in the initiation and progres-

From: *Methods in Molecular Medicine, Vol. 117: Fibrosis Research: Methods and Protocols*
Edited by: J. Varga, D. A. Brenner, and S. H. Phan © Humana Press Inc., Totowa, NJ

sion of fibrosis ***(5)***, as well as the abnormal accumulation of fat that can occur in tissues such as the orbit ***(6)***.

The notion of fibroblast heterogeneity is now well documented as occurring in a variety of tissues that include the lung, reproductive tract, orbit, and gingiva ***(5,7–14)***. In this regard, fibroblasts not only differ among organ systems, but also within a given anatomical site. Traditional methods of identifying fibroblast subsets have relied on morphology, size, proliferative potential, response to inflammatory mediators, biosynthetic capacity (i.e., collagen production), and cell surface characteristics ***(15–18)*** such as C1q ***(18)*** and Thy-1 expression ***(11,12)***. Using ligands directed against surface markers in conjunction with flow cytometry and fluorescence-activated cell sorting (FACS) allows for the separation and characterization of fibroblast subsets. Surface markers in concert with a cell separation strategy allows for the precise and reproducible separation of a heterogeneous population of cells. Once separated, fibroblast subsets can then be experimentally manipulated using standard in vitro cell culture techniques. As highlighted herein, the identification of lung fibroblast subsets on the basis of Thy-1 expression will illustrate the methods utilized to isolate and characterize fibroblast phenotypes. The approaches described in this chapter can easily be applied to any human tissue, as well as those from rodents and other species.

2. Materials

1. Culture medium: minimum essential medium (MEM) supplemented with 2 m*M* glutamine (Invitrogen, Carlsbad, CA) and 10% fetal bovine serum (FBS) (Hyclone Labs, Logan UT); RPMI 1640 media (Invitrogen).
2. Eight-well glass chamber slides (BD Biosciences, San Diego, CA).
3. Confocal or standard immunofluorescence microscope.
4. Flow cytometer (FACS Calibur, BD Biosciences).
5. CellQuest software (BD Biosciences).
6. Fluorescence-activated cell sorter (BD Biosciences).
7. Cell culture vessels: (25 cm^2 and 75 cm^2) (BD Biosciences).
8. Phosphate-buffered saline (PBS).
9. Trypsin/ethylenediaminetetraacetic acid (EDTA) solution (Invitrogen/Sigma Chemical Co.).
10. Anti-Thy-1 capture antibody: mouse immunoglobulin $(Ig)G_1$ anti-human Thy1 hybridoma supernatant (Clone F15-421-5); this solution should be sterile filtered before use in the bead separation procedure; storage is at 4°C.
11. Anti-human α-smooth muscle actin (SMA) antibody (Sigma, St. Louis, MO).
12. Isotype control for αSMA antibody mouse IgG2a (Caltag, Burlingame, CA).
13. Isotype control for Thy-1 antibody: mouse IgG_1 (Caltag).
14. Biotinylated horse anti-mouse IgG antibody (heavy and light chain) (Vector Labs, Burlingame, CA).

15. Streptavidin-conjugated horseradish peroxidase (SA-HRP) (Jackson Immunoresearch Labs, West Grove, PA).
16. Aminoethyl-carbazole (AEC) chromogen (Zymed, South San Fransisco, CA).
17. Immu-mount (Shanndon, Pittsburgh, PA).
18. Fluoromount-G (Southern Biotech., Birmingham, AL).
19. 2% paraformaldehyde (in PBS).
20. Magnetic beads: CELLection™ Pan Mouse IgG kit (cat. no. 155.19, Dynal, Oslo, Norway).
21. Dynal MPC magnet (can be refrigerated prior to use to keep the cells and suspensions cold during capture) (Dynal).
22. Beading buffer (BB) (PBS/0.1% bovine serum albumin [BSA]); sterile filtered and stored at 4°C.
23. PAB: PBS containing 1% BSA and 0.1% sodium azide.
24. DNase releasing buffer, prepared according to manufacturer's instructions (aliquot 30-µL portions and store at –20°C).
25. 5% Normal horse serum.
26. 5% Normal goat serum.
27. Fluorescein isothiocyanate conjugated goat anti-mouse Ig (Sigma).
28. Truncated, filtered pipet tips.
29. Monoclonal anti-collagen Type 1 antibody (cat. no. C2456, Sigma).
30. Monoclonal anti-cytokeratin peptide 18 (cat. no. C8541, Sigma).
31. Anti-LCA CD45 antibody (DAKO N-series).

3. Methods

The methods described in this chapter outline (1) the explant procedure used to initiate and establish fibroblast strains from tissue, (2) fibroblast characterization using fibroblast markers and morphological features, (3) immunofluorescence and flow cytometry for Thy-1 expression, and (4) fibroblast subset separation on the basis of Thy-1 expression using magnetic beading and/or FACS. **Figure 1** provides an overview of the procedures.

3.1. Fibroblast Strain Derivation

The establishment of fibroblast strains is described in this section and includes information on (a) the initial cultivation of cells from tissue explants and (b) the propagation and maintenance of the newly isolated fibroblast strains.

3.1.1. Tissue Explants

1. Fibroblast cultures are initiated from lung explants (or other tissue; *see* **Note 1**) by placing the tissue on the bottom of a sterile plastic tissue culture dish and mechanically disrupting using a scalpel (for other methods of dissociation; *see* **Note 2**). During excision and once explants are obtained, aseptic techniques should be adhered to (including performing all of the techniques in cell culture hoods), thereby minimizing contamination of the primary culture.

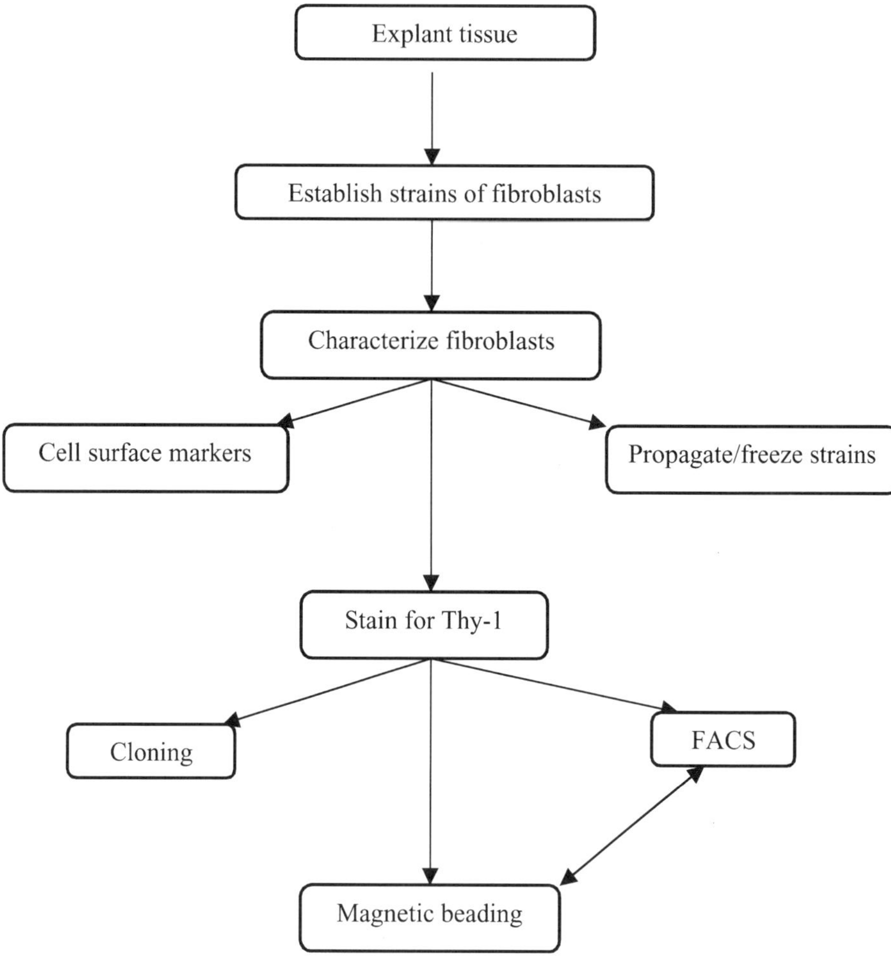

Fig. 1. Overview of the strategies used to establish, characterize and separate lung fibroblasts. Separation of Thy-1 fibroblast subsets is used to illustrate the various techniques that can be used. A detailed description for each of the protocols is included in the text of this chapter.

2. The disrupted explants are allowed to adhere to the bottom of the culture plates before covering them with Richter's improved MEM insulin (RPMI) cell culture medium supplemented with penicillin/streptomycin (1:100) and gentamicin (50 µg/mL), 20% FBS, nonessential amino acids (0.1 m*M*), sodium pyruvate (1 m*M*), L-glutamine (2 m*M*), *N*-2-hydroxyethylpiperazine-*N*'-2-ethanesulfonic acid (HEPES) (10 m*M*), and β-mercaptoethanol (50 µ*M*). Cultures are maintained in a 37°C, humidified incubator with 7% CO_2-enriched atmosphere.

3. Media should be changed once or twice each week for a period of approx 2 wk.
4. During this period, care should be taken not to disturb the explants; failure of the tissue to adhere to the bottom of the culture dish will result in an absence of fibroblast proliferation. To prevent this, sterile glass cover slips may be used to cover the tissue and prevent its dissociation from the substratum. Here, a small amount of sterile vacuum grease may be used to secure the cover slip to the bottom of the culture dish.

3.1.2. Establishment, Propagation, and Maintenance of Primary Fibroblast Strains

During the first 2 wk of culture, most nonfibroblast cells (i.e., epithelial and endothelial cells) perish while the fibroblasts continue to proliferate and become established as the predominant cell type. This allows for the generation of a strain of fibroblasts adequate for propagation and subsequent characterization of their purity as well as sorting into Thy-1$^+$ and Thy-1$^-$ strains.

1. Once the fibroblasts are outgrown (**Fig. 2**), the remaining tissue pieces are removed, the monolayer of cells washed once with sterile PBS and disrupted using 1:1 0.05% trypsin:0.1% EDTA solution at room temperature. If the cells are resistant to detachment, they can be incubated in the detachment solution at 37°C. However, the trypsin:EDTA solution should not be left on the cells for longer then 5 min.
2. Once the cells have separated from the plate, they are resuspended in an equal volume of complete cell culture media (MEM supplemented with glutamine and 10% FBS; the FBS will neutralize the trypsin) and centrifuged at 200*g* for 5 min.
3. The cells from one culture dish are then replated into either 25-cm^2 or 75-cm^2 cell culture flasks containing cell culture media (typically RPMI or MEM). If desired, the fibroblasts may be counted according to standard cell culture methods and seeded at a density of 10,000 cells/cm^2.
4. Once established, media should be replaced twice weekly and the cultured cells used between passages 3 and 15, because primary fibroblast strains have a finite life span. Additionally, cells should be allowed to reach confluency (80–100%) before subculturing and should be passaged at a ratio of 1:3 or 1:4.
5. Once the cultures have become established, fibroblasts should be maintained and subcultured in MEM supplemented with 10% FBS and glutamine. If so desired, fibroblasts at an early passage may be frozen and stored indefinitely in liquid nitrogen (*see* **Note 3**).

3.2. Fibroblast Characterization: Immunohistochemistry

Cultures derived from the tissue explants typically consist of fibroblasts only. Nonetheless, it is important to document the purity of each strain. The usual strategy involves assessing the presence of cell markers and phenotypic

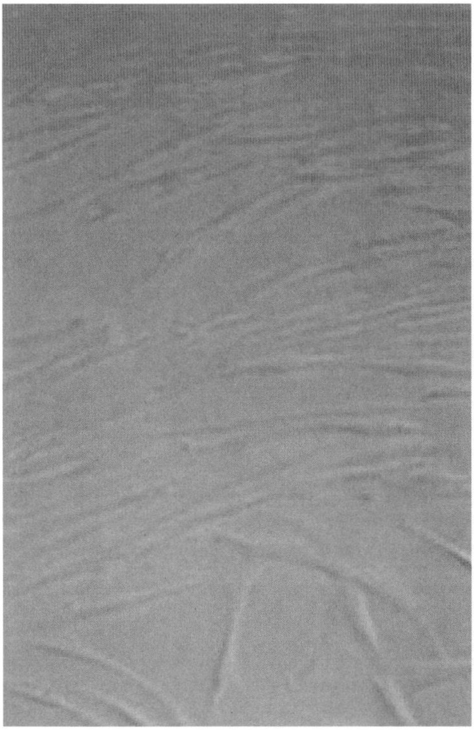

Fig. 2. Establishment of primary fibroblasts strains derived from tissue explants. Tissue was disrupted, allowed to adhere to cell culture dishes and incubated for 2 wk in cell culture media. Cells can be observed growing out from the tissue within a couple of days and by the end of the 2 wk, few cells other than fibroblasts remain, as seen here.

properties of fibroblasts. Typically, fibroblasts exhibit a characteristic morphology. They are flat, elongated cells with oval nuclei. They express vimentin and collagen; in contrast, cytokeratin, a prominent epithelial cell marker, α-smooth muscle actin, expressed by myofibroblasts and smooth muscle cells, and CD45 are typically absent in fibroblasts. The methods described in this section outline the immunostaining procedures that are useful in distinguishing fibroblasts from other cell types.

1. Inoculate fibroblasts onto glass chamber slides (20,000 cells per well) in culture medium (MEM). Allow fibroblasts to adhere and check for approx 50 to 75% confluency (approx 24–48 h) at 37°C before conducting experiments.
2. Remove culture media. Gently rinse twice with PBS. Fix with fresh 2% paraformaldehyde for 5 min.
3. Rinse once with PBS. Rinse with PBS-Tween twice for 5 min each.

4. Incubate with 3% hydrogen peroxide (diluted in methanol) for 10 min to block peroxidase activity. Rinse with PBS-Tween twice for 5 min at room temperature.
5. Incubate with 5% normal horse serum in PBS/0.1% BSA to block nonspecific binding for 1 h at room temperature.
6. To stain the cells for collagen, cytokeratin, or αSMA, incubate cultures with anti-collagen type 1 antibody (1:2000), anti-cytokeratin peptide 18 (1:800), or anti-human αSMA antibody (1:800), respectively, overnight at 4°C. As a negative control, some cultures should be incubated with the appropriate isotype: mouse IgG1 (for collagen and cytokeratin) or mouse IgG2a (αSMA). To assess collagen production, it may prove necessary to incubate cultures with ascorbic acid (*see* **Note 4**).
7. CD45 (leukocyte common antigen) can be detected by staining cultures with monoclonal anti-LCA CD45 antibody (DAKO N-series). The primary antibody is available as a prepared solution. Cover monolayers completely with this solution in the slide chamber. An incubation time of 10 min at room temperature appears optimal.
8. For vimentin staining, cover monolayer with DAKO EPOS anti-vimentin/HRP (U 7034). This reagent is supplied as ready to use. Incubate for 60 min at room temperature. The negative control is the DAKO EPOS Immunoglobulin-HRP. **Note:** blocking is unnecessary when using the DAKO-EPOS system.
9. Incubate with PBS-Tween three times for 5 min at room temperature.
10. Add secondary antibody (biotinylated horse anti-mouse) at a dilution of 1:200 for 2 h at 4°C.
11. Rinse with PBS-Tween three times.
12. Add SA-HRP at a dilution of 1:1000 in PBS/0.1% BSA for 1 h at room temperature.
13. Rinse three times with PBS. Add two drops of AEC solution per sample. Allow color development for 30 min at RT (5–15 min for vimentin). Rinse with distilled water. Counterstain if desired and cover slip with Immu-Mount.

3.3. Detection of Thy-1 Expression

3.3.1. Immunofluorescence

Distinguishing fibroblast subsets on the basis of Thy-1 expression can be accomplished by immunofluorescence. Fibroblasts are seeded into eight-well chamber slides as previously described. They are then allowed to proliferate to a subconfluent state. This is important because distinguishing individual fibroblasts will allow clear-cut assessment of Thy-1 fluorescence. Confluent cell layers can also "roll up" during the washing procedures, resulting in a loss of cells.

To stain for Thy-1:

1. Rinse the fibroblasts twice with PAB and fix in 2% paraformaldehyde/PBS for 10 min at 4°C.
2. Rinse twice for 5 min each with PAB.

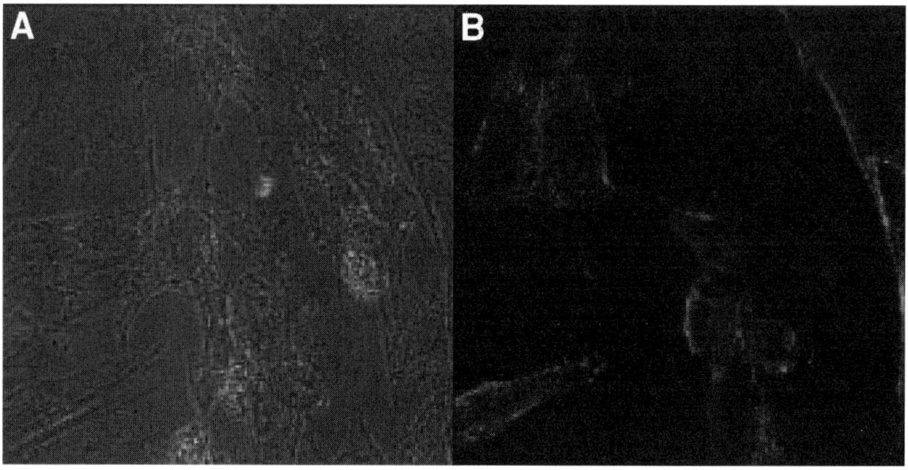

Fig. 3. Thy-1^+ fibroblasts are easily detected using immunofluorescence. Primary fibroblast cultures were incubated with anti-human Thy-1 and fluorescein isothiocyanate-conjugated goat-anti-mouse and then visualized with a confocal microscope. Bright-field image **(A)** and immunofluorescent image of Thy-1^+ fibroblasts **(B)**. Note that not all fibroblasts are Thy-1^+.

3. Incubate for 1 h at 4°C with normal goat serum (5% in PAB)
4. Incubate for 45 min with the mouse IgG_1 anti-human Thy-1 antibody F15-421-5 or the isotype control antibody (10 µg/mL in PAB) at 4°C.
5. Rinse three times with PAB.
6. Incubate with goat anti-mouse Ig conjugated with fluorescein isothiocyanate as a secondary antibody for 45 min at 4°C.
7. Rinse three times with PAB.
8. Cover slip with Fluoromount-G.
9. Thy-1^+ cells (**Fig. 3**) are easily detected with either conventional fluorescent light or confocal microscope.

3.3.2. Flow Cytometry

As an alternative to immunohistochemistry, flow cytometry is a quantitative tool that can be used to assess Thy-1 expression.

1. Monolayers of confluent fibroblasts are dissociated as previously described.
2. Suspend one million cells per sample in PAB and incubate with the primary anti-Thy-1 antibody followed by rinses in PAB and incubation with the fluorescein isothiocyanate (FITC)-conjugated secondary antibody for the time points indicated in **Subheading 3.3.**

3. Following incubation with the secondary antibody, wash the cells three times and resuspend (using truncated, filtered pipet tips) in 1 mL of PAB. Fibroblasts are delicate and care should be taken when washing or suspending the cells.
4. Resuspended samples can then undergo analysis by flow cytometry.

3.4. Thy-1 Subset Separation Using FACS and Magnetic Beads

Detection of Thy-1 expression on isolated fibroblasts by immunohistochemistry and flow cytometry gives an indication of the relative abundance of those cells displaying the glycoprotein in primary fibroblast strains. Because Thy-1^+ and Thy-1^- subsets may be functionally distinct *(12)*, it is sometimes advantageous to separate them. Obtaining subpopulations of cells can be accomplished by using a variety of techniques, including FACS, magnetic beading, and clonal expansion (*see* **Note 5** and **Fig. 1**). The methods outlined here describe the procedures for sorting the cells by using FACS or by magnetic beading. In addition, these procedures may be used in conjunction with one another, ensuring separation purity greater than 99%.

3.4.1. FACS

Using FACS to separate cells from a complex mixture can prove highly reproducible *(15)*. One disadvantage to this technique relates to the fragile nature of some cells that may become damaged during the sorting process. Another concerns the low yield. However, FACS is an effective tool for separating fibroblasts on the basis of Thy-1 expression. The same primary anti-human Thy-1 antibody used for immunofluorescence and flow cytometry can be employed in this procedure. Following FACS, cells can undergo several rounds of magnetic beading.

3.4.2. Magnetic Beading

Magnetic beading also allows for the separation of cell subsets on the basis of surface markers, but without the need for specialized equipment. For this procedure, perform all operations at 4°C (or on ice) except where indicated. Use truncated filtered pipet tips to reduce mechanical shearing of the cells except where indicated.

1. Harvest fibroblasts into a 15-mL centrifuge tube as previously described and count total number of cells by standard methods using a hemocytometer.
2. Centrifuge cells at 200*g* to pellet. Aspirate the supernatant and resuspend in 1.5 mL BB and transfer to a 2.0-mL microcentrifuge tube.
3. Centrifuge at 200*g* for 5 min at 4°C to wash the cells.
4. Carefully remove the supernatant and resuspend the cells in a solution containing the anti-Thy-1 antibody (100 µL of undiluted antibody solution per 1×10^6 cells). Incubate for 30 min with gentle mixing by inversion every 10-min interval.

5. While incubating with the coating antibody, calculate the number of beads necessary, wash the beads to remove the azide, and calculate the binding volume (*see* **Notes 6–8**). Use at least 10 beads per cell and keep the binding volume such that there are greater than 3×10^7 beads/mL.
6. Add 1.5 mL of BB to the antibody-coated cells and centrifuge at 1800 rpm in a microcentrifuge for 5 min.
7. Remove the supernatant and resuspend in 2 mL of BB and repeat **step 6** three times.
8. Resuspend the cells in the volume of BB calculated in **Note 8**.
9. Add the washed beads to antibody-coated cells and mix by pipetting up and down several times.
10. Place microcentrifuge tube on a tilting rocker and gently rock for 30 min.
11. Add MEM supplemented with 10% FBS to the suspension for a total volume of 1.0 mL and place the microcentrifuge tube in the magnet and capture the bead/cell rosettes.
12. Carefully remove the nonrosetted cells in suspension away from the bead/cell rosettes. This is the Thy-1^- population. Transfer this cell suspension to a 15-mL centrifuge tube at 4°C. While removing the Thy-1^- cells, care should be taken to leave the bead/cell rosettes captured on the wall of the tube undisturbed.
13. Remove the microcentrifuge tube from the magnet, resuspend the bead/cell rosettes, and repeat capturing of the rosettes. Pool the Thy-1^- cells, bring to a volume of 5 mL and plate the cells (*see* **Note 9**).
14. To isolate the Thy-1^+ cells, resuspend the bead/cell rosettes in 1 mL of BB. Replace the tube in the magnet to capture the bead cell rosettes. Remove the washing solution and discard. Repeat to a total of six washes.
15. Resuspend the bead/cell rosettes in room temperature MEM with 1% FBS at a bead density of 5×10^7 beads/mL, based on the original number of beads used.
16. Bead/cell rosettes can be monitored by transferring a small aliquot to a hemocytometer. The majority of cells should be surrounded by several beads. All cells should have at least a few beads. If bead-free cells are found, more washing is necessary.
17. Add 10 μL of DNAse releasing buffer for each 10^7 beads used. Ensure that the concentration of DNAse in solution is 2500 U/mL (50 μL/mL) and there are at least 50 U of DNAse/10^6 beads.
18. Place microcentrifuge tube on a tilting rocker at room temperature for 90 min. Every 15-min, aseptically pipet the bead/cell rosettes up and down 10 times using a regular filtered pipet tip. This is necessary to shear the beads off cells.
19. Add complete media at 4°C to bring the volume to 1 mL and place the microcentrifuge tube in the magnet and capture the released beads. Carefully remove the suspended cells and transfer to a 15-mL centrifuge tube.
20. Remove the tube from the magnet and resuspend the beads in 1 mL of media. Replace the tube in the magnet to capture the beads. Remove suspended cells and pool into the same 15-mL tube. Repeat a total of four times
21. Place the tube with the Thy-1^+ cells in the magnet to capture the residual beads as describe for Thy-1 cells in **Note 9**.

4. Notes

1. Primary fibroblast cultures may be initiated from various organs including, but not limited to, the lung, orbit, myometrium, endometrium, gingival tissue, periodontium, spleen *(7)*, and bone marrow.
2. Alternative methods to mechanically disrupting tissue include enzymatic dissociation using collagenase and/or dispase.
3. To freeze the fibroblasts, cells should be counted and resuspended in freezing media (complete MEM media supplemented with 50% FBS and 10% dimethylsulfoxide) and frozen in isopropanol freezing containers at –80°C. For long-term storage, vials of frozen cells should be maintained in liquid nitrogen.
4. In order to enhance collagen production, fibroblasts may need to be incubated with ascorbic acid at a concentration of 50 µg/mL ***(19)***.
5. One method for generating clones is limiting dilution followed by clonal expansion (the reader is referred to **refs.** ***7*** and ***8*** for more technical information). Cells can be seeded at a low density (as low as 1 cell/well) and allowed to proliferate for 2 wk. At this point, selected wells are harvested and expanded. Thy-1 expression can then be assessed by immunofluorescence and flow cytometry.
6. The number of beads used is based on the percentage of Thy-1^+ cells in the initial population. For less than 20% Thy-1^+ cells, use 15 µL of bead suspension (6×10^6 beads) per 1×10^6 cells; between 20 and 80%, use 25 µL and more than 80%, use 35 µL of bead suspension.
7. To wash the beads, resuspend them in a supplied stock tube, transfer the necessary volume to a microcentrifuge tube, and add 1 mL of BB. Capture the beads in the magnet and aspirate the supernatant. Repeat and resuspend the beads in 100 µL of BB and store at 4°C.
8. It is necessary to keep the density of the beads in BB at 30×10^6 beads per mL during binding of the beads to the target cells. From the total number of beads being used in the separation (from **Note 6**), calculate the total volume of BB to use minus 100 µL (the volume in which to suspend the washed beads).
9. To complete the Thy-1^- isolation, place the 15-mL tube on the magnet and let set for 3 min to capture any residual beads from the suspension of cells. Gently pour into a second tube. Add 5 mL of media, centrifuge, aspirate the media, and resuspend the cells in 2 to 5 mL of media. The cells should be counted and 90% of the cells plated into a 75-cm^2 culture flask and 10% into a single well of a six-well plate to be used for flow cytometric analysis of Thy-1 expression of cells.

Acknowledgments

This work was supported by USPHS grants ES01247, HLO78603, DE11390, EY08976, EY11708, EY014564; WRHR K12HD01332-04; Howard Hughes Biomedical Support; EPA PM Center; Philip Morris External Research Program; The Endometriosis Association; The Cystic Fibrosis Foundation; and an American Lung Association fellowship (CJB).

References

1. Korn, J. H., Thrall, R. S., Wilbur, D. C., Kream, B. E., and Piela-Smith, T. H. (1992) Fibroblast heterogeneity: clonal selection of fibroblasts as a model for fibrotic disease. In: Phipps, R. P., ed. *Pulmonary Fibroblast Heterogeneity.* CRC, Boca Raton: pp. 119–133.
2. Agostini, C. and Semenzato, G. (1996) Immunology of idiopathic pulmonary fibrosis. *Curr. Opin. Pulm. Med.* **2,** 364–369.
3. Phan, S. H. (2002) The myofibroblast in pulmonary fibrosis. *Chest* **122,** 286S–289S.
4. Karmiol, S. and Phan, S. H. (1992) Phenotypic changes in lung fibroblast populations in pulmonary fibrosis. In: Phipps, R. P., ed. *Pulmonary Fibroblast Heterogeneity.* CRC, Boca Raton: pp. 1–26.
5. Penney, D. P., Keng, P. C., Derdak, S., and Phipps, R. P. (1992) Morphologic and functional characteristics of subpopulations of murine lung fibroblasts grown in vitro. *Anat. Rec.* **232,** 432–443.
6. Smith, T. J., Koumas, L., Gagnon, A., et al. (2002) Orbital fibroblast heterogeneity may determine the clinical presentation of thyroid-associated ophthalmopathy. *J. Clin. Endocrinol. Metab.* **87,** 385–392.
7. Borrello, M. A. and Phipps, R. P. (1996) Differential Thy-1 expression by splenic fibroblasts defines functionally distinct subsets. *Cell Immunol.* **173,** 198–206.
8. Fries, K. M., Blieden, T., Looney, R. J., et al. (1994) Evidence of fibroblast heterogeneity and the role of fibroblast subpopulations in fibrosis. *Clin. Immunol. Immunopathol.* **72,** 283–292.
9. Hagood, J. S., Miller, P. J., Lasky, J. A., et al. (1999) Differential expression of platelet-derived growth factor-alpha receptor by Thy-1(-) and Thy-1(+) lung fibroblasts. *Am. J. Physiol.* **277,** L218–L224.
10. Koumas, L., Smith, T. J., Feldon, S., Blumberg, N., and Phipps, R. P. (2003) Thy-1 expression in human fibroblast subsets defines myofibroblastic or lipofibroblastic phenotypes. *Am. J. Pathol.* **163,** 1291–1300.
11. Koumas, L., Smith, T. J., and Phipps, R. P. Fibroblast subsets in the human orbit: Thy-1^+ and Thy-1^- subpopulations exhibit distinct phenotypes. *Eur. J. Immunol.* **32,** 447–485.
12. Koumas, L., King, A. E., Critchley, H. O. D. , Kelly, R. W., and Phipps, R. P. (2001) Existence of functionally distinct Thy 1+ and Thy1- human female reproductive tract fibroblasts. *Am. J. Pathol.* **159,** 925–935.
13. Phipps, R. P., Borrello, M. A., and Blieden, T. M. (1997) Fibroblast heterogeneity in the periodontium and other tissues. *J. Periodontal. Res.* **32,** 159–165.
14. Phipps, R. P., Penney, D. P., Keng, P., et al. (1989) Characterization of two major populations of lung fibroblasts: distinguishing morphology and discordant display of Thy 1 and class II MHC. *Am. J. Respir. Cell Mol. Biol.* **1,** 65–74.
15. Froncek, M. J., Derdak, S., Felch, M. E., Silvera, M. R., Watts, H. B., and Phipps, R. P. (1992) Cellular and molecular characterization of Thy-1+ and Thy-1- murine lung fibroblasts. In: Phipps, R. P., ed. *Pulmonary Fibroblast Heterogeneity.* CRC, Boca Raton: pp. 135–198.

16. Hagood, J. S., Mangalwadi, A., Guo, B., MacEwen, M. W., Salazar, L., and Fuller, G. M. (2002) Concordant and discordant interleukin-1-mediated signaling in lung fibroblast thy-1 subpopulations. *Am. J. Respir. Cell Mol. Biol.* **26,** 702–708.
17. Raghow, R. (1992) Heterogeneity and plasticity of extracellular matrix gene expression in fibroblasts: a pulmonary fibrosis perspective. In: Phipps, R. P., ed. *Pulmonary Fibroblast Heterogeneity.* CRC, Boca Raton: pp. 79–104.
18. Bordin, S., Kolb, W. P., and Page, R. C. (1983) C1Q receptors on cultured human gingival fibroblasts: analysis of binding properties. *J. Immunol.* **130,** 1871–1875.
19. Sansilvestri-Morel, P., Rupin, A., Jaisson, S., et al. (2001) Synthesis of collagen is dysregulated in cultured fibroblasts derived from skin of subjects with varicose veins as it is in venous smooth muscle cells. *Circulation* **106,** 479–483.

7

Methods for Measuring Type I Collagen Synthesis In Vitro

David C. Rishikof, Ping-Ping Kuang, Mangalalaxmy Subramanian, and Ronald H. Goldstein

Summary

The excess accumulation of type I collagen within tissues leads to organ dysfunction and occurs as a result of an imbalance between synthesis and degradation. This chapter outlines several methods to assess the in vitro production of type I collagen that are employed in our laboratory. We describe Western immunoblotting of intact α1(I) collagen using antibodies directed to α1(I) collagen amino and carboxyl propeptides. The measurement of α1(I) collagen mRNA levels using real-time polymerase chain reaction is then outlined. Finally, methods to determine the transcriptional regulation of α1(I) collagen using a nuclear run-on assay are described.

Key Words: Type I collagen; Western immunoblot; real-time PCR; nuclear run-on assay.

1. Introduction

The production of type I collagen is complex and tightly regulated. Type I collagen is a heterotrimeric protein consisting of two α1 chains and one α2 chain. In humans, the α1 chain is encoded on chromosome 17 and the α2 chain on chromosome 7. Following posttranslational modifications, the chains are assembled into a triple helical structure and secreted *(1–3)*. In the extracellular space, amino and carboxyl peptides are cleaved from procollagen molecules that are subsequently assembled into fibrils and then into fibers. Type I collagen is also regulated by processes that control gene transcription and by posttranscriptional mechanisms such as mRNA stability *(4–6)*. An overall increase in collagen synthesis can result from increases in the rate of transcription, increases in the stability of the mRNA, alterations in processing, or decreases in collagen degradation. This chapter outlines several methods to measure the expression of α1(I) collagen mRNA and protein in vitro that are currently employed in our laboratory.

From: *Methods in Molecular Medicine, Vol. 117: Fibrosis Research: Methods and Protocols*
Edited by: J. Varga, D. A. Brenner, and S. H. Phan © Humana Press Inc., Totowa, NJ

1.1. Western Immunoblotting of α1(I) Collagen

Type I collagen production requires the coordinated activity of several chaperones and enzymes to ensure its appropriate secretion *(1,2)*. The carboxyl terminus of two α1(I) procollagen chains and one α2(I) procollagen chain associate within the endoplasmic reticulum in a process involving protein-disulfide isomerase *(7,8)*. Procollagen production is also regulated by its interaction with the endoplasmic reticulum resident heat stress protein Hsp47 *(9)*. The assembly of the trimeric protein proceeds from the carboxyl to amino terminus and is dependent on the hydroxylation of proline residues by prolyl-4-hydroxlase for stability *(10)*. Ascorbic acid is a cofactor for the enzymatic activity of prolyl-4-hydroxylase. The absence of ascorbic acid results in the accumulation of underhydroxylated, nonhelical procollagen within the endoplasmic reticulum that is secreted at a slower rate or targeted for degradation *(11–15)*.

Prior to secretion, up to 30% of newly synthesized collagen is degraded intracellularly *(16,17)*. Although the mechanism of basal intracellular degradation is incompletely understood, it may occur in nonlysosomal compartments *(18,19)*. In several model systems, cells can be induced to synthesize increased levels of improperly folded collagen thereby increasing its intracellular degradation *(15,18,20)*. In these systems, the increase in intracellular degradation above the basal level appears to occur in lysosomes.

Collagen protein levels can be detected using hydroxyproline as a marker for collagen. Hydroxyproline accounts for approx 30% of the amino acid residues in the repeating amino acid triplet that comprises the collagen helix. Hydroxyproline content can be assessed by various means including high-pressure liquid chromatography, amino acid analysis, and colorimetric assay. These methods all require the assumption that the hydroxylation of proline moieties is not affected by the treatment procedure. The cellular trafficking of type I collagen has been facilitated by the production of synthetic peptide antisera directed against the amino and carboxyl terminus of the α1(I) collagen propeptide *(21,22)*. In our laboratory, we have successfully used antisera LF-39 and LF-41 to detect human α1(I) collagen amino propeptide and human α1(I) collagen carboxyl propeptide, respectively, by Western immunoblot analysis (**Fig. 1**).

1.2. Real-Time PCR to Measure α1(I) Collagen

The expression of α(1)I collagen mRNA may be evaluated by real-time polymerase chain reaction (PCR) using SYBER Green. SYBER Green is a minor groove binding dye that is specific for double-stranded DNA. Real-time PCR monitors the fluorescence emitted by SYBER Green during the reaction

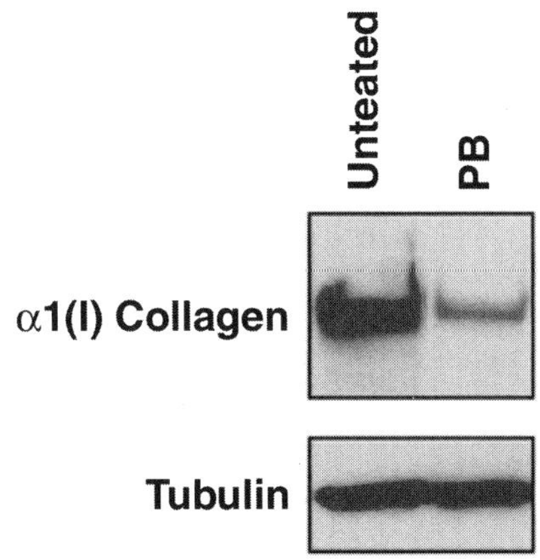

Fig. 1. Western immunoblot using LF-41 antisera to detect α1(I) collagen carboxyl propeptide. IMR-90 human embryonic lung fibroblasts were left untreated or treated with phenylbutyrate (PB) an inhibitor of type I collagen production.

as an indicator of amplicon production for each PCR cycle. This is in contrast with end point detection by conventional quantitative PCR methods.

Using SYBER Green obviates the need for target-specific fluorescent probes, but its specificity is determined entirely by the primers used in the reaction. As the presence of any double-stranded DNA generates fluorescence, reverse transcription (RT) PCR product verification is achieved by plotting fluorescence as a function of temperature to generate a melting curve of the amplicon *(23)*. A characteristic peak at the melting temperature of the amplicon distinguishes it from amplification artifacts that melt at lower temperatures in broader peaks.

1.3. Nuclear Run-On Transcription Assay of α1(I) Collagen

Type I collagen mRNA is abundantly expressed in most mesenchymal cells and can be readily measured by Northern blotting. Several bands are usually identified using this method, reflecting multiple polyadenylation sites on the mRNA *(24–26)*. The synthesis of intact type I collagen protein is generally related to the levels of α1(I) collagen and α2(I) collagen mRNA, and the detection of these two mRNA species provides an estimate of overall type I collagen production. The α1(I) collagen and α2(I) collagen genes are usually, but not always, coordinately regulated *(27)*.

Transcriptional regulation of type I collagen genes is mediated by interactions between *cis*-acting DNA sequences and *trans*-acting protein factors *(28)*. Regulatory sequences within the α1(I) collagen and α2(I) collagen gene pro-

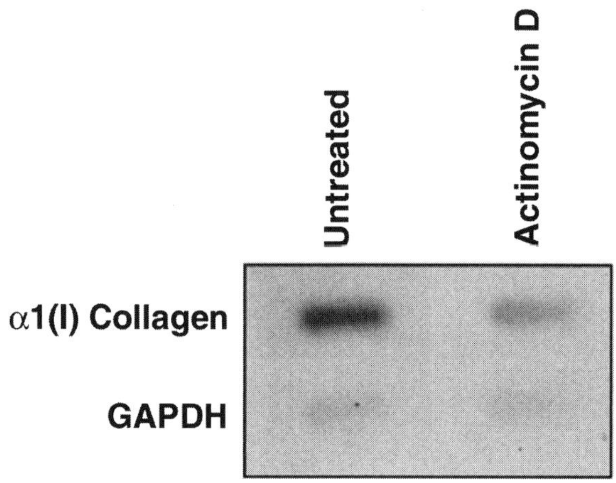

Fig. 2. Nuclear run-on transcription assay demonstrating the effect of the transcriptional inhibitor Actinomycin D on α1(I) collagen mRNA transcription.

moters have been identified using transfection studies of different promoter segments controlling a reporter gene. Although promoter activity has been used as a surrogate measure of transcriptional activity, the promoter activity in transient transfection experiments may not accurately reflect the endogenous transcriptional activity because of the need for additional *cis*-acting regulatory elements within other regions of the gene. Furthermore, chromatin structure is an essential regulator of endogenous gene transcription, but does not alter promoter activity in transient transfection studies. The transcriptional rate of the α1(I) collagen gene can be more precisely measured using a nuclear run-on assay (**Fig. 2**).

2. Materials

2.1. Western Immunoblotting of α1(I) Collagen

1. Phosphate-buffered saline (PBS) (Invitrogen).
2. Radioimmunoprecipitation (RIPA) buffer: 1% NP-40, 0.5% sodium deoxycholate, 0.1% sodium dodecyl sulfate (SDS), in PBS.
3. Complete protease inhibitor cocktail tablet (Roche Molecular Biochemicals).
4. Protein assay (Bio-Rad Laboratories).
5. NuPAGE 4% to 12% gradient Bis-Tris gel (Invitrogen).
6. Rainbow molecular weight markers (Amersham Biosciences).
7. Nitrocellulose membrane.
8. Nonfat evaporated milk.
9. Tween-20.

10. LF-39, LF-41 antisera (Provided by Larry W. Fisher, National Institutes of Health).
11. Mouse anti-α-tubulin antibody (Sigma).
12. Goat anti-rabbit antibody conjugated to horseradish peroxidase, goat anti-mouse antibody conjugated to horseradish peroxidase (Promega).
13. Enhanced chemiluminescence kit (PerkinElmer).

2.2. Real-Time PCR to Measure α1(I) Collagen

1. Spectrophotometer.
2. Oligo dT_{18} (IDT).
3. Master mix: 1 μL 200 U/μL M-MLV RT, 0.5 μL 40 U/μL RNase inhibitor, 4 μL M-MLV 5X RT buffer, 1 μL 25 m*M* dNTP (all from Promega), 1.5 μL nuclease-free water.
4. PTC-150 MiniCycler (PerkinElmer).
5. Syber Green (Applied Biosystems).
6. ABI PRISM 7700 sequence detector (PerkinElmer/Applied Biosystems).
7. cDNA primers (IDT).
8. cDNA primer sequences:
   - Human a1(I) collagen forward primer: 5'-CAAAAGACTCTGTACCTATTTGTATGTGTATAA-3'
   - Human α1(I) collagen reverse primer: 5'-AGCAATCAAAATAATTAAAAACATCTCAA-3'
   - GAPDH forward primer: 5'-CACAAGAGGAAGAGAGAGACCCTC-3'
   - GAPDH reverse primer: 5-TGAGTGTGGCAGGGACTCC-3

2.3. Nuclear Run-On Transcription Assay of α1(I) Collagen

1. PBS.
2. Tris buffer: 10 m*M* Tris-HCl, pH 7.4, 3 m*M* $CaCl_2$, 2 m*M* $MgCl_2$.
3. Lysis buffer: 1% NP-40 in Tris buffer.
4. Dounce tissue grinder fitted with a tight pestle (Thomas Scientific).
5. Storage buffer: 50 m*M* Tris-HCl, pH 8.3, 40% glycerol, 5 m*M* $MgCl_2$, 0.1 m*M* ethylenediaminetetraacetic acid (EDTA).
6. Liquid nitrogen.
7. Reaction buffer (2X): 10 m*M* Tris-HCl, pH 8.0, 5 m*M* $MgCl_2$, 0.3 *M* KCl, 5 m*M* dithiothreitol (DTT), 2 m*M* ATP, CTP, GTP (Invitrogen), 100 U RNasine (Promega), 20 μL α-^{32}P-UTP 3000 μCi/ml (NEN).
8. Stop buffer: 100 U of RNase-free DNase (Promega), 2 m*M* $CaCl_2$,10 m*M* $MgCl_2$.
9. Protease K (Invitrogen).
10. Protease K buffer (2X): 0.2 *M* Tris-HCl, pH 7.5, 0.44 *M* NaCl, 2% SDS, 25 m*M* EDTA.
11. Water-saturated phenol (American Bioanalytical).
12. Phenol/chloroform/ether (24:24:1).
13. Chloroform (Sigma-Aldrich).

14. 2 *M* Sodium acetate, pH 4.0 (Sigma-Aldrich).
15. Ethanol.
16. Dry ice.
17. TE buffer: 10 m*M* Tris-HCl, 0.1 m*M* EDTA, pH 7.6.
18. NaOH.
19. 1 *M* acid-free N-2-hydrroxyethylpiperazine-N'-2-ethansulfanic acid (HEPES) (Sigma).
20. NucTrap probe purification column (Stratagene).
21. Scintillation counter.
22. Minifold II slot-blotter (Schleicher & Schuell).
23. cDNA plasmids: elastin, α1(I) collagen, glyceraldehyde-3-phosphate dehydrogenase (GAPDH), pBluescript vector (Stratagene).
24. Restriction enzymes: *Eco*RI, *Pst*I, *Eco*RI, and *Hin*dIII.
25. 20X Saline-sodium citrate (SSC).
26. Nitrocellulose membrane.
27. Vacuum oven.
28. 6 cm × 2 cm glass tubes (VWR).
29. Hybridization solution: X5 Denhardt's solution, X5 SSC, 0.5% SDS, 50 m*M* sodium phosphate buffer, pH 6.5, 250 μg/mL yeast tRNA (Invitrogen), 50% formamide (American Bioanalytical).
30. Hybridization oven (VWR).
31. 20% SDS.
32. Autoradiography film (Kodak).

3. Methods

3.1. Western Immunoblotting of α1(I) Collagen

3.1.1. Preparing the Cell Lysate

1. Wash adherent cells twice with ice-cold PBS (**Note 1**).
2. Add 600 μL of ice-cold RIPA buffer containing protease inhibitors to a 100-mm tissue culture dish and incubate on ice for 5 min.
3. Scrape adherent cells off the dish with a plastic cell scraper. Transfer the cell suspension to a microcentrifuge tube using a syringe fitted with a 22-gage needle and incubate on ice for 15 min.
4. Centrifuge the cell suspension at 14,000*g* for 20 min at 4°C. Transfer the supernatant to a new microcentrifuge tube and discard the pellet.
5. Determine the protein concentration using the colorimetric assay. The sample can be divided into aliquots and stored at –20°C.

3.1.2. Western Immunoblotting

1. Perform SDS-polyacrylamide gel electrophoresis (PAGE). Load 50 to 100 μg of each sample and a colored molecular weight protein marker onto the gel.
2. Transfer the proteins to a nitrocellulose membrane. Wash the nitrocellulose membrane twice with distilled water (**Note 2**).

3. Block the nitrocellulose membrane in freshly prepared 5% nonfat evaporated milk in PBS containing 0.1% Tween-20 for 1 h at room temperature with constant agitation.
4. Dilute the primary antibody LF-39 (human α1[I] collagen amino propeptide) or LF-41 (human α1[I] collagen carboxyl propeptide) 1 μg/mL PBS containing 0.1% Tween-20. Incubate the nitrocellulose membrane in the primary antibody solution overnight at 4°C with constant agitation.
5. Wash the nitrocellulose membrane three times for 5 min each with PBS containing 0.1% Tween-20.
6. Incubate the nitrocellulose membrane for 1 h at room temperature in a 1:5000 secondary antibody solution of goat anti-rabbit antibody conjugated to horseradish peroxidase in PBS containing 0.1% Tween-20 with constant agitation.
7. Wash the nitrocellulose membrane three times for 5 min each with PBS containing 0.1% Tween-20.
8. Rinse the nitrocellulose membrane three times in water. Detect proteins using the enhanced chemiluminescence kit.
9. In order to confirm equal loading of each protein sample onto the gel, the nitrocellulose membrane may then be stripped and incubated in a 1:3000 solution of mouse anti-α-tubulin antibody followed by a 1:5000 solution of goat anti-mouse antibody conjugated to horseradish peroxidase.

3.2. Real-Time PCR to Measure α1(I) Collagen

3.2.1. Synthesizing cDNA

1. Determine the RNA concentration of each sample by absorbance measurement using a spectrophotometer.
2. Mix 1 or 2 μg of each RNA sample with 5 μ*M* of Oligo dT_{18} (IDT) in a final volume of 12 μL. Centrifuge the mixture briefly and heat at 75°C for 3 min in order to melt any secondary structure that could impede the reverse transcription reaction. A maximum temperature of 85°C may be used in cases where targets are GC-rich or have a high degree of secondary structure. Centrifuge the mixture again briefly and place on ice.
3. Add 8 μL of the master mix to each sample.
4. Centrifuge the mixture briefly and incubate at 42°C for 60 min (RT reaction) and then at 92°C for 10 min (RT inactivation). The reactions are carried out in the PTC-150 minicycler.
5. Store sample mixtures at –20°C.

3.2.2. Performing Real-Time PCR

1. Create PCR reaction mixtures for each sample in triplicate by combining 0.2 μL cDNA, 0.25 μ*M* of each α1(I) collagen primer, and 12.5 μL 2X Syber Green. Add water to a final volume of 25 μL.
2. Create PCR reaction mixtures for amplification of an endogenous control such as GAPDH in separate to standardize the amount of sample cDNA added to a reaction.

3. In order to exclude the presence of fluorescence contaminants in the sample or in the heating block of the thermal cycler, at least three No Amplification Controls (NAC) as well as three No Template Controls (NTC) are run in each plate. NAC contain sample and no enzyme.
4. The threshold cycle (C_T) value is used for quantification. The C_T is detected when a significant increase in the signal associated with an exponential growth of PCR product occurs during the log-linear phase. The higher the initial amount of genomic DNA, the sooner the accumulated product is detected, and the lower the C_T value. A C_T value of 40 is interpreted as no amplification and this value is not included in subsequent calculations.

3.2.3. Interpreting Results

1. Obtain the difference (ΔC_T) between the C_T values of the target and the normalizer:

$$\Delta C_T = C_T \text{ (target)} - C_T \text{ (normalizer)}$$

The value calculated for each sample is greater than zero unless the target is expressed at a higher level than the normalizer. The untreated (control) sample is used as a reference for each comparison (**Note 3**).

2. The comparative ΔC_T calculation involves finding the difference between the ΔC_T of each sample and the baseline ΔC_T. The ΔC_T values are either less than or greater than zero depending on whether the level of expression increases or decreases.
3. Transform comparative values to absolute values using the formula:

$$\text{Comparative expression level} = 2^{-\Delta CT}$$

3.3. Nuclear Run-On Transcription Assay of α1(I) Collagen

3.3.1. Isolating Nuclei

1. Remove medium from a 150-mm tissue culture dish (four dishes per experimental condition) and wash twice with 10 mL of PBS. Scrape adherent cells off the dishes with a plastic cell scraper in 51 mL of PBS per dish. Transfer the cell suspension to a 50-mL conical tube (**Note 4**).
2. Centrifuge the cell suspension at 500*g* for 5 min. Discard the supernatant and resuspend the cell pellet in 20 mL of ice-cold Tris-HCl buffer by vortexing at half-maximal setting for 5 s.
3. Centrifuge the cell suspension again at 500*g* for 5 min. Discard the supernatant and resuspend the cell pellet in 2 mL of ice-cold lysis buffer by vortexing at half-maximal setting for 5 s.
4. Homogenize the sample with 12 strokes of a Dounce tissue grinder fitted with a tight pestle. At this point, the efficiency of nuclei release may be monitored by phase-contrast microscopy.
5. Transfer the homogenized cell lysate to a 15-mL conical tube and centrifuge at 500*g* for 5 min. Discard the supernatant and resuspend the nuclei (approx 4×10^7

nuclei) in 250 μL of storage buffer by pipetting up and down six times without generating air bubbles.

6. Transfer the nuclei to a microcentrifuge tube. Immediately freeze the sample in a liquid nitrogen bath and store in a liquid nitrogen tank.

3.3.2. Synthesizing and Purifying Nascent RNA

1. Remove the microcentrifuge tube containing the nuclei from the liquid nitrogen tank and thaw on ice in the cold room for 15 min.
2. Start the run-on reaction by adding equal volumes of nuclei and reaction buffer to a microcentrifuge tube. Gently mix the suspension by pipetting up and down three times. Incubate the reaction mixtures in a 30°C heating block for 30 min.
3. Stop the run-on reaction by adding stop buffer and incubating at 37°C for 30 min.
4. Add protease K and protease K buffer and incubate at 42°C for 15 min.

3.3.3. Extracting Newly Synthesized RNA

1. Add an equal volume of water-saturated phenol to the protease K-digested lysate and vortex at maximal speed for 10 s.
2. Centrifuge at maximal speed for 2 min. Transfer the supernatant to a new microcentrifuge tube.
3. Add an equal volume of phenol/chloroform/ether, vortex at maximal speed for 10 s, centrifuge at maximal speed for 2 min, and transfer the supernatant to a new microcentrifuge tube. Repeat.
4. Add 0.1 vol of chloroform, vortex at maximal speed for 10 s, centrifuge at maximal speed for 2 min, and transfer the supernatant to a new microcentrifuge tube.
5. Precipitate the RNA by adding 0.1 vol of 2 *M* NaAcetate and 2.5 vol of 100% ethanol. Vortex at maximal speed for 5 s and incubate in dry ice-ethanol bath for 15 min. Centrifuge at maximal speed for 20 min. Discard the supernatant.
6. Wash the RNA pellet by adding 1 mL 70% ethanol and centrifuging at maximal speed for 5 min. Discard the supernatant.
7. Dissolve the RNA pellet in 90 μL of TE buffer by a combination of vortexing and centrifuging four times at room temperature.
8. Denature RNA by adding 10 μL of 2 *N* NaOH and incubating on ice for 10 min. Neutralize the solution by adding 10 μL of 1 *M* acid-free HEPES.
9. Remove the unincorporated α-^{32}P-UTP in the RNA sample solution using a NucTrap probe purification column according to the manufacturer's protocol.
10. Use 5 μL of the sample to determine the concentration of ^{32}P-labeled RNA using a scintillation counter. Equal counts (10^7 cpm) of ^{32}P-labeled RNA from each experimental condition were used in the slot blot hybridization.

3.3.4. Binding cDNA Plasmids to Nitrocellulose Strips

1. Use 10 μg of cDNA plasmid per slot of the Minifold II slot-blotter.
2. Linearize the cDNA plasmids of elastin, α1(I) collagen, GAPDH, and the pBluescript vector using the restriction enzymes *Eco*RI, *Pst*I, *Eco*RI, and *Hin*dIII, respectively.

3. Denature the digested plasmids by adding 0.1 vol of 3 *N* NaOH and incubating at 65°C for 1 h. After cooling to room temperature, add 20X SSC to a final concentration of 6X SSC. Further dilute the cDNA plasmids to 10 μg per 200 μL with X6 SSC.
4. Apply the sample onto the nitrocellulose membrane using the Minifold II slot-blotter according to the manufacturer's protocol.
5. Mark the edge of the nitrocellulose membrane with a pencil and air-dry overnight.
6. Immobilize the DNA using a vacuum oven set at 80°C for 2 h.
7. Trim the narrow strip of the slot blot containing elastin, α1(I) collagen, GAPDH, and the pBluescript vector along the marked edges.

3.3.5. Hybridization Analysis

1. Place each strip of the slot blot into a 6 × 2 cm RNase-free glass tube with 2 mL of hybridization solution.
2. Prehybridize in a rotating hybridization oven at 42°C for 16 h.
3. For hybridization, remove 0.5 mL hybridization solution from each tube, mix with the RNA probe, and add back to the tube. Incubate at 42°C for 72 h.
4. Wash the slot blots twice with 2X SSC/0.1% SDS at room temperature for 15 min then once with 0.1X SSC/0.1% SDS at 42°C for 30 min. Monitor background radioactivity on the slot blots using a Geiger counter.
5. Dry the slot blots briefly and expose to autoradiography film for 24 to 72 h. If the background noise is unacceptably high, then digestion with DNase-free RNase may be carried out to decrease nonspecific binding.

4. Notes

1. The cell lysate is prepared with the tissue culture dish placed on ice.
2. If the nitrocellulose membrane is allowed to dry, background staining will increase.
3. Results are interpreted by the comparative C_T method (ΔC_T) for relative quantification of gene expression.
4. Isolation of nuclei is performed in a 4°C room using precooled materials.

Acknowledgments

This work was supported by the National Institutes of Health grants K08-HL04232 and R01-HL66547 and the VA Research Enhancement Award Program.

References

1. Prockop, D. J., Kivirikko, K. I., Tuderman, L., and Guzman, N. A. (1979) The biosynthesis of collagen and its disorders (second of two parts). *N. Engl. J. Med.* **301(2),** 77-85.
2. Prockop, D. J., Kivirikko, K. I., Tuderman, L., and Guzman, N. A. (1979) The biosynthesis of collagen and its disorders (first of two parts). *N. Engl. J. Med.* **301(1),** 13–23.

3. Vuorio, E. and de Crombrugghe, B. (1990) The family of collagen genes. *Annu. Rev. Biochem.* **59,** 837–872.
4. Raghow, R., Lurie, S., Seyer, J. M., and Kang, A. H. (1985) Profiles of steady state levels of messenger RNAs coding for type I procollagen, elastin, and fibronectin in hamster lungs undergoing bleomycin-induced interstitial pulmonary fibrosis. *J. Clin. Invest.* **76(5),** 1733–1739.
5. Penttinen, R. P., Kobayashi, S., and Bornstein, P. (1988) Transforming growth factor beta increases mRNA for matrix proteins both in the presence and in the absence of changes in mRNA stability. *Proc. Natl. Acad. Sci. USA* **85(4),** 1105–1108.
6. Stefanovic, B., Hellerbrand, C., Holcik, M., Briendl, M., Aliebhaber, S., and Brenner, D. A. (1997) Posttranscriptional regulation of collagen alpha1(I) mRNA in hepatic stellate cells. *Mol. Cell Biol.* **17(9),** 5201–5209.
7. Doege, K. J. and Fessler, J. H. (1986) Folding of carboxyl domain and assembly of procollagen I. *J. Biol. Chem.* **261(19),** 8924–8935.
8. Wilson, R., Lees, J. F., and Bulleid, N. J. (1998) Protein disulfide isomerase acts as a molecular chaperone during the assembly of procollagen. *J. Biol. Chem.* **273(16),** 9637–9643.
9. Rocnik, E. F., van d, V., Cao, H., Hegele, R. A., and Pickering, J. G. (2002) Functional linkage between the endoplasmic reticulum protein Hsp47 and procollagen expression in human vascular smooth muscle cells. *J. Biol. Chem.* **277(41),** 38,571–38,578.
10. Kivirikko, K. I., Myllyla, R., and Pihlajaniemi, T. (1989) Protein hydroxylation: prolyl 4-hydroxylase, an enzyme with four cosubstrates and a multifunctional subunit. *FASEB J.* **3(5),** 1609–1617.
11. Berg, R. A., Steinmann, B., Rennard, S. I., and Crystal, R. G. (1983) Ascorbate deficiency results in decreased collagen production: under-hydroxylation of proline leads to increased intracellular degradation. *Arch Biochem. Biophys.* **226(2),** 681–686.
12. Rowe, L. B. and Schwarz, R. I. (1983) Role of procollagen mRNA levels in controlling the rate of procollagen synthesis. *Mol. Cell Biol.* **3(2),** 241–249.
13. Schwarz, R. I. (1985) Procollagen secretion meets the minimum requirements for the rate-controlling step in the ascorbate induction of procollagen synthesis. *J. Biol. Chem.* **260(5),** 3045–3049.
14. Fitzgerald, J., Lamande, S. R., and Bateman, J. F. (1999) Proteasomal degradation of unassembled mutant type I collagen pro-alpha1(I) chains. *J. Biol. Chem.* **274(39),** 27,392–27,398.
15. Rishikof, D. C., Ricupero, D. A., Poliks, C. F., and Goldstein, R. H. (1999) Amino acid availability regulates type I procollagen accumulation in human lung fibroblasts. *J. Cell Biochem.* **75(1),** 130–137.
16. Bienkowski, R. S. (1984) Collagen degradation in human lung fibroblasts: extent of degradation, role of lysosomal proteases, and evaluation of an alternate hypothesis. *J. Cell Physiol.* **121(1),** 152–158.
17. Rennard, S. I., Stier, L. E., and Crystal, R. G. (1982) Intracellular degradation of newly synthesized collagen. *J. Invest. Dermatol.* **79(Suppl 1),** 77s–82s.

18. Berg, R. A., Schwartz, M. L., and Crystal, R. G. (1980) Regulation of the production of secretory proteins: intracellular degradation of newly synthesized "defective" collagen. *Proc. Natl. Acad. Sci. USA* **77(8),** 4746–4750.
19. Barile, F. A., Guzowski, D. E., Ripley, C., Siddiqi, Z. A., and Bienkowski, R. S. (1990) Ammonium chloride inhibits basal degradation of newly synthesized collagen in human fetal lung fibroblasts. *Arch Biochem. Biophys.* **276(1),** 125–131.
20. Berg, R. A., Schwartz, M. L., Rome, L. H., and Crystal, R. G. (1984) Lysosomal function in the degradation of defective collagen in cultured lung fibroblasts. *Biochemistry* **23(10),** 2134–2138.
21. Fisher, L. W., Stubbs, J. T., III, and Young, M. F. (1995) Antisera and cDNA probes to human and certain animal model bone matrix noncollagenous proteins. *Acta. Orthop. Scand.* **266 (Suppl),** 61–65.
22. Fisher, L. W., Lindner, W., Young, M. F., and Termine, J. D. (1989) Synthetic peptide antisera: their production and use in the cloning of matrix proteins. *Connect Tissue Res.* **21(1–4),** 43–48.
23. Ririe, K. M., Rasmussen, R. P., and Wittwer, C. T. (1997) Product differentiation by analysis of DNA melting curves during the polymerase chain reaction. *Anal. Biochem.* **245(2),** 154–160.
24. Barsh, G. S., Roush, C. L., and Gelinas, R. E. (1984) DNA and chromatin structure of the human alpha 1 (I) collagen gene. *J. Biol. Chem.* **259(23),** 14,906–14,913.
25. Pfarr, D. S., Rieser, L. A., Woychik, R. P., Rottman, F. M., Rosenberg, M., and Reff, M. E. (1986) Differential effects of polyadenylation regions on gene expression in mammalian cells. *DNA* **5(2),** 115–122.
26. Maatta, A., Ekholm, E., and Penttinen, R. P. Effect of the 3'-untranslated region on the expression levels and mRNA stability of alpha 1(I) collagen gene. *Biochim. Biophys. Acta* **1260(3),** 294–300.
27. Fine, A., Matsui, R., Zhan, X., Poliks, C. F., Smith, B. D., and Goldstein, R. H. (1992) Discordant regulation of human type I collagen genes by prostaglandin E2. *Biochim. Biophys. Acta* **1135(1),** 67–72.
28. Rossert, J., Terraz, C., and Dupont, S. (2000) Regulation of type I collagen genes expression. *Nephrol. Dial Transplant.* **15(Suppl 6),** 66–68.

8

Methods for Assessing the Molecular Mechanisms Controlling Gene Regulation

Richard A. Rippe and Branko Stefanovic

Summary

Regulation of gene expression is a complex process that can be controlled at several steps, including transcription, pre-mRNA splicing and export, mRNA stability, translation, protein modification, and protein half-life. Because transcriptional regulation often involves DNA–protein interactions, several techniques are used, including nuclear run-off assays, DNase I footprinting analysis, and mobility shift assays. Together these assays can determine transcriptional rates, as well as locate, identify, and characterize DNA–protein interactions. Functional analyses to assess the role of specific regulatory regions in gene regulation often requires the introduction of reporter genes under the control of regulatory elements being investigated into mammalian cells. This is often accomplished using transient transfections or, more recently, adenovirally mediated gene delivery. Adenovirus-mediated gene delivery is useful for cells that are difficult to transfect with conventional methods, such as hepatic stellate cells, and when close to 100% of transfection efficiency is needed. Posttranscriptional regulation is often involved in regulating gene expression and may involve mRNA stabilization or translational regulation. Together, these techniques can provide information about which step a particular gene is predominantly regulated. This chapter will detail common methodology used to assess molecular mechanisms involved in controlling gene regulation.

Key Words: Gene expression; gene regulation; mRNA; mRNA stability; transcription; DNase I footprinting; nuclear run-off; mobility shift assay; adenovirus construction; gene delivery; transient transfection; nuclear extract; RNase protection assay; hybridization; actinomycin D; reporter genes.

1. Introduction

Gene expression is a complex process that can be regulated at the level of transcription, pre-mRNA splicing and export, mRNA stability, translation, protein modifications, and/or protein half-life *(1)*. Expression of all genes is probably regulated at most of these steps; however, for some genes one level of regulation is more important and predominant over the others *(2–6)*. Measure-

From: *Methods in Molecular Medicine, Vol. 117: Fibrosis Research: Methods and Protocols*
Edited by: J. Varga, D. A. Brenner, and S. H. Phan © Humana Press Inc., Totowa, NJ

ment of steady-state level of an mRNA by Northern blot, RNase protection assay or reverse transcription polymerase chain reaction (RT-PCR) is one of the most common procedures *(7–9)*. Very often, researchers wrongfully assume that an increase in mRNA observed in these assays is evidence for transcriptional upregulation. Steady-state level of an mRNA is a balance between the rate of synthesis and degradation ***(10)***, so no conclusions about the mechanisms of gene regulation should be made unless direct measurement of the transcriptional rate and mRNA stability are made. The classical assay for determining the transcription rate of a gene is the nuclear run-off assay ***(11,12)***. It is based on freezing transcriptional complexes in isolated nuclei that are already loaded on the genes and then allowing them to complete one round of elongation in presence of radiolabeled UTP. All nascent transcripts get labeled; however, transcripts from the gene under study are assayed by selective hybridization and subsequently quantified. Blocking transcription with Actinomycin D or 5,6-dichloro-1-β-D-ribofuranosylbenzimideazole (DRB) ***(13)*** and measuring the steady-state level of mRNA after several time points measures mRNA stability ***(14)***.

Regulation of gene expression is primarily controlled by specific protein–nucleic acid interactions. A great deal of the work involved in understanding the molecular mechanisms of gene regulation is aimed at locating and characterizing the sites on the nucleic acid where regulatory proteins interact and at identifying the proteins which interact at these sites. Initially, studies are directed at locating general regions involved in gene regulation. Regulatory regions have been located within the 5'-flanking region, introns, and 3'-flanking regions of genes. Additional regulatory elements can be located at considerable distances from the transcription start site of a gene. Initial steps to analyze the molecular mechanisms that control gene regulation involve linking the promoter region of the gene of interest to a reporter gene (i.e., green fluorescent protein [GFP], red fluorescent protein [RFP], luciferase, chloramphenicol acetyltransferase [CAT], β-galactosidase, to mention a few). Subsequently, reporter gene constructs are prepared containing progressive 5' deletions of the promoter region that are used to identify general regions that either positively or negatively influence promoter activity. There are several methods that can be used to generate progressive deletions of the 5' flanking region; however, the utilization of convenient restriction endonuclease sites is the most convenient and commonly used method. Once prepared, the reporter gene plasmids are transiently introduced into cultured cells by a variety of methods. The method outlined as follows describes a lipid-based reagent (of which several commercial forms are available); however, other methods to introduce DNA into cultured cells include calcium phosphate co-precipitation, electroporation, viral transduction (adenoviruses, adeno-associated viruses, retroviruses, lentiviruses), and receptor-mediated endocytosis. Generally, cells are more receptive to one method over another, and optimization of each method is generally required for maximum transfection efficiency. Relevant *cis*-regulatory elements may also be detected as areas of DNase I hypersensitivity in native chromatin. DNase I footprinting analysis is subsequently used to locate the precise location of DNA–protein interactions within the identified regulatory regions. The detection, isolation, and characterization of the proteins that interact with these regulatory regions are further investigated using various modifications of the mobility shift assay.

The inability to efficiently introduce genes into quiescent hepatic stellate cells (HSCs) has limited studies of gene expression in this cell type. However, delivery of genes using adenoviral vectors represents a dramatic advancement in the study of gene expression in HSCs. Adenoviral gene delivery represents a receptor-mediated process and infection with equal multiplicity of infection (MOI) into a given population of cells results in uniform and reproducible gene transfer. Using this technology, we were able to successfully study gene expression in quiescent HSCs only one day after isolation ***(15,16)***. We have shown that using a MOI of 500 more than 95% of HSCs are transduced ***(15,16)***.

The protocols described below have been successfully used in our laboratory to analyze the regulatory regions of several genes ***(17–24)***. This chapter describes protocols for the nuclear run-off assay, mRNA stability determination, transient transfections, and the mobility shift assay as applied to HSCs and the α1(I) collagen gene.

2. Materials

The materials used for the procedures detailed as follows are typically found in most laboratories. A standard microcentrifuge is required along with waterbaths. All electrophoresis equipment, including power supplies, can be obtained from CBS Scientific Company, Inc., Del Mar, CA. An electroporator, available from several companies, is also required for adenoviral construction.

2.1. Nuclear Run-Off Transcription

1. pGEM3zf+ vector (Promega, Madison, WI).
2. pGEM3zf- vector (Promega).
3. Rat α1(I) collagen cDNA.
4. Rat glyceraldehyde-3-phosphate dehydrogenase (GAPDH) cDNA (Ambion, Inc., Austin, TX).
5. Luria broth (LB) medium: 10 g tryptone, 5 g yeast extract, 10 g NaCl; bring to 1 L with water and adjust pH to 7.5. Autoclave.
6. Agarose.
7. Plastic wrap.

8. Hybond-N membrane, (Amersham, Piscataway, NJ).
9. Helper phage R408, (Promega).
10. PEG/NaCl solution: 20% PEG, 1.5 *M* NaCl.
11. Slot or dot blot apparatus.
12. Sodium dodecyl sulfate (SDS)/prot K solution: 2% SDS, 10 m*M* Tris-HCL, pH 7.6, 20 mg/mL proteinase K (Sigma-Aldrich, St. Louis, MO).
13. 20X Saline-sodium citrate (SSC): 3 *M* NaCl, 0.3 *M* sodium citrate.
14. Nuclei isolation buffer A: 10 m*M* Tris-HCl (pH 7.4), 3 m*M* $CaCl_2$, 2 m*M* $MgCl_2$, 1 m*M* dithiothreitol (DTT), 0.1 m*M* phenylmethylsulfonylfluoride, 50 U of RNasin (Promega) per mL, 0.4% NP-40.
15. Nuclei isolation buffer B: 1 *M* Tris-HCl (pH 7.4), 10 m*M* NaCl, 3 m*M* $MgCl_2$.
16. Nuclei storage buffer: 50 m*M* Tris-HCl (pH 8.3), 5 m*M* $MgCl_2$, 0.1 m*M* EDTA, 40% glycerol, 1 m*M* DTT, 0.1 m*M* phenylmethylsulfonyl fluoride, 50 U RNasin per m*L*.
17. 2X Transcription buffer: 300 m*M* KCl, 12.5 m*M* $MgCl_2$, 6.25 m*M* DTT, 0.25 m*M* EDTA, 2 m*M* each ATP, CTP, GTP, 0.5 mCi [^{32}P]α-UTP (3000 Ci/mmol) (*see* **Note 1**).
18. Proteinase K buffer: 2% SDS, 20 m*M* Tris-HCl (pH 7.5), 10 m*M* EDTA.
19. Proteinase K, 20 mg/mL (Sigma-Aldrich).
20. RNase-free DNase I (Roche, Indianapolis, IN).
21. Phenol-chloroform-isoamyl alcohol, 25:24:1.
22. 100% ethanol.
23. 7.5 *M* sodium acetate.
24. DNase I buffer: 10 m*M* Tris-HCl (pH 7.4), 10 m*M* NaCl, 5 m*M* $MgCl_2$, 1 m*M* $CaCl_2$.
25. Hybridization buffer: 50 m*M* piperazine-*N*,*N*9-*bis*-(2-ethanesulfonic acid) (PIPES); pH 6.5, 100 m*M* NaCl, 50 m*M* sodium phosphate (pH 7.0), 1 m*M* EDTA, 5% SDS.
26. Washing buffer A: 5% SDS, 13X SSC.
27. Washing buffer B: 0.1% SDS, 0.13X SSC.

2.2. mRNA Stability

1. Radiolabeled antisense riboprobes to α1(I) collagen mRNA and GAPDH mRNA.
2. RNase A, 10 mg/mL (Sigma).
3. RNase T1 (Sigma) (*see* **Note 2**).
4. Actinomycin D (Sigma) (*see* **Note 3**).
5. RNase buffer: 10 m*M* Tris-HCl, pH 7.5, 5 m*M* EDTA, 300 m*M* NaCl, 40 μg/mL RNase A, 6000 U/mL RNase T1.
6. Diethylpyrocarbonate (DEPC) treated water ***(9)***.
7. RPA hybridization buffer: mix 0.1 vol 10X hybridization buffer (400 m*M* PIPES, pH 6.4, 4 *M* NaCl, 10 m*M* EDTA), 0.1 vol water, 0.8 vol deionized formamide.
8. Yeast t-RNA (10 mg/mL).
9. Solution D: dissolve 25 g of guanidine isothiocyanate, 0.37 g sodium citrate, and 0.25 g sarcosyl in 25 mL DEPC water.
10. Loading dye: 95% formamide, 10 m*M* EDTA, bromophenol blue, xylene cylenol.

2.3. Transient Transfections

1. Purified plasmid DNA.
2. Lipofect-Amine reagent (Gibco-BRL, Gaithersburg, MD).
3. Optimem media (Gibco-BRL).

2.4. Mobility Shift Assays

2.4.1. Preparation of Nuclear Extracts

1. Stock solutions:

Solution	Storage	Sterilization
1 *M* HEPES, pH 7.6	Room temperature (RT)	Autoclave
2 *M* KCl	RT	Autoclave
0.2 *M* EDTA	RT	Autoclave
1 *M* DTT	–20°C	
100 m*M* paramethylsulfonyl fluoride (PMSF) (in isopropanol)	–20°C	
1 *M* Na_2MoO_4	RT	
50% glycerol	RT	Autoclave
1 *M* $MgCl_2$	RT	Autoclave
4 mg/mL aprotinin	–20°C	
4 mg/mL leupeptin	–20°C	
4 mg/mL bestatin	–20°C	

2. Add stock solutions of DTT, sodium molybdate, and the protease inhibitors PMSF, aprotinin, leupeptin, and bestatin, just before using the buffer.
3. Dignam A buffer: 10 m*M* 4-(2-hydroxyethyl)-1-piperazine ethanesulfonic acid (HEPES), pH 7.6, 1.5 m*M* $MgCl_2$, 10 m*M* KCl, 0.5 m*M* DTT, 0.5 m*M* PMSF, 2 µg/mL aprotinin, 0.5 µg/mL leupeptin, 40 µg/mL bestatin, 10 m*M* Na_2MoO_4. Make Dignam A buffer fresh prior to each use and keep on ice.
4. Dignam C buffer: 10 m*M* HEPES, pH 7.6, 25% glycerol, 420 m*M* NaCl, 1.5 m*M* $MgCl_2$, 0.2 m*M* EDTA, 0.5 m*M* DTT, 0.5 m*M* PMSF, 2 µg/mL aprotinin, 0.5 µg/mL leupeptin, 40 µg/mL bestatin and 10 m*M* Na_2MoO_4. Make Dignam C buffer fresh prior to each use and keep on ice.
5. Final concentrations of phosphatase inhibitors for all buffers: 10 m*M* paranitrophenylphosphate (PNPP) (make a 2 *M* stock solution in water), 20 m*M* β-glycerolphosphate (make a 1 *M* stock solution in water), 10 m*M* sodium orthovanadate (for preparation boil a 0.2 *M* stock solution in water until it becomes translucent, pH to 10.0). Phosphatase inhibitors can be obtained from Roche, Indianapolis, IN. Store all stock solutions at –20°C.
6. 10% NP-40 (Sigma) in water.
7. Disposable pestle (cat. no. K749521-1590, Fisher Scientific).

2.4.2. Mobility Shift Assay

1. Single-strand or double-stranded oligonucleotide.
2. 10X Kinase Buffer: 0.5 *M* Tris-HCl, pH 7.5, 0.1 *M* $MgCl_2$, 0.05 *M* DTT.
3. T4 polynucleotide kinase.
4. 10 mg/mL yeast tRNA.
5. 5 *M* ammonium acetate.
6. 75% and 100% ethanol.
7. $[^{32}P]\gamma$-dATP; 6000 Ci/mmol (or 3000 Ci/mmol).
8. 10X Reverse Transcriptase Buffer: 0.5 *M* Tris-HCl, pH 8.3, 0.5 *M* NaCl, 50 m*M* $MgCl_2$, 20 m*M* DTT.
9. 5 m*M* dNTP mix prepared fresh and diluted in water from 100 m*M* stock solutions. Use each of the bases except for the radiolabeled base in the nucleotide mix.
10. $[^{32}P]\alpha$-dCTP, 3000 Ci/mmol.
11. Reverse transcriptase (20 U M-MLV; 10 U AMV) (Gibco-BRL).
12. 10 mg/mL yeast tRNA.
13. Phosphate-buffered saline (PBS): 8 g NaCl, 0.2 g KCl, 1.44 g Na_2HPO_4, 0.24 g KH_2PO_4 in 800 mL water. pH to 7.4, bring volume to 1 L, autoclave.
14. 100 m*M* EDTA.
15. 5 *M* ammonium acetate.
16. 75% and 100% cold ethanol.
17. 30% acrylamide solution (29:1).
18. 0.4X TBE: (1X TBE): 89 m*M* Tris-borate, 2 m*M* EDTA.
19. 10% ammonium persulfate.
20. *N,N,N',N'*-tetramethylethylenediamine (TEMED).
21. Radiolabeled double-stranded oligonucleotide probe (or short DNA fragment).
22. 5 mg/mL poly[d(I-C)] (cat. no. 219 847, Roche) dissolved in water.
23. Cold competitor DNA, either 100 ng/mL or 10 ng/mL (depending on the specific activity of the probe and the amount of competitor desired in the reaction).
24. Nuclear extract (**Subheading 3.7.2.**).
25. Dye mixture: 10 m*M* HEPES, pH 7.6, 10% glycerol, 0.01% bromophenol blue.

2.4.3. Adenovirally Mediated Gene Delivery

2.4.3.1. Construction of Adenoviruses

1. pADTRACK, pADTRACK-CMV, pShuttle, pShuttle-CMV vectors (Stratagene) (*see* **Note 22**).
2. pAdEasy-1 or pAdeasy-2 adenoviral backbone plasmids (Stratagene) (*see* **Note 23**).
3. 293 cells (ATCC).
4. Electrocompetent BJ5183 *Escherichia coli* cells (Stratagene).
5. Chemically competent DH5α *E. coli* cells, subcloning efficiency (Life Technologies).
6. Lipofectamine transfection reagent (Life Technologies).
7. Dulbecco's modified Eagle's medium (DMEM) supplemented with 10% fetal calf serum (FCS).

8. PBS supplemented with 5 m*M* $MgCl_2$.
9. LB and kanamycin LB agar plates.
10. QIAquick PCR purification kit (Qiagen).

3. Methods

The methods described below include making single-stranded DNA for hybridization, slot/dot blotting, nuclear run-off transcription, hybridization of nascent transcripts, and determination of mRNA stability.

3.1. Making of Single-Stranded DNA

*3.1.1. Cloning of Rat α1(I) Collagen cDNA and Rat GAPDH cDNA into Vector for Making Single-Stranded DNA (ss-DNA) (see **Note 4**)*

The 375-nt *Pst*I–*Ava*I fragment from rat α1(I) collagen cDNA (clone py1R1; a gift from David Rowe) was cloned into *Hin*cII–*Pst*I sites of the pGEM 3zf+ (for making sense strand ss-DNA) and pGEM3zf- vector (for making antisense ss-DNA). A 340-nt *Eco*RI–*Hin*dIII fragment of rat GAPDH cDNA was cloned into plasmids pGEM 3zf+ and pGEM 3zf-, respectively (*see* **Note 5**). Antisense ss-DNA (–) binds to transcripts from α1(I) collagen and GAPDH genes. GAPDH is used to normalize the signals in determining the transcription rate. Sense ss-DNA (+) is used as a negative control. The clones were made by standard cloning techniques ***(25)***.

3.1.2. Making ss-DNA

1. Inoculate one tube with 10 mL of LB medium containing 100 μg/mL ampicillin with a single colony from each of the above clones and shake at 37°C for 6 h at 300 rpm.
2. Inoculate four fresh tubes with 5 mL LB medium containing 100 μg/mL ampicillin with 0.5 mL of the first culture of each clone and incubate at 37°C for 1 h at 300 rpm.
3. Add 40 mL of helper phage R408 (2×10^{11} pfu/mL) into each tube and grow at 37°C overnight with vigorous aeration.
4. Pour culture in eppendorf tubes and spin for 10 min at 16,000*g*, pour supernatant in new tube and repeat the spin.
5. Collect the supernatant into new tube and add 300 μL polyethyloene glycol (PEG)/NaCl solution. Incubate 30 min on ice and spin down for 10 min at 16,000*g* (phage pellet containing ss-DNA should be visible).
6. Discard supernatant with suction, spin at 16,000*g* for 1 min and carefully remove all residual liquid. Dissolve pellet by vortexing in 300 μL SDS/Prot.K solution and incubating at 37°C for 1 h, or at room temperature overnight.
7. Check ss-DNA on 1% agarose gel (load 10 μL aliquot).

3.2. Slot/Dot Blotting

1. Place Hybond-N membrane in the blot apparatus, wet with X20 SSC.
2. Mix 2.5 µg of ssDNA containing antisense or sense sequence of α1(I) collagen cDNA and GAPDH cDNA with 200 µL of X20 SSC and blot onto the membrane (*see* **Note 6**).
3. Allow to air dry for up to 1 h or dry at 80°C for 10 min.
4. Wrap Hybond-N+ in plastic wrap and cross-link the DNA to the membrane by placing the membrane DNA-side down on a transilluminator for 2 to 5 min at 312 nm wavelength (*see* **Note 7**). Store the membrane at 4°C until use.

3.3. Nuclear Run-Off Transcription

Nuclei are prepared from 2×10^7 quiescent or activated HSCs (*see* **Note 8**). Purifying nuclei over a sucrose cushion ***(26)*** is not necessary for the nuclear run-off assay. We employed the simple protocol below. Typically, quiescent HSCs result in 5.6×10^6 cpm of radiolabeled transcripts generated, whereas activated HSCs result in approx 6.1×10^6 cpm of radiolabeled transcripts generated (*see* **Note 9**). These are typical yields, although other cell types can produce more or less cpm of radiolabeled transcripts.

1. Incubate the cells for 10 min on ice in 5 mL of nuclei isolation buffer A, transfer into 10 mL Dounce homogenizer and homogenize with 20 to 30 strokes (*see* **Note 10**).
2. Mix samples with 4 vol of nuclei isolation buffer B and centrifuge for 10 min at 500*g*.
3. Suspended the nuclear pellet in 0.4 mL of nuclei storage buffer, flash freeze in liquid N_2, and store at –80°C.
4. Mix 0.4 mL of nuclei (thawed on ice) with 0.4 mL of 2X transcription buffer. Incubate at 30°C for 30 min.
5. Treat the nuclei with 40 U of RNase-free DNase I (Roche, Indianapolis, IN) at 37°C for 15 min.
6. Add 0.8 mL of proteinase K buffer and 16 µL of proteinase K (20 mg/mL) and continue incubation for additional 30 min.
7. Extract the samples with phenol-chloroform, collect the aqueous phase, and precipitate the radiolabeled RNA with 0.5 vol of 7.5 *M* ammonium acetate and 2.5 vol of ethanol at –20°C for at least 1 h. Spin at 16,000*g* for 5 min and wash the pellet with 70% ethanol.
8. Suspend the pellet in 2 mL of DNase I buffer and digest with 200 U of RNase-free DNase I at 37°C for 60 min.
9. Extract with phenol-chloroform and ethanol precipitate as previously described.
10. Dissolve the samples in hybridization buffer and measure radioactivity.

3.4. Hybridization

We use aqueous hybridization buffer, although formamide-based hybridization buffer can be used ***(11,12)***. If the background signals are high, the filter can be incubated with 10 mg/mL RNase A and 350 U/ml RNase T1 which digests unhybridized single stranded RNA resulting in dramatically reduce background signals (*see* **Note 11**).

1. Prehybridize membranes, from **Subheading 3.2., step 4**, at 65°C for 2 h in 2 mL of hybridization buffer. Discard the buffer.
2. Add equal number of counts of quiescent and activated HSC nascent transcripts from the nuclear run-off transcription reactions (**Subheading 3.3.1., step 10**) in 0.2 mL hybridization buffer (*see* **Note 12**).
3. Hybridize in 0.2 mL of hybridization buffer at 65°C for 3 d.
4. Wash membranes once at room temperature for 15 min in washing buffer A.
5. Wash membranes twice at 65°C for 30 min in washing buffer B.
6. Expose membranes to X-ray film at –80°C for 3 to 5 d using an intensifying screen.

3.5. Measurement of mRNA Stability

We use RNase protection assays to quantitate mRNAs because this assay is not sensitive to minor degradation of RNA, unlike Northern blot analysis which is sensitive to mRNA degradation *(7,27)*. The same plasmids used for making ss-DNA can be used for making riboprobes for the RNase protection assay. The probes are made according to standard protocols for in vitro transcription *(28)* and are not described here. Isolation of total RNA is also done according to standard protocols *(25)*. We routinely use Actinomycin D to block transcription and describe the protocol here; however, at 67 μ*M* DRB *(29)* can also be used (*see* **Note 13**).

3.5.1. Treatment of Cells With Actinomycin D

1. Incubate freshly isolated HSCs in suspension with 25 μg/mL of Actinomycin D (*see* **Note 14**) or add Actinomycin D to activated HSCs grown in culture. Prepare as many tubes or plates of cells as the number of time points you want to analyze (*see* **Note 15**). Use at least 3×10^6 cells per time point.
2. Incubate the cells with Actinomycin D for desired time points. Pellet quiescent HSCs by centrifugation at 1500*g* for 2 min and dissolve the cell pellet in 0.5 mL of Solution D. Scrape activated HSCs from the plate, spin as above and dissolve in 0.5 mL Solution D (*see* **Note 16**).
3. Extract total RNA according to standard protocols and measure RNA concentration *(25)*.

3.5.2. RNase Protection Assay

1. Transfer 25 μg of total RNA to an Eppendorf tube, add 10^5 cpm each of α1(I) collagen and GAPDH riboprobes to the same tube and dry in speed-vac (*see* **Note 17**).
2. Dissolve the pellet in 30 μL of RPA hybridization buffer, heat at 95°C for 10 min, and transfer to 50°C water-bath and incubate overnight.
3. Add 300 μL of RNase buffer and incubate at 37°C for 1 h.

4. Add 3 μL of 20% SDS and 3 μL of proteinase K and continue incubation at 37°C for 30 min.
5. Add 10 μg yeast t-RNA. Extract with an equal volume of phenol/chloroform and ethanol precipitate with the addition of 1.0 mL 100% ethanol. Incubate at –20°C for 1 h, centrifuge the sample at 16,000*g* for 10 min, decant the supernatant, and wash the pellet once with 70% ethanol and dissolve in 7 μL of loading dye.
6. Heat at 95°C for 10 min, chill on ice and load on 6% sequencing gel. Load 500 cpm of undigested probes and radiolabeled size markers. Run for 2 h at 1800 V.
7. Expose to X-ray film at –80°C overnight using an intensifying screen or expose the gel to a phosphorimager screen. Quantitate the signal from α1(I) collagen mRNA relative to the signal obtained from GAPDH mRNA in the same lane (*see* **Note 18**).

3.6. Transient Transfections

The introduction of nucleic acid (plasmid DNA) into mammalian cells can be accomplished by several methods, including calcium phosphate precipitation, lipid-based systems, electroporation, and others. The efficiency for each cell type varies and each system will require optimization that entails modifying plasmid DNA concentration, cell density, and vehicle concentration. For HSCs we have successfully introduced plasmid DNA using a commercially available lipid-based system, Lipofect-Amine (Life Technologies, Gaithersburg, MD). In the protocol detailed below 2.5 mL of transfection mix is prepared containing 6 to 8 μg of plasmid DNA (4–6 μg of reporter gene, 2 to 4 μg of plasmid DNA to normalize for transfection efficiency) along with 32 μg of Lipofect-Amine reagent is added per 60-mm dish. Two dishes per plasmid or condition are typically used (*see* **Note 19**). Therefore, 2.5X the amount of transfection mix, 6.25 mL, should be prepared for two 60-mm dishes.

1. Seed 60-mm dishes with 1.5×10^5 HSCs/dish the day before transfection.
2. Make 2.5X transfection mix needed. For two 60-mm dishes, you need 6.25 mL transfection mix containing 15 to 20 μg total plasmid DNA and 80 μg Lipofect-Amine reagent.
3. In two polystyrene tubes, add 3.125 mL of Optimem media (Invitrogen).
4. To one tube, add plasmid DNA.
5. To the second tube, add 40 μL of Lipofect-Amine reagent.
6. Mix the contents of each tube well.
7. Add the contents of the tube containing the Lipofect-Amine reagent to the DNA containing tube.
8. Mix the tube well but gently.
9. Incubate at room temperature for 30 min.
10. Wash cells twice with 5 mL (each wash) with Optimem media.
11. Add 2.5 mL of the transfection mix to the cells.
12. Incubate at 37°C for 8 h.

13. Aspirate transfection mix, add fresh growth media (you do not need to wash the cells), and continue incubating the cells at 37°C.
14. Harvest cell for reporter gene activity after 36 to 48 h.
15. Perform reporter gene assays. The amount of cell lysate to use will depend on the reporter gene assay being used. For luciferase activity, we lyse the cells in 125 µL of cell lysis solution and assay 50-µL aliquots for luciferase activity according to the manufacturer's recommended protocol.

3.7. Mobility Shift Assay

3.7.1. Preparation of Nuclear Extracts

Below is a detailed protocol modified from Schreiber et al. ***(30)*** describing the preparation of nuclear extracts from cultured cells. The method is easily adapted to small pieces of tissue by placing the tissue in an Eppendorf tube and using a disposable Dounce homogenizer to grind the tissue in Dignam A or Dignam C (for whole cell extracts) buffer. If using larger portions of tissue, the procedure describe elsewhere is recommended ***(31)***.

3.7.2. Nuclear Extract Preparation

3.7.2.1. Nuclear Extracts From Cultured Cells

Adherent cells can be grown in tissue culture dishes ranging from 24-well size to 150-mm diameter dishes. Cells grown in suspension can be cultured in volumes ranging from 50 mL to liters. For most applications the use of protease inhibitors (PMSF, aprotinin, bestatin, leupeptin) in the buffers is adequate. If the extracts are to be used for in vitro kinase assays, or if phosphorylation of the protein of interest is important for binding activity, the addition of phosphatase inhibitors (*see* **Subheading 2.4.1.**) to all buffers is required.

1. Remove all but approx 0.5 mL of the growth medium from the cells and scrape the cells from the tissue culture dish using a cell lifter (cat. no. 3008; Costar, Cambridge, MA). Transfer the cell suspension to a microfuge tube. Centrifuge the cells at 1500*g* at 4°C for 5 min. If using nonadherent cells, centrifuge the cell suspension at 1500*g* at 4°C for 5 min. Wash the cells once with PBS and pellet the cells by centrifugation at 1500*g* at 4°C for 5 min. Do not trypsinize the cells as residual trypsin may damage the integrity of the proteins in the nuclear extract.
2. Measure the packed cell volume (PCV) by comparing the volume to a precalibrated microfuge tube, and then decant the supernatant.
3. If the PCV is less than or equal to 100 µL, add 400 µL of ice-cold Dignam A Buffer to the pellet and suspend the cells by pipetting. If the PCV is greater than 100 µL, suspend the cells using a proportional amount of ice-cold Dignam A Buffer.
4. Allow the cells to swell on ice for 15 min.
5. Add 25 mL 10% NP-40 per 400 mL of swelled cells and vortex the tube for 10 s.
6. Immediately centrifuge the cellular homogenate in a microfuge at 16,000*g* at room temperature for 30 s.

7. Discard the supernatant (this contains cytoplasm and RNA; this fraction may be saved for other analysis).
8. The nuclear pellet is lysed by adding 50 µL (or approximately an equal volume of the pelleted nuclei) ice-cold Dignam C Buffer and gently rocking the tube at 4°C for 15 min. To obtain a nuclear extract with a higher protein concentration, use less Dignam C buffer (*see* **Note 20**).
9. Centrifuge the nuclear extract in a microfuge at 16,000*g* at 4°C for 5 min.
10. Collect the supernatant and aliquot into several tubes to prevent repeated freezing and thawing, as this will damage some proteins. Store aliquots at –80°C.
11. Determine the protein concentration of 1 to 4 µL of the extract using the Bradford assay (Bio-Rad Laboratories, Hercules, CA). Typical protein concentrations range from 1 to 10 µg/µL.

3.7.2.2. Nuclear Extracts From Tissue

1. Mince liver on glass plate sitting on ice with a razor blade.
2. Place minced liver into Eppendorf tube with 200 µL of Dignam A Buffer.
3. Homogenize liver with a disposable pestle (Fisher, cat. no. K749521-1590).
4. Allow the cells to swell on ice for 10 min.
5. Add 25 µL of 10% NP-40 and vortex for 10 s.
6. Centrifuge (16,000*g*) at room temperature for 30 s.
7. Discard supernatant (contains cytoplasm and RNA).
8. Lyse the nuclear pellet using 200 µL of Dignam C (volume will vary with pellet size) by incubating for 15 to 30 min on ice (*see* **Note 20**).
9. Centrifuge (16,000*g*) at 4°C for 5 min.
10. Collect supernatant, measure protein concentration, and store at –80°C.

3.7.3. Mobility Shift Assay

3.7.3.1. Probe Preparation

Probes used for the mobility shift assay should be relatively small, to give better separation of DNA–protein complexes from one another and from the free DNA probe in the resolving gel. Short double-stranded oligonucleotides (15–50 bp) are used, but DNA fragments (<200 bp) are also used. Double-stranded oligonucleotides can be labeled using several methods. If the ends of the oligonucleotides are blunt-ended or contain 3'-overhangs, they may be kinased with [^{32}P]γ-dATP using T4 polynucleotide kinase. Double-stranded oligonucleotide with 5'-overhangs may be labeled with [^{32}P]γ-dATP in the same way or by filling in using Klenow fragment or M-MLV or AMV reverse transcriptase (*see* **Subheading 3.7.3.3.**). To label an oligonucleotide using T4 polynucleotide kinase, either single-stranded or double-stranded oligonucleotides may be used in the labeling reaction. Once labeled, single-stranded oligonucleotides can be annealed to the complementary strand prior to use in the mobility shift assay.

3.7.3.2. Labeling Probe Using T4 Polynucleotide Kinase

1. In an Eppendorf tube, add:

   200 ng of double-stranded or single-stranded oligonucleotide
   5 µL [^{32}P]γ-dATP (6000 Ci/mmol [or 3000 Ci/mmol])
   4 µL 10X Kinase Buffer
   1 µL T4 polynucleotide kinase (10 U)
   Water to 39 mL
2. Incubate the reaction at 37°C for 45 min.
3. After incubation, precipitate the reaction mixture with the addition of 1 µL 10 mg/mL yeast tRNA, 40 µL 5 *M* ammonium acetate, 200 µL 100% ethanol.
4. Set at –20°C for 10 min.
5. Centrifuge at 16,000*g* in a microfuge at room temperature for 10 min, then decant the supernatant.
6. Dissolve the pellet in 50 µL water and precipitate again by adding of 50 µL 5 *M* ammonium acetate, and 250 µL 100% ethanol.
7. Incubate at –20°C for 10 min, then centrifuge the tube at 16,000g in a microfuge at room temperature for 10 min. Decant the supernatant, and wash the pellet twice with 1.0 mL 75% ethanol.
8. Dry the pellet in a Speed-Vac, then dissolve it in 100 µL water.
9. Count 1 µL in a scintillation counter.

3.7.3.3. Labeling Probe Using the Fill-In Reaction

This procedure can be used to radiolabel double-stranded oligonucleotides containing 5'-overhangs with either reverse transcriptase (M-MLV or AMV) or Klenow fragment. By precipitating the radiolabeled oligonucleotide with ammonium acetate, free isotope is selectively eliminated from the radiolabeled product.

1. In an Eppendorf tube, add:

   200 ng of double-stranded oligonucleotide
   6 µL [α^{32}P]-dCTP, 3000 Ci/mmol,
   (or other labeled base, depending on the nucleotide sequence of the overhang)
   3 µL 10X RT buffer
   1 µL RT (20 U M-MLV; 10–20 U AMV)
   3 µL 5 m*M* dNTP mix (if label = dCTP, then use dATP, dGTP, dTTP)
   water to 30 µL
2. Incubate the reaction mixture at 37°C for 45 min.
3. After incubation, precipitate the radiolabeled oligonucleotide with the addition of 2 µL 10 mg/mL yeast tRNA, 3 µL 100 m*M* EDTA, 25 µL water, 60 µL 5 *M* ammonium acetate, and 300 µL 100% ethanol.

4. Set the reaction mixture at –20°C for 10 min.
5. Pellet the radiolabeled oligonucleotide by centrifugation at 16,000*g* in a microfuge at room temperature for 10 min, then decant the supernatant.
6. Repeat the precipitation by dissolving the pellet in 60 μL water and adding 60 μL 5 *M* ammonium acetate and 300 μL 100% ethanol to the tube and repeating **steps 4** and **5**.
7. Wash the pellet twice with 1.0 mL 75% ethanol, then briefly dry the pellet.
8. Dissolve in 100 μL TE (10 m*M* Tris-HCl, 1 m*M* EDTA) or water.
9. Count 1 μL in a scintillation counter.

3.7.3.4. Gel Preparation

1. Clean and assemble glass plates (approx w = 165–200 mm; l = 200 mm) using 1.0- to 1.5-mm-thick spacers.
2. Use a 4% native polyacrylamide gel (probes 150–300 bp in size) or a 5% native gel (probes 18–150 bp in size).
3. Use the following table to prepare a gel mixture:

	5% gel	4% gel
30% acrylamide (29:1)	10 mL	8 mL
10X TBE	2.4 mL	2.4 mL
Water	47.2 mL	49.2 mL
10% ammonium persulfate	400 μL	400 μL
TEMED	60 μL	60 μL

4. Quickly pour the gel mixture between the glass plates and let the gel polymerize for 1 to 2 h.
5. Pre-electrophorese the gel using 0.4X TBE as the running buffer for approx 1 h at 200 V, constant voltage. The amperage usually starts out at approx 35 mA, when it drops about in half, to about 15 to 20 mA, the gel is ready to run.
6. After prerunning the gel, discard the running buffer and replace with fresh 0.4X TBE.

3.7.3.5. Binding Reaction

The presence and concentration of $MgCl_2$ and other salts is dependent on the DNA binding protein being assessed. Generally, proteins usually require an optimal salt concentration to bind to DNA between 50 and 200 m*M* KCl/NaCl that needs to be empirically determined. Poly[d(I-C)] in the binding reaction is to capture nonspecific DNA binding proteins from the extract; if using purified protein, omit this. A 10- to 200-fold molar excess of cold competing oligonucleotide is used to confirm the specificity of complex formation. For supershift assays, used to confirm the identity of a protein forming a specific complex, add the antibody after adding the probe (*see* **Note 21**).

1. Prepare an 18 μL binding reaction that contains 2 to 20 μg nuclear extract, 1 to 5 μg poly [d(I-C)], 10 m*M* HEPES, pH 7.6, 50 to 150 m*M* KCl, 0.1 m*M*

EDTA, 1 m*M* DTT, 10% glycerol, 0 to 5 m*M* $MgCl_2$. Mix the reaction mixture after adding each component using a pipet tip; avoid bubbles, as this may damage proteins. Do not vortex binding reactions.
2. Incubate the binding reaction on ice for 10 min.
3. Add 2 μL (20,000 CPM) of the radiolabeled probe diluted in water.
4. Incubate the reaction mixture on ice for 20 min.
5. Add 1.5 μL of dye mixture to each tube.
6. Load 20 μL of the reaction mixture on the nondenaturing pre-run acrylamide gel.

3.7.3.6. Gel Electrophoresis

The low ionic strength of the running buffer (0.4X TBE) increases the affinity and hence the stability of most DNA–protein interactions resulting in longer associations between the two. Pre-electrophorese the gel at 200 V until the initial mA drop in half, then change the running buffer prior to loading the binding reaction samples on the gel. The gel should be run at a constant voltage, 200 V, until the gel dye migrates to approximately three-quarters down the gel (this is dependent on the size of the probe; larger probes can be run longer to allow separation of the complexes). The buffers from the upper and lower compartments should be mixed every 30 min during electrophoresis to keep the pH constant; DNA–protein complexes are very pH-dependent. After electrophoresis, dry the gel and expose gel to X-ray film using an intensifying screen at –80°C overnight.

3.8. Construction of Recombinant Adenoviruses Expressing Gene of Interest

1. Clone the gene of interest into either pAd-TRACK or pAd-Shuttle vector of choice using standard cloning techniques. Plate on Kanamycin containing plates.
2. Verify successful cloning by restriction analysis, PCR, or DNA sequencing.
3. Linearize the clone with *Pme*I restriction enzyme. Verify that the plasmid is cut to completion (*see* **Note 24**).
4. Remove the restriction endonuclease enzyme and buffer from the reaction using QIAquick PCR purification kit (*see* **Note 25**).
5. Mix 0.1 μg of supercoiled pAdEasy-1 and 0.5 to 1.0 μg of linearized pAd-TRACK (or pAd-Shuttle) plasmids in total volume of 6 μL. Add 20 μL of electrocompetent BJ5183 cells and electroporate in 2-mm cuvets at 2.5 kV, 200 ohms, and 25 μF (*see* **Note 26**).
6. Add 1 mL of LB broth, incubate at 37°C for 30 min, centrifuge briefly to pellet bacterial cells, suspend the bacterial pellet in 200 μL of LB, and spread aliquots of the electroporated sample on at least four Kanamycin containing plates. Incubate the plates overnight at 37°C.
7. Pick the 10 smallest growing colonies and incubate in liquid LB with Kanamycin at 37°C overnight.

8. Prepare plasmid minipreps and run aliquots in a 0.8% agarose gel. Run pAd-TRACK plasmid as a control. Select several clones that contain larger plasmids than pAd-TRACK.
9. Verify that these clones contain your gene by PCR analysis. Transform correct plasmids into competent *E. coli* DH5α bacterial cells and plate aliquots of the transformation mixture on Kanamycin containing plates and incubate the plates at 37°C overnight (*see* **Note 27**).
10. Prepare plasmid minipreps from at least two colonies and repeat agarose gel analysis and PCR as described in **step 9**.
11. Cut 4 μg of the selected clones with *Pac*I and transfect the linearized plasmid into 50 to 70% confluent 293 cells grown in 25 cm^2 flasks using LipofectAmine reagent (*see* **Subheading 3.6.**).
12. Incubate the cells at 37°C for 7 to 10 d until plaques expressing GFP appear (*see* **Note 28**).
13. Amplify the adenovirus using standard techniques ***(32,33)*** and verify expression of your protein by Western blot analysis.

3.8.1. Adenoviral Transduction of HSCs

1. Isolate HSCs as previously described ***(20)*** and culture for desired period of time (*see* **Note 29**).
2. Dialyze adenovirus against PBS containing 5 m*M* $MgCl_2$ before adding to the cells.
3. Estimate viral titer by diluting viral stock 1:20 in 0.1% SDS and measuring $OD_{260.}$ One A_{260} unit represents approx 10^{12} virions. There are generally 100 to 300 virions per pfu; therefore, one A_{260} unit contains approx 0.3 to 1.0×10^{10} pfu ***(32)***.
4. Add adenovirus at a MOI of 500 to HSCs (*see* **Note 30**) and incubate for desired period of time.

4. Notes

1. It is critical to use high specific activity [^{32}P]α-UTP.
2. Not all commercially available RNase T1 preparations work in the RNase protection assay. We have had good results with RNase T1 obtained from Sigma.
3. Actinomycin D often comes with impurities. After dissolving in ethanol, measure OD_{460} and calculate the concentration based on the molar extinction coefficient for Actinomycin D. Actinomycin D also tends to precipitate upon storage. Repeat the assessment of the concentration if this happens.
4. Single-stranded DNA hybridizes much stronger to RNA than denatured dsDNA. We strongly recommend making single stranded DNA for run-off assays with HSCs.
5. pGEM3zf+ and pGEM3zf- vectors are identical except that the f1 origin of replication is in opposite orientation. The orientation of the cloned insert relative to the orientation of f1 determines which ss-strand will be produced.
6. Denaturing is not necessary.
7. Alternatively, bake in an oven at 80°C for 2 h.
8. This is a minimal number of nuclei for successful experiment. Do not attempt the assay if you have less nuclei. The more nuclei you use, the better.

9. This is typical yield per 2×10^7 nuclei. If you obtain less cpm, repeat the transcription reaction.
10. Check cell lysis microscopically, if needed; homogenize more until free nuclei are visible. It is helpful to compare the homogenized preparation with a small aliquot of unhomogenized sample to view cell lysis and nuclei release.
11. If the background signals are high, this can be reduced by rinsing the membranes in 100 m*M* sodium phosphate (pH 7.2) and digesting with 10 mg of RNase A and 350 U of RNase T1 per mL at 37°C for 30 min. Then, perform a final rinse of the filter in 100 m*M* sodium phosphate and re-expose the filter to X-ray film or phosphorimager analysis.
12. It is necessary to add equal number of counts. This normalizes the signal to the total transcription rate.
13. For reliable results, it is best to do the experiment using both drugs.
14. Working concentrations of Actinomycin D are from 5 to 25 μg/mL. We have obtained identical results with HSCs using either 10 μg/mL or 25 μg/mL Actinomycin D.
15. Time points must be determined empirically. Collagen mRNA is stable in activated HSCs and fibroblasts, so time points up to 24 h should be taken. GAPDH also decays very little within 24 h. We do not recommend incubation with Actinomycin D longer than 24 h, because of general toxicity to the cells. The same is true for DRB.
16. Trizol reagent can be used instead of Solution D.
17. Both probes are added to the hybridization reaction at the same time. GAPDH serves as a control for the amount, integrity and recovery of the samples.
18. GAPDH mRNA shows almost no decay in HSCs within 24 h of Actinomycin D treatment. It should be used to normalize collagen mRNA signal for quiescent HSCs cells. For activated HSCs, decay of α1(I) collagen mRNA is similar to decay of GAPDH mRNA and the ratio should remain constant.
19. It is best to use at least two plates per condition and average the results obtained from the reporter gene assay.
20. Dislodge the nuclear pellet by sharply flicking the tube with your finger. Do this several times to assure that the pellet is well dislodged to allow for complete nuclear lysis. Alternatively, you can suspend the nuclear pellet in the residual Dignam A buffer by pipetting, then add the Dignam C buffer. It is important to make sure that the nuclear pellet is well disrupted to allow for efficient nuclear lysis. Do not vortex the tube, as this may damage protein integrity.
21. For supershift assays, add 1 to 2 μL of antibody (add more if needed, depending on concentration of the antibody used and the binding affinity of the antibody to the protein being assayed) to the binding reaction 10 min after adding the probe. Incubate the binding reaction containing the antibody for an additional 30 to 60 min on ice. Then add the dye mixture and load the samples on the nondenaturing acrylamide gel. Some antibodies will disrupt complex formation, whereas others will alter the mobility of the DNA–protein complex in the gel, resulting in a "supershifted" complex. Additionally, some antibodies may require pre-incubation with the nuclear extract prior to the addition of the radiolabeled probe.

22. pAd-TRACK vector is used to express gene of interest using its own promoter. pAdTRACK-CMV is used to express promoter-less gene of interest using constitutive cytomegalovirus promoter supplied by the vector. Both vectors express also GFP as an independent transcription unit, which greatly facilitate tracking of viral packaging. pShuttle and pShuttle-CMV are equivalents of the pAd-TRACK vectors, but do not have GFP expression cassette *(3)*. We strongly recommend using pAd-TRACK vectors, because without GFP expression it is difficult to observe generation of a productive virus.
23. pAdEasy-1 allows insertion of genes up to 5.9 kB and propagates in 293 or 911 cells. pAdEasy-2 allows insertion of genes up to 8.6 kB and propagates in 911E4 cells *(3)*. We routinely use pAdEasy-1.
24. It is important that cutting is complete and no supercoiled plasmid remains as this will result in an unacceptable background level of nonrecombinant plasmids after **step 5**.
25. Failure to remove salts from the cutting reaction will cause arching during electroporation.
26. Time constant should be around 4.
27. It is very difficult to grow large amount of recombinant adenoviral backbone plasmids extracted from BJ5183 cells or cut them with restriction enzymes.
28. You must look at the cells with ultraviolet microscope to see GFP expression. Plaques are not clearly discernable under visible light.
29. We successfully transduced HSCs as early as 24 h after isolation *(4)*.
30. Sometimes it is difficult to estimate viral MOI. A pilot experiment where progressively more virus is added to a constant number of cells and assist in determining the percentage of cells that express GFP is useful.

References

1. Lindquist, J. N., Marzluff, W. F., and Stefanovic, B. (2000) Fibrogenesis. III. Posttranscriptional regulation of type I collagen. *Am. J. Physiol. Gastrointest. Liver Physiol.* **279,** G471–476.
2. Stefanovic, B., Hellerbrand, C., and Brenner, D. A. (1999) Regulatory role of the conserved stem-loop structure at the 5' end of collagen alpha1(I) mRNA. *Mol. Cell Biol.* **19,** 4334–4342.
3. Stefanovic, B., Hellerbrand, C., Holcik, M., Briendl, M., Aliebhaber, S., and Brenner, D. A. (1997) Posttranscriptional regulation of collagen alpha1(I) mRNA in hepatic stellate cells. *Mol. Cell Biol.* **17,** 5201–5209.
4. Stefanovic, B., Lindquist, J., and Brenner, D. A. (2000) The 5' stem-loop regulates expression of collagen alpha1(I) mRNA in mouse fibroblasts cultured in a three-dimensional matrix. *Nucleic Acids Res.* **28,** 641–647.
5. Stefanovic, B. and Brenner, D. A. (2003) 5' stem-loop of collagen alpha 1(I) mRNA inhibits translation in vitro but is required for triple helical collagen synthesis in vivo. *J. Biol. Chem.* **278,** 927–933.
6. Stefanovic, B., Schnabl, B., and Brenner, D. A. (2002) Inhibition of collagen alpha 1(I) expression by the 5' stem-loop as a molecular decoy. *J. Biol. Chem.* **277,** 18,229–18,237.

7. Porchet, N. and Aubert, J. P. (2000) Northern blot analysis of large mRNAs. *Methods Mol. Biol.* **125,** 305–312.
8. Joyce, C. (2002) Quantitative RT-PCR. A review of current methodologies. *Methods Mol. Biol.* **193,** 83–92.
9. Henttu, P. (2001) Quantification of mRNA levels using ribonuclease protection assay. *Methods Mol. Biol.* **169,** 65–79.
10. Ross, J. (1996) Control of messenger RNA stability in higher eukaryotes. *Trends Genet.* **12,** 171–175.
11. Li, L. and Chaikof, E. L. (2002) Quantitative nuclear run-off transcription assay. *Biotechniques* **33,** 1016–1017.
12. Srivastava, R. A. and Schonfeld, G. (1998) Measurements of rate of transcription in isolated nuclei by nuclear "run-off" assay. *Methods Mol. Biol.* **86,** 201–207.
13. Chodosh, L. A., Fire, A., Samuels, M., and Sharp, P. A. (1989) 5,6-Dichloro-1-beta-D-ribofuranosylbenzimidazole inhibits transcription elongation by RNA polymerase II in vitro. *J. Biol. Chem.* **264,** 2250–2257.
14. Blaxall, B. C. and Port, J. D. (2000) Determination of mRNA stability and characterization of proteins interacting with adrenergic receptor mRNAs. *Methods Mol. Biol.* **126,** 453–465.
15. Stefanovic, B., Hellerbrand, C., and Brenner, D. A. (1999) Regulatory role of the conserved stem-loop structure at the 5' end of collagen alpha1(I) mRNA. *Mol. Cell Biol.* **19,** 4334–4342.
16. Lang, A., Brenner, D. A., and Rippe, R. A. (2000) Role of NF-kB in hepatic stellate cell activation. *J. Hepatol.* **33,** 49–58.
17. Rippe, R. A., Lorenzen, S.-I., Brenner, D. A., Breindl M. (1989) Regulatory elements in the 5' flanking region and the first intron contribute to transcriptional control of the mouse alpha 1 type I collagen gene. *Mol. Cell. Biol.* **9,** 2224–2227.
18. Brenner, D. A., Rippe, R. A., Veloz, L. (1989) Analysis of the collagen a1(I) promoter. *Nucl. Acids Res.* **17,** 6055–6064.
19. Nehls, M. C., Rippe, R. A., Veloz, L., Brenner, D. A. (1991) Transcription factors NF-I and Sp1 interact with the murine collagen alpha 1(I) promoter. *Mol. Cell. Biol.* **11,** 4065–4073.
20. Rippe, R. A., Almounajed, G., and Brenner, D. A. (1995) Sp1 binding activity increases in activated Ito cells. *Hepatology* **22,** 241–251.
21. Rippe, R. A., Kimball, J., Breindl, M., and Brenner, D. A. (1997) Binding of USF-1 to an E-box in the 3' flanking region stimulates a1(I) collagen gene expression. *J. Biol. Chem.* **272,** 1753–1760.
22. Tugores, A., Magness, S. T., and Brenner, D. A. (1994) A single promoter directs both housekeeping and erythroid preferential expression of the human ferrochelatase gene. *J. Biol. Chem.* **269,** 30,789–30,797.
23. Yata, Y., Scanga, A. E., Gillian, A., Breindl, M., Brenner, D. A., and Rippe, R. A. (2003) The role DNase I hypersensitive sites in a1(I) collagen gene expression following an *in vivo* fibrogenic stimulus. *Hepatology* **37,** 267–276.
24. Reif, S., Lang, A., Lindquist, J. N., Gäbele, E., Scanga, A., Brenner, D. A., and Rippe, R. A. (2003) The role of FAK-PI3-K-Akt signaling in hepatic stellate cell proliferation and type I collagen expression. *J. Biol. Chem.* **278,** 8083–8090.

25. Sambrook, J., Fritsch, E. F., and Maniatis, T. (eds.) (1989) *Molecular Cloning: A Laboratory Manual.* 2nd ed. Cold Spring Harbor Laboratory Press, Cold Spring Harbor, NY.
26. Marzluff, W. F., Jr. (1978) Transcription of RNA in isolated nuclei. *Methods Cell Biol.* **19,** 317–332.
27. Srivastava, R. A. and Schonfeld, G. (1994) Quantification of absolute amounts of cellular messenger RNA by RNA-excess solution hybridization. *Methods Mol. Biol.* **31,** 273–279.
28. Gurevich, V. V., Pokrovskaya, I. D., Obukhova, T. A., and Zozulya, S. A. (1991) Preparative in vitro mRNA synthesis using SP6 and T7 RNA polymerases. *Anal. Biochem.* **195,** 207–213.
29. Zandomeni, R., Mittleman, B., Bunick, D., Ackerman, S., and Weinmann, R. (1982) Mechanism of action of dichloro-beta-D-ribofuranosylbenzimidazole: effect on in vitro transcription. *Proc. Natl. Acad. Sci. USA* **79,** 3167–3170.
30. Schreiber, E., Matthias, P., Muller, M. M., and Schaffner, W. (1989) Rapid detection of octamer binding proteins with 'mini-extracts', prepared from a small number of cells. *Nucl. Acids Res.* **17,** 6419.
31. Rippe, R. A., Brenner, D. A., and Tugores, A. (2001) Techniques to measure nucleic acid-protein binding and specificity: nuclear extract preparations, DNase I footprinting and mobility shift assays, in *Nuclease Methods and Protocols* (Schein, C., ed.), Humana , Totowa, NJ: pp. 459–479.
32. Graham, F. L. and Prevec, L. (1992) Adenovirus-based expression vectors and recombinant vaccines. *Biotechnology* **20,** 363–390.
33. He, T. C., Zhou, S., da Costa, L. T., Yu, J., Kinzler, K. W., and Vogelstein, B. (1998) A simplified system for generating recombinant adenoviruses. *Proc. Natl. Acad. Sci. USA* **95,** 2509–2514.

9

Methods for Measuring TGF-β Using Antibodies, Cells, and Mice

Vladimir Jurukovski, Branka Dabovic, Vesna Todorovic, Yan Chen, and Daniel B. Rifkin

Summary

The transforming growth factor (TGF)-βs are essential in pre- and postnatal development, differentiation and morphogenesis of higher organisms. Quantitation of the levels of TGF-β synthesis, secretion, and activation are crucial for grasping the mechanisms that control these events and ultimately control TGF-β action. Rather than presenting a single method, we describe several methods for measuring active TGF-β in different experimental situations. This is possible as a result of advances in transgenic mice technology that allow in vivo TGF-β measurements in addition to the more established in vitro approaches.

Key Words: TGF-β; measurement; mink lung epithelial assay; luciferase; GFP; ELISA; immunohistochemistry; Smad; transgenic mice.

1. Introduction

Members of the transforming growth factor (TGF)-β super family play significant and important roles in development, cell differentiation, and tissue morphogenesis both in embryonic and adult organisms *(1,2)*. The canonical superfamily members, TGF-β1, -β2, and -β3 *(3–5)*, are the subject of this chapter in which several methods for their measurement are presented.

Unlike most cytokines, mature TGF-β is secreted in an inactive form, and extracellular activation is necessary for the cytokine to exert its biological effects *(6)*. TGF-βs are synthesized as homodimeric proproteins (proTGF-β). Within the trans Golgi, a furin-like protease cuts at a residue approx two-thirds from the N-terminal end of the proprotein, creating two homodimeric peptides that remain noncovalently associated in what is called the small latent complex (SLC) *(7–9)*. This cleavage is referred to as processing to distinguish it from the later release of the active TGF-β from the latent complex, a process we call activation. The smaller peptide is the mature TGF-β, and the larger

From: *Methods in Molecular Medicine, Vol. 117: Fibrosis Research: Methods and Protocols*
Edited by: J. Varga, D. A. Brenner, and S. H. Phan © Humana Press Inc., Totowa, NJ

peptide is the propeptide, also known as the latency-associated peptide (LAP), which has a dual role: to keep TGF-β in an inactive form and to allow binding of the SLC to one of the latent TGF-β binding proteins (LTBP-1, -3, or -4) ***(10–14)***. Disulfide bonds between LAP and the third cysteine rich domain of a single LTBP-1, -3, or -4 results in the formation of a trimeric complex consisting of TGF-β, LAP, and LTBP. This complex is called large latent complex (LLC). Most TGF-β is secreted bound to LTBP as LLC. LTBP targets TGF-β to the extracellular matrix (ECM), sequestering it for later release and activation. The release of mature TGF-β from its latent complex is often called activation, a process that is still not completely understood.

The activation of latent TGF-β is strictly regulated and is critical in the control of the biological activity of the cytokine ***(15)***. Various mechanisms of activation have been described and the activating molecules include proteases, integrins, thrombospondin and reactive oxygen ***(6,16–19)***. As a result of the activation processes, TGF-β is liberated from the latent complex and binds to its receptors, thus triggering a cascade of intracellular signaling events. TGF-β signaling through its receptors is achieved through intracellular phosphorylation of Smad molecules that ultimately enter the nucleus and regulate the expression of specific genes ***(20–22)***. Measurement of TGF-β activity is essential in understanding the intricate processes involved in the regulation of TGF-β activation. However, quantification of TGF-β levels is difficult for several reasons: the molecule is formed in low amounts at the site of action; TGF-β is probably not formed in solution and may never have a very long half-life in its soluble phase; and TGF-β is sticky and can be lost by binding to different surfaces and different extracellular proteins. Here we present several methods for TGF-β quantitation that are reproducible, sensitive, and relatively easy to establish in the lab.

1.1. Detection of Active TGF-β

A number of methods have been developed for the detection and measurement of the active form of TGF-β. These methods were developed based on the known effects of TGF-β on cell behavior, on changes in the phosphorylation status of Smads, and on gene expression. The presence of TGF-β in the extracellular milieu generates cellular responses in culture similar to its effects in normal tissue, thereby creating the possibility for quantification based on cellular assays. Methods developed to quantify TGF-β activation include measurements of decreased epithelial cell proliferation ***(23,24)***, inhibition of endothelial cell migration ***(25)***, decreased plasminogen activator activity ***(26)***, decreased receptor availability, and increased production of plasminogen activator inhibitor (PAI)-1 ***(27)***. Whereas in vitro quantification of TGF-β is relatively simple and precise, reliable measurement of TGF-β levels in tissues is more difficult. In an attempt to provide information on the activity of TGF-β in tissues, several methods have been developed to visualize the presence of active TGF-β either using specific antibodies to the active form of the cytokine or antibodies that recognize the phosphorylated forms of Smad 2 and 3 (pSmad 2/3), which are responsible for the transfer of the TGF-β signal to the nucleus. Finally, the generation of transgenic mice that contain a transgene consisting of the green fluorescent protein (GFP) under control of the TGF-β-responsive element $(CAGA)_{12}$ ***(28)*** provides animals in which TGF-β levels can be visualized directly or indirectly in organs and tissues throughout the animal by measuring GFP expression. These latter methods are semiquantitative but are useful when the activity of TGF-β has to be detected in vivo.

In this chapter, we provide details on several methods used in our laboratory to assess and measure TGF-β activity and distribution. The methods we will discuss are:

1. The mink lung epithelial cell (MLEC) luciferase assay.
2. Immunohistochemical assay for active TGF-β.
3. Immunohistochemical assay for pSmad.
4. Transgenic GFP mice.
5. Enzyme-linked immunosorbent assay (ELISA) for detection of TGF-β.

With both the MLEC luciferase assay and the transgenic GFP mouse assay, changes in TGF-β activity are translated into specific increases or decreases of unique gene products, luciferin or GFP, regulated by PAI-1 promoter elements. These promoter elements contain DNA response sequences that are positively regulated by TGF-β signaling ***(29,30)***. In the individual assays, activation of the promoter drives expression of either luciferase (MLEC assay) ***(31)*** or GFP (GFP mouse assay) ***(30)***. In the in vitro-based MLEC assay, the increase of luciferase expression can be quantified by using standard curves obtained by incubation of the MLEC cells with increasing amounts of recombinant active TGF-β. The measurement of GFP intensities in the transgenic mice, however, are semiquantitative comparisons between the experimental and control animals.

When measuring active TGF-β in cell culture medium, one should keep in mind that usually the detectable levels will be very low, as active TGF-β may be concentrated on the cell surface, where activation occurs ***(12,32,33)***, or may be bound to its receptors and/or ECM. These conditions create low levels of soluble cytokine. The MLEC luciferase assay can partially circumvent the problem of measuring "immobilized" TGF-β as the MLEC can be cocultured with the cells of interest ***(12,34)***. The close proximity of activating and reporter cells reduces, but does not eliminate, some of the aforementioned problems.

Immunohistochemical assays for both pSmad and active TGF-β yield only semi-quantitative measurements of the TGF-β levels in cells and tissues. In the case of antibodies against active TFG-β *(35,36)*, comparisons between the experimental and control samples are assessed by differences in the intensity of staining in individual tissue sections. This method works well in cases where there are significant changes in TGF-β synthesis, secretion, or activation. On the one hand, this method is not recommended for assessing active TGF-β in cells grown on slides, because it is difficult to prevent TGF-β diffusion. On the other hand, assays using anti-pSmad antibodies can be used with both tissue sections and cells grown on slides because of the intracellular nature of the assay—measurement of phosphorylation of Smads—and their translocation to the cell nucleus. Simple counting and comparison of stained nuclei in experimental and control samples provides information on the presence of active TGF-β capable of triggering intracellular signaling.

ELISA assay for detection of TGF-β is a simple method to perform. The availability of "ready-to-use" ELISA plates from several companies makes this technique relatively easy to establish and reproducible in addition to its high sensitivity. The method is based on a quantitative sandwich immunoassay procedure that employs primary antibody to immobilize TGF-β and a secondary antibody to TGF-β that is conjugated with horseradish peroxidase as a reporter molecule.

In all of the above measurements, it is important to include appropriate controls. The measurement of TGF-β must be shown to be specific. In culture systems, and sometimes in whole animals, TGF-β neutralizing antibodies must be included to verify that the measured effect is not the result of other factors present in the system. TGF-β isoform-specific neutralizing antibodies can provide information on the activity of individual TGF-β members. Also, the measurement of increased levels of active TGF-β can be the result of increased TGF-β production and secretion as well as increased TGF-β activation. To distinguish between these possibilities, measurement of the total TGF-β (active + latent) should be done. This measurement is easiest to perform when determining the total TFG-β in conditioned media. The latent TGF-β can be activated by heating *(36)* or by acidification *(32)* of the media, thereby permitting measurement of total TGF-β present.

2. Materials

2.1. General

1. Phosphate-buffered saline (PBS) pH approx 7.3, 137 m*M* NaCl, 2.7 m*M* KCl, 4.3 m*M* Na_2HPO_4, 1.4 m*M* KH_2PO_4. Filter-sterilize and store at 4°C.
2. 100% and 70% ethanol for general tissue culture disinfection and immunohistochemistry.
3. Xylene.

2.2. For Tissue Culture

1. Minimum essential medium (αMEM). Store at 4°C.
2. Dulbecco's modified Eagle's medium (DMEM). Store at 4°C.
3. Fetal calf serum (FCS), store sterile at –20°C. Keep at 4°C after thawing.
4. Bovine serum albumin (BSA). Store at 4°C.
5. Penicillin-streptomycin-L-glutamine (PSG) stock (100X): 20 g/L streptomycin, 50×10^6 U/L penicillin G. 29.2 g/L L-glutamine. Filter-sterilize and store aliquots at –20°C. Keep at 4°C after thawing.
6. Trypsin solution pH 7.2: 0.25% trypsin, 1 m*M* ethylenediamine tetraacetic acid (EDTA). Filter-sterilize and store aliquots at –20°C. Keep at 4°C after thawing.
7. Recombinant TGF-β (R&D cat. no. 240-B-002) stock solution: 5 m*M* HCl, 0.1% BSA, 2 mg/mL TGF-β. Store at 4°C.
8. Neutralizing anti-TGF-β antibodies (R&D cat. no. mAb1835) and nonimmune immunoglobulin (Ig)G. Store as aliquots at –30°C. Keep at 4°C after thawing.
9. Control medium (serum-free medium): to avoid effects of serum constituents, most experiments are conducted in the absence of serum. Serum-free medium contains αMEM or DMEM, depending on the cell type used in each assay, 0.1% BSA, and 1X PSG. Filter-sterilize and store at 4°C.
10. Preparation of test cell conditioned medium: (a) cells are plated at subconfluence in regular growth medium and allowed to attach at 37°C for 2 to 4 h; (b) cells are washed twice with PBS; (c) serum-free medium is added and the cells are incubated at 37°C for 24 h; (d) medium is collected and centrifuged to remove cell debris. The conditioned medium prepared in this way is ready to be tested for the presence and levels of total active TGF-β (*see* **Notes 1–4**).
11. Acid- or heat-activated conditioned medium. Acidification: (a) Acidify the conditioned medium to pH 2.0 with 1 *M* HCl; (b) incubate 1 h at room temperature; (c) neutralize with 1 *N* NaOH. Use immediately. Heat treatment: (a) incubate the conditioned medium for 10 min at 80°C; (b) let the medium cool to 37°C. Use immediately (*see* **Notes 5** and **6**).
12. MLEC permanently transfected with the expression construct p800neoLUC *(29)*.
13. Geneticin stock solution (Invitrogen, Carlsbad, CA): 80 mg/mL in PBS. Filter-sterilize and store at –20°C.
14. Lysis buffer 3X stock solution (Analytical Luminescence, San Diego, CA: Dilute the stock solution 1:3 with dH_2O. Prepare fresh.
15. Assay buffer: prepare fresh from the following stock solutions: 5X luciferin buffer (1 *M* tricine, 5.35 m*M* $[MgCO_3]_4Mg[OH]_2$, 13.35 m*M* MgSO4, 0.5 m*M* EDTA, 166.5 m*M* DTT); 50X ATP (37.5 m*M*); 20X luciferin (16 m*M*). Keep luciferin in the dark (luciferin is rapidly oxidized by exposure to light). Store stock aliquots at –30°C.
16. Luminometer.

2.3. For Immunohistochemistry

1. Tissue fixation: 10% neutral buffered formalin stored at room temperature or 4% paraformaldehyde stored at 4°C (*see* **Note 7**),

2. For frozen sections:
   a. 18% sucrose in water.
   b. Optimal cutting temperature (OCT) compound.
3. Xylene for deparafinizing and dehydrating.
4. Tris-buffered saline (TBS), pH 7.4; 10 m*M* Tris-Hcl, 0.85% NaCl.
5. Bovine testicular hyaluronidase for antigen retrieval (Sigma H-3884). Keep at – 20°C. Prepare fresh at 1 mg/mL in 100 m*M* sodium actetate pH 5.5, 0.85% NaCl.
6. Normal goat serum. Store at –20°C in small aliquots. Keep at 4°C after thawing.
7. BSA (fraction V). Keep at 4°C.
8. Hydrogen peroxide 30% for quenching endogenous peroxidase activity. Keep at 4°C. Prepare 0.6% solution in methanol for quenching before use.
9. Anti-TGF-β antibody LC-30 for detection of extracellular TGF-β at 5 to 10 mg/ mL TBS/1% BSA (*see* **Notes 8** and **9**). Store in small aliquots at –20°C, keep at 4°C after thawing.
10. Polyclonal rabbit anti pSmad2/3 antibody (Santa Cruz Biotechnology) at 1:100 to 1:200 dilutions in TBS. Same storage conditions as for the other antibodies (*see* **Note 8**).
11. Polyclonal rabbit anti-GFP antibody (Invitrogen Life Biotechnology).
12. Vectastain Elite biotinylated goat anti-rabbit IgG kit (Vector Laboratories). Keep at 4°C.
13. ABC reagent provided in the anti-rabbit IgG kit or purchased separately (Vector Laboratories). Prepare fresh at least 30 min before application.
14. Peroxidase substrate 3,3'-diaminobenzidine (DAB). Several premeasured kits are on the market (Sigma DAB tablets, cat. no. D5905 and Vectastain DAB kit, cat. no. sk-4100). The composition of the DAB solution is 0.05% DAB, 0.1% hydrogen peroxide in water, prepared fresh before use.
15. Mayer's hematoxylin for counterstaining (*see* **Note 10**).
16. Permount for slide embedding.

3. Methods

3.1. Cell Culture for MLEC Luciferase Assay

This assay is based on the ability of TGF-β to upregulate PAI-1. A truncated PAI-1 promoter fused to the firefly luciferase reporter gene as the expression construct p800neoLUC was permanently transfected into MLEC *(31)*. The specificity and sensitivity of the assay are a result of the regions in the promoter that produce maximal response to TFG-β *(29)*.

MLEC are grown in DMEM containing 10% FCS, 1X PSG, and 250 μg/mL Geneticin (Invitrogen).

3.1.1. Standard Luciferase Assay (31)

1. Detach MLEC using trypsin and re-suspend at 3×10^5 cells/mL in complete growth medium.

2. Plate in triplicate 50 μL/well (1.5 × 10^4 cells) in 96-well plate (*see* **Note 11**).
3. Allow the cells attach to the plate for 3 to 4 h.
4. Depending on the experimental design, replace the medium with 50 μL of each of the following:
   a. Control medium—to determine the basal levels of TGF-β produced by the transfected MLEC.
   b. Control medium containing increasing concentrations of recombinant TGF-β—to generate a standard curve; this assay can be used to measure TGF-β levels in the 0.2 to 30 pM range ***(31)***.
   c. Conditioned medium from the experimental culture—to measure TGF-β.
   d. Acid- or heat-activated conditioned medium—to measure total (latent plus active) TGF-β.
   e. Conditioned medium with neutralizing anti-TGF-β antibodies or non-immune IgG—to test the specificity of the PAI-1-luciferase induction.
5. Incubate the MLEC for 16 to 20 h at 37°C (*see* **Note 12**).
6. Wash the cells two times with PBS and aspirate all the PBS after the second wash.
7. Luciferase activity can be measured by various assays. In all protocols, cells transfected with the expression plasmid are lysed to release the reporter luciferase protein. ATP and luciferin are added to the lysate in a luminometer. The enzyme catalyzes the ATP-dependent oxidation of the substrate thus emitting light. Below, we describe the protocol used in our laboratory using LumiStar Galaxy Luminometer (BMG Labtechnologies, Inc.) (30). Lyse the cells with 35 μL of 1X cell lysis buffer (Analytical Luminescence, San Diego, CA) for 20 min at room temperature.
8. Transfer 30 μL of the cell extract to an opaque 96-well plate.
9. Two seconds after injection of 100 μL of freshly prepared luciferin buffer containing 800 mM luciferin and 750 μ*M* ATP, emitted light is measured for 3 s (*see* **Note 13**).
10. The luciferase activity is recorded as relative light units (RLU). RLU values are converted to TFG-β activity (pg/mL) using the TGF-β standard curve.

3.1.2. Coculture Assay

1. Detach MLEC and test cells with trypsin and resuspend them separately in complete growth medium at 3 × 10^5 cells.
2. For each sample, plate 4 to 6 wells of MLEC 50 μL/well (1.5 × 10^4 cells) in 96-well plate.
3. Add 50 μL/well (2.5 × 10^4 cells) of test cells (*see* **Notes 14–16**).
4. Add neutralizing anti-TGF-β antibodies to one set of wells to test the specificity of the PAI-1-luciferase induction (*see* **Note 17**).
5. Incubate the coculture for 16 to 20 h at 37°C.
6. Wash the cells two times with PBS and aspirate all of the PBS after the second wash.
7. Lyse the cells and measure TGF-β activity as described in the standard luciferase assay.
8. The luciferase activity is recorded as relative light units (RLU). RLU values are converted to TFG-β activity (pg/mL) using the TGF-β standard curve. The TGF-

β activity in co-culture is compared with the TGF-β activity of the MLEC alone. TGF-β activity induced by different test cells can also be compared.

3.2. Immunohistochemical Measurements

The immunohistochemical assays presented here detect either the active, secreted form of TGF-β, a phosphorylated form of Smad, which correlates with the intensity of the signal coming from TGF-β receptors, or the amount of GFP induced by TGF-β in mouse tissues. The first assay detects active TGF-β regardless of the competency of the cell to respond to TGF-β, because not all cells possess the receptors for proper signal transduction. The detection of pSmad and GFP will identify the subset of cells that have the receptors and successfully transfer the signal to the nucleus. All of the assays have similarities and there is flexibility in their execution depending on the type and source of tissue, fixative used, and the source of the antibody. The protocols presented here can be used as described, but also can be modified or optimized for the specific needs of the investigator.

Because the staining protocols for detection of active TGF-β, pSmad and GFP are comparable, the following protocol is applicable for all antibodies. The antibody LC-30 was developed for detection of active TGF-β *(35)* (*see* **Note 9**). The antibody against pSmad is commercially available from several companies. The conditions described here are for the rabbit polyclonal pSmad2/3 antibody from Santa Cruz Biotechnology (cat. no. sc-11769R). The GFP is detected with rabbit polyclonal antibody (Invitrogen, cat. no. R970-01).

3.2.1. Tissue Fixation

1. Rinse blood from tissues with PBS before fixation.
2. Fix the tissue with either 10% neutral buffered formalin for at least 24 h at room temperature, or with 4% paraformaldehyde overnight at 4°C (*see* **Notes 18–20**).
3. Rinse twice in 70% ethanol and store in 70% ethanol until tissue processing and paraffin embedding.
4. Cut 5-μm sections and place on microscopic slides.

3.2.2. Staining Protocol

1. Deparaffinize the sections for 10 min in xylene (2X) and hydrate them for 3 min each in 100% ethanol (2X), 95% ethanol (1X), 80% ethanol (1X), 70% ethanol and in water.
2. Block endogenous peroxidase by incubating the sections in 0.6% hydrogen peroxide in methanol for 30 min at room temperature (*see* **Note 21**).
3. Quickly rinse the slides four times in distilled water followed by three 3-min washes in TBS/0.1% BSA.
4. Remove as much liquid as possible and circle the sections with a hydrophobic pen (Pap pen, Kiyota International, Inc.).

5. Antigen retrieval: place slides in a humidified chamber and cover the sections with bovine testicular hyaluronidase for 30 min at 37°C (*see* **Notes 22** and **23**).
6. Rinse slides three times for 3 min in TBS.
7. Remove excess fluid and incubate the slides in 1.5% normal goat serum in TBS for 30 min at 37°C in humidified chamber.
8. Remove the blocking solution and apply the antibody diluted in TBS/0.1% BSA at 5 to 10 µg/mL and incubate overnight at 4°C in a well-sealed humidified chamber. Control section should be incubated with normal rabbit serum IgG (*see* **Notes 24–26**).
9. The next day, move the slides to room temperature, check that all of the slides remained moist during the incubation, and wash four times quickly and four times for 3 min in TBS.
10. Remove excess liquid and incubate the slides in humidified box for 1 h at room temperature with the biotinilated goat anti-rabbit IgG secondary antibody prepared according to the instructions of Vectastain Elite Kit. Briefly, 75 µL of normal goat serum and 25 µL of the secondary antibody are added to 5 mL of TBS (no BSA).
11. During this incubation, prepare the ABC reagent by mixing 90 µL each ABC-A and ABC-B (provided with the kit) in 5 mL TBS. This solution should stand at room temperauture at least 30 min before applying to the sections.
12. Wash the slides three times for 3 min in TBS.
13. Remove excess fluid and incubate the slides with the prepared ABC reagent in humidified box for 1 h at room temperature.
14. Wash slides three times for 3 min in TBS.
15. Prepare the DAB solution.
16. Incubate the slides with DAB solution for 2 to 10 min. The development of color should be monitored carefully with a microscope until the desired color intensity is achieved, at which time the slide should be placed in distilled water to stop the reaction.
17. Counterastain with Mayer's hematoxylin for 1 to 2 min (*see* **Note 10**).
18. Put the slides under running water for 5 min.
19. Dehydrate slides by sequential incubation 2 min each in 70% ethanol, 80% ethanol, 95% ethanol, twice in 100% ethanol, and twice in xylene.
20. Cover slip with Permount.

3.3. Assay Using GFP Transgenic Mice

Changes in TGF-β activation and signaling can be directly visualized and quantified in GFP transgenic mice. The availability of transgenic animals in which the GFP gene is under the regulation of TGF-β-sensitive promoter affords the possibility to analyze TGF-β actions in vivo. Because the GFP construct is present throughout the animal, levels of GFP expression can potentially reflect TGF-β action in all organs of the mouse.

Several experimental designs are possible when using the GFP animal model. The simplest is to have TGF-β neutralizing antibodies or chemical compounds that affect TGF-β activation or secretion delivered systemically in experimental GFP animals and compare the changes in fluorescence intensity with the control GFP animals. The second possibility is to breed GFP mice with other genetically modified mice and obtain wild-type, heterozygous, and homozygous animals for the modified gene(s) that at the same time express GFP. This approach will provide information on the consequences of deletion or increased expression of different genes (transgenes) on TGF-β activity in vivo.

A brief description of tissue preparation for direct observation of GFP is presented. This approach can be used in addition or conjunction with the immunohistochemical approach for GFP detection previously described.

1. Mice are sacrificed and tissues of interest collected.
2. Tissues are fixed in 4% paraformaldehyde overnight at 4°C.
3. Subsequently submerge tissues in 18% sucrose for 2 to 3 h (*see* **Note 27**).
4. Embed the tissues in an OCT compound.
5. Cut 5-µm tissue sections.
6. Cover slip with Fluoromount G (Southern Biotechnology, cat. no. 0100-01) (*see* **Notes 28** and **29**).
7. Observe under fluorescent microscope, using a filter with absorbance maximum of 395 nm and emission maximum of 508 nm. Photograph.
8. The quantification of the signal can be preformed visually or by using specialized image analysis software.

3.4. ELISA for TGF-β Measurement

TGF-β levels can be measured by using ELISA assays that are sensitive and reproducible. This method can detect low levels of TGF-β in conditioned medium, serum, and plasma. Availability of pre-made plates form several companies (R&D Systems; Promega Corporation) make the assay reproducible and simple to establish. At the current time, there are ELISA assays available for detection of human, mouse, porcine, and rat TGF-β isoforms. A disadvantage of the assay is that the biological activity of the detected antigen is uncertain.

The assay employs quantitative sandwich enzyme immunoassay technique. The wells of a microplate are coated with either anti-TGF-β antibody or TGF-β soluble receptor type II protein. This represents the immobilized component of the ELISA assay that captures TGF-β from the samples analyzed. After applying the secondary antibody conjugated with reporter enzyme, substrate is added, color is developed, and the intensity of the color is measured and quantified. Because protocols from various companies vary slightly, the protocol described here is based on R&D System's Quantikine® TGF-β1 immunoassay.

1. Prepare all reagents, samples, and standards; activate TGF-β in the samples by acid or heat treatment described above (*see* **Note 30**).
2. Add 200 µL of sample or standard in appropriate diluent per well. Cover with adhesive strip and incubate 3 h at room temperature (*see* **Note 31**).

3. Aspirate each well and wash with 400 μL wash buffer three times. Removal of the wash buffer after each wash improves the performance of the procedure. After the last wash, aspirate wash buffer completely or blot the plate against paper towel.
4. Add 200 μL of TGF-β antibody conjugate in appropriate diluent to each well. Cover with a new adhesive strip and incubate 1.5 h at room temperature.
5. Repeat the aspiration/wash procedure as in **step 3**.
6. Add 200 μL of substrate solution to each well and incubate 20 min at room temperature away from light.
7. Add 50 μL of stop solution to each plate and tap the plate to ensure proper mixing.
8. Determine the intensity of color in a plate reader at 450 nm. Correction readings should be taken at 540 nm and 570 nm to compensate for plate imperfections. These readings should be subtracted from the 450 nm reading. If this correction is not done, the readings at 450 nm may be higher and less accurate.

4. Notes

1. The number of cells and the incubation times needed to produce the conditioned medium may vary according to the experiment and may need to be optimized.
2. Depending on the amount of active TGF-β produced by the cells, the conditioned medium may be concentrated or diluted with fresh control medium for optimal reading within the range of the assay. It should be noted that concentration of the samples can result in loses of mature TGF-β or activation of latent TGF-β.
3. When comparing several samples, normalization of the conditioned medium to either the cell number or cell extract concentration in the culture used to prepare the media is needed.
4. The medium should be used immediately or kept at 4°C for only a short period of time. Repeated freezing and thawing could result in activation of latent TGF-β.
5. The amount of TGF-β in the conditioned medium after acidification or heating may be high (50–200 times the amount of active TGF-β produced by cells). Samples should be diluted in fresh serum-free medium in order to achieve concentrations in the optimal range of the assay.
6. Although heat inactivation is easier to perform, this process can result in protein precipitation.
7. Depending on the tissue and the source of antibody, different fixation agents may give better results.
8. The optimal dilution of the antibody should be determined.
9. Another antibody reported to detect active TGF-β is antigen purified chicken anti-TGF-β1 from R&D Systems, cat. no. AF-101-NA (**37,38**).
10. Other counterstains such as Giemsa, methyl green, or May Grunwald can be used.
11. For statistical purposes each measurement should be done in triplicate.
12. The incubation times should be kept under 20 h to avoid complications in interpretation of the results owing to effects of TGF-β on MLEC proliferation.
13. Both delay and measurement times should be optimized.
14. For statistical purposes, each measurement should be done in triplicate.
15. The optimal ratio of test cells and MLEC should be determined experimentally.
16. Plating the test cells 24 to 48 h in advance may be needed.

17. Different test cells can nonspecifically induce or suppress MLEC luciferase activity.
18. The choice of fixative can affect the specificity of the staining. Therefore, if the use of another fixative is required, optimization of the procedure is necessary.
19. The fixation time with buffered formalin should be increased or decreased depending on the type and size of tissue sample.
20. Bone needs to be decalcified before embedding.
21. This step is necessary when using biotin-labeled secondary antibody and the ABC system. If the secondary antibody is fluorochrom-conjugated or the use of fluorochrom labeled avidin or sreptavidin is planned, this step can be omitted.
22. This step is not always required and depends on the nature of the antigen and the antibody used.
23. Other methods of antigen retrieval can be used, such as microwaving samples in citrate buffer for 10 min.
24. The concentration of the normal rabbit serum IgG should be the same as the concentration of the TGF-β antibody.
25. This step can be performed for 1 h at 37°C, with the possibility that the background staining may increase.
26. The sections should never be allowed to dry, because this may increase nonspecific staining.
27. This step removes excess water that can affect the morphology and quality of tissue sections after freezing. This step can be skipped if the tissue of interest has relatively low water content.
28. This compound has antifade properties that prevent fast bleaching of GFP.
29. Samples should be analyzed shortly after mounting since the GFP signal can fade with time.
30. Serum present in conditioned media contains high levels of latent TGF-β that can result in readings above those of the standards. Dilutions of the samples or use of serum free media can circumvent this problem.
31. The length of incubation differs depending on the system used.

Acknowledgments

This work was supported by grants from the National Institutes of Health.

References

1. Massagué, J. (1990) The transforming growth factor-beta family. *Annu. Rev. Cell Biol.* **6,** 597–641.
2. Tiapale, J., Saharinen, J., and Keski-Oja, J. (1998) Extracellular matrix-associated transforming growth factor-beta: role in cancer cell growth and invasion. *Adv. Cancer Res.* **75,** 87–134.
3. Derynck, R., Jarret, J. A., Chen, E. Y., et al. (1985) Human transforming growth factor-beta complememtary DNA sequence and expression in normal and transformed cells. *Nature* **381,** 701–705.

4. de Martin, R., Haendler, B., Hofer-Warbinek, R., et al. (1987) Complementary DNA for human glioblastoma-derived T cell suppressor factor, a novel member of the transforming growth factor-beta gene family. *EMBO J.* **6,** 3673–3677.
5. ten Dijke, P., Hansen, P., Iwata, K. K., Pieler, C., and Foulkes, J. G. (1988) Identification of another member of the transforming growth factor type beta gene family. *Proc. Natl. Acad. Sci USA* **85,** 4715–4719.
6. Lawrence, D. A. (1991) Identification and activation of latent transforming growth factor beta. *Methods Enzymol.* **198,** 327–336.
7. Lawrence, D. A., Pircher, R., Kryceve-Martinerie, C., and Julien, P. (1984) Normal embryo fibroblasts release transforming growth factor in a latent form. *J. Cell Physiol.* **121,** 184–188.
8. Lawrence, D. A., Pircher, R., and Julien, P. (1985) Conversion of high molecular weight latent beta-TGF from chicken embryo fibroblasts into low molecular weight active beta-TGF under acidic conditions. *Biochem. Biophys. Res. Commun.* **133,** 1026–1034.
9. Gentry, L. E., Lioubin, M. N., Purchio, A. F., and Marquardt, H. (1988) Molecular events in processing of recombinant type 1 pre-transforming growth factor beta to mature polypeptide. *Mol. Cell. Biol.* **8,** 4162–4168.
10. Miyazono, K., Hellman, U., Wernstedt, C., and Heldin, C.-H. (1988) Latent high molecular weight complex of transforming growth factor beta 1. Purification from human platelets and structural characterization. *J. Biol. Chem.* **263,** 6407–6415.
11. Kanzaki, T., Olofsson, A., Moren, A., et al. (1990) TGF-beta 1 binding protein: a component of the large latent complex of TGF-beta 1 with multiple repeat sequences. *Cell* **61,** 1051–1061.
12. Tsuji, T., Okada, F., Yamaguchi, K., and Nakamura, T. (1990) Molecular cloning of the large subunit of transforming growth factor type beta masking protein and expression of the mRNA in various rat tissues. *Proc. Natl. Acad. Sci. USA* **87,** 8835–8839.
13. Yin, W., Smiley, E., Germiller, J., et al. (1995) Isolation of a novel latent transforming growth factor-beta binding protein gene (LTBP-3). *J. Biol. Chem.* **270,** 10147–10160.
14. Giltay, R., Kostka, G., and Timpl, R. (1997) Sequence and expression of a novel member (LTBP-4) of the family of latent transforming growth factor-beta binding proteins. *FEBS Lett.* **411,** 164–168.
15. Theodorescu, D., Caltabiano, M., Greig, R., Reiman, D., and Kerbel, R. S. (1991) Reduction of TGF-beta activity abrogates growth promoting tumor cell-cell interactions in vivo. *J. Cell Physiol.* **148,** 380–390.
16. Munger, J. S., Huang, X., Kawakatsu, H., et al. (1999) The integrin alpha v beta 6 binds and activates latent TGF beta 1: a mechanism for regulating pulmonary inflammation and fibrosis. *Cell* **96,** 319–328.
17. Gleizes, P. E., Munger, J. S., Nunes, I., Harpel, J. G., Mazzieri, R., Noguera, I., and Rifkin, D. B. (1997) TGF-beta latency: biological significance and mechanisms of activation. *Stem Cells* **15,** 190–197.

18. Rifkin, D. B., Gleizes, P. E., Harpel, J,. Nunes, I., Munger, J., Mazzieri, R., and Noguera, I. (1997) Plasminogen/plasminogen activator and growth factor activation. *Ciba Found Symp.* **212,** 105–115; discussion 116–118.
19. Kawabata, M., Imamura, T., Inoue, H., et al. (1999) Intracellular signaling of the TGF-beta superfamily by Smad proteins. *Ann. NY Acad. Sci.* **886,** 73–82.
20. Kawabata, M., Inoue, H., Hanyu, A., Imamura, T., and Miyazono, K. (1998) Smad proteins exist as monomers in vivo and undergo homo- and hetero-oligomerizatian upon activation by serine/threanine kinase. *EMBO J.* **17,** 4056–4065.
21. Stroschein, S. L., Wang, W., and Luo, K. (1999) Cooperative binding of Smad proteins to two adjacent DNA elements in the plasminogen activator inhibitor-1 promoter mediates transforming growth factor beta-induced Smad-dependent transcriptional activation. *J. Biol. Chem.* **274,** 9431–9441.
22. Heimark, R. L., Twardzik, D. R., and Schwartz, S. M. (1986) Inhibition of endothelial regeneration by type-beta transforming growth factor from platelets. *Science* **233,** 1078–1080.
23. Sato, Y. and Rifkin, D. B. (1988) Autocrine activities of basic fibroblast growth factor: regulation of endothelial cell movement, plasminogen activator synthesis, and DNA synthesis. *J. Cell Biol.* **107,** 1199–1205.
24. Danielpour, D., Dart, L. L., Flanders, K. C., Roberts, A. B., and Sporn, M. B. (1989) Immunodetection and quantitation of the two forms of transforming growth factor-beta (TGF-beta 1 and TGF-beta 2) secreted by cells in culture. *J. Cell. Physiol.* **138,** 79–86.
25. Saksela, O., Moscatelli, D., and Rifkin, D. B. (1987) The opposing effects of basic fibroblast growth factor and transforming growth factor beta on the regulation of plasminogen activator activity in capillary endothelial cells. *J. Cell Biol.* **105,** 957-963.
26. Thalacker, F. W. and Nielsen-Hamilton, M. (1992) Opposite and independent actions of cyclic AMP and transforming growth factor beta in the regulation of type 1 plasminogen activator inhibitor expression. *Biochem. J.* **287,** 855–862.
27. Neptune, E. R., Frischmeyer, P. A., Arking, D. E., et al. (2003) Dysregulation of TGF-beta activation contributes to pathogenesis in Marfan syndrome. *Nature Genet.* **33,** 405–411.
28. Keeton, M. R., Curriden, S. A., van Zonneveld, A. J., and Loskutoff, D. J. (1991) Identification of regulatory sequences in the type 1 plasminogen activator inhibitor gene responsive to transforming growth factor beta. *J. Biol. Chem.* **266,** 23,048–23,052.
29. Dennler, S., Itoh, S., Vivien, D., ten Dijke, P., Huet, S., and Gauthier, J. M. (1998) Direct binding of Smad3 and Smad4 to critical TGF beta-inducible elements in the promoter of human plasminogen activator inhibitor-type 1 gene. *EMBO J.* **17,** 3091-3100.
30. Abe, M., Harpel, J. G., Metz, C. N., Nunes, I., Loskutoff, D. J., and Rifkin, D. B. (1994) An assay for transforming growth factor-beta using cells transfected with a plasminogen activator inhibitor-1 promoter-luciferase construct. *Anal. Biochem.* **216,** 276–284.

31. Dennis, P. A. and Rifkin, D. B. (1991). Cellular activation of latent transforming growth factor beta requires binding to the cation-independent mannose 6-phosphate/insulin-like growth factor type II receptor. *Proc. Natl. Acad. Sci. USA* **88,** 580–584.
32. Sato, Y., Tsuboi, R., Lyons, R., Moses, H., and Rifkin, D. B. (1990) Characterization of the activation of latent TGF-beta by co-cultures of endothelial cells and pericytes or smooth muscle cells: a self-regulating system. *J. Cell Biol.* **111,** 757–763.
33. Crawford, S. E., Stellmach, V., Murphy-Ullrich, J. E., et al. (1998) Thrombospondin-1 is a major activator of TGF-β1 in vivo. *Cell* **93,** 1159–1170.
34. Flanders, K. C., Thompson, N. L., Cissel, D. S., et al. (1989) Transforming growth factor-beta 1: histochemical localization with antibodies to different epitopes. *J. Cell Biol.* **108,** 653–660.
35. Brown, P. D., Wakefield, L. M., Levinson, A. D., and Sporn, M. B. (1990) Physicochemical activation of recombinant latent transforming growth factor-beta's 1, 2, and 3. *Growth Factors* **3,** 35–43.
36. Ehrhart, E. J., Segarini, P., Tsang, M. L., Carroll, A. G., and Barcellos-Hoff, M. H. (1997) Latent transforming growth factor beta1 activation *in situ*: quantitative and functional evidence after low-dose gamma-irradiation. *FASEB J.* **11,** 991–1002.
37. Barcellos-Hoff, M. H., Ehrhart, E. J., Kalia, M., Jirtle, R., Flanders, K., and Tsang, M. L. (1995) Immunohistochemical detection of active transforming growth factor-beta *in situ* using engineered tissue. *Am. J. Path.* **147,** 1228–1237.
38. Chong, H., Vodovotz, Y., Cox, G. W., and Barcellos-Hoff, M. H. (1999) Immunocytochemical localization of latent transforming growth factor-β1 activation by stimulated macrophages. *J. Cell Phys.* **178**, 275–283.

III

Studying Fibrosis Using Animal Models

10

Morphological Methods for Assessment of Fibrosis

Rakesh K. Kumar

Summary

Morphological methods can provide valuable spatial information about the development and progression of fibrosis, as well as facilitating efficient assessment of the response to interventions. Morphologically based techniques such as immunohistochemistry and *in situ* hybridization can also contribute to understanding the relationship between cellular expression of mediators and the development of fibrosis. This chapter focuses on simple histological staining methods and morphometric techniques to quantify fibrosis in specific tissue compartments. Issues related to sampling and the use of interactive computer-assisted measurement are discussed, and pitfalls associated with automated measurement are examined.

Key Words: Fibrosis; morphometry; point counting; computer-assisted measurement; Sirius Red stain; reticulin stain.

1. Introduction

Morphological methods are integral to studies of the pathogenesis of fibrosis and the assessment of responses to interventions. Histological examination using appropriate stains for collagen can provide valuable spatial information about the pattern of response, whereas the use of quantitative methods facilitates sensitive assessment of fibrosis within specific compartments of complex tissues. When properly used, apparently simple morphometric techniques can efficiently yield reproducible data that are not easily obtained by other methods *(1)*. Further information may be available using immunohistochemical methods, which permit reliable identification—and thus quantification—of subtypes of collagen or of other matrix components within tissues *(2–4)*. In addition, immunohistochemistry permits assessment of the expression of mediators relevant to fibrosis *(5,6)* and thus provides a link between form and function. Parallel assessment of messenger RNA by *in situ* hybridization can further contribute to understanding the relationship between cellular expression of mediators and the development of fibrosis *(7–9)*. Other morphological

From: *Methods in Molecular Medicine, Vol. 117: Fibrosis Research: Methods and Protocols*
Edited by: J. Varga, D. A. Brenner, and S. H. Phan © Humana Press Inc., Totowa, NJ

methods such as laser capture microdissection can facilitate functional assessment within specific tissue compartments, permitting selective collection of populations of responding cells for further study using, e.g., molecular biological or proteomics techniques *(10–12)*. This chapter focuses on simple methods for quantifying fibrosis.

2. Materials

Picro-Sirius Red solution: dissolve 0.5 g Sirius Red F3B (also known as Direct Red 80, CI 35780) in 500 mL saturated aqueous picric acid. (**Caution:** When dry, picric acid may explode as a result of shock, friction, or fire. It forms unstable salts with many metals. Solutions should be prepared with appropriate precautions and should not be allowed to dry out.)

Modified Harris' hematoxylin: dissolve 100 g potassium alum $AlK(SO_4)_2 \cdot 12H_2O$ in 1000 mL warm distilled water in a large beaker. Dissolve 5 g hematoxylin (CI 75290) in 50 mL absolute ethanol, then add to alum solution and bring rapidly to the boil. (**Caution:** ethanol is flammable. Appropriate precautions must be taken when heating an ethanolic solution.) Add 0.37 g sodium iodate $NaIO_3$ and cool rapidly in an ice bath. When cold, add 40 mL glacial acetic acid. Filter before use. Formation of a precipitate indicates deterioration of the stain.

Scott's Blue: dissolve 3.5 g sodium bicarbonate $NaHCO_3$ and 20 g magnesium sulfate $MgSO_4$ in 1000 mL distilled water.

3. Methods

This section describes a procedure for staining collagens with Sirius Red and introduces basic principles of morphometry.

3.1. Sirius Red Staining for Collagen in Tissue Sections

This technique *(13)* is one of the simplest among the various histological staining methods available for collagens in tissue sections (*see* **Note 1**).

1. Dewax and rehydrate sections through 100% ethanol and 70% ethanol to water.
2. Stain with Picro-sirius red solution for 1 h.
3. Wash with 0.01 *N* hydrochloric acid for 2 min.
4. Wash well with water.
5. Optionally, counterstain with modified Harris' hematoxylin for 1 min, wash in Scott's Blue for 30 s, then wash well with water (*see* **Note 2**).
6. Dehydrate with ethanol, clear with xylene or other appropriate clearing agent, and mount.

Collagen stains bright red (**Fig. 1A**) and exhibits birefringence under polarized light (**Fig. 1B**).

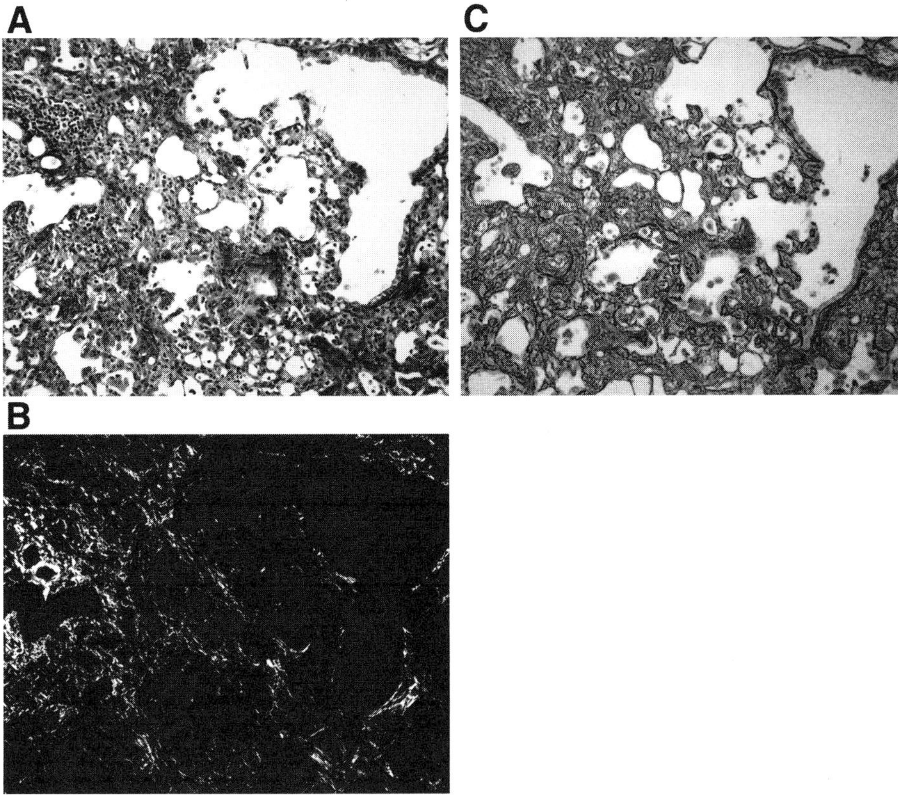

Fig. 1. Pulmonary fibrosis 3 wk after experimental administration of bleomycin to a susceptible strain of mice. (**A**) Sirius Red staining reveals accumulation of multiple foci of collagen fibers. (**B**) Examination of the same section under polarized light is more sensitive and reveals more widespread accumulation of collagen. (**C**) A consecutive section stained with Gordon and Sweet's reticulin stain also demonstrates extensive early fibrosis.

3.2. Quantifying Fibrosis Using Point Counting

Despite the widespread availability of digital image capture and computer-assisted morphometric analysis, point counting remains a valuable and relevant technique for quantifying fibrosis (*see* **Note 3**).

3.2.1. Sampling

Specimen preparation and the approach to sampling are crucial to any quantitative microscopic assessment. As discussed in detail by Weibel, systematic sampling with a random start ensures superior data collection ***(14)***.

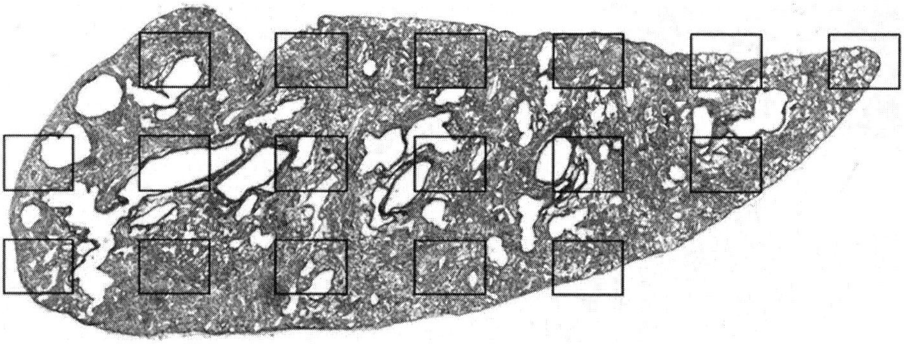

Fig. 2. Low-power micrograph of bleomycin-induced pulmonary fibrosis demonstrating an approach to systematic sampling for morphometry. Each rectangle represents an image examined at high magnification for, e.g., point counting for assessment of fibrosis or enumeration of immunoreactive cells.

For each sample to be examined, a random section and starting position should be selected, followed by sampling of fields at regular intervals, at a suitable magnification to permit observation of the features of interest and a suitable interval to ensure that the entire specimen is sampled within a manageable number of fields (say 10–20). An example of the approach is shown in **Fig. 2** and will work equally well for a patchy or a diffuse process. This approach to sampling is facilitated by a motor-driven stage, but the latter is not a necessity because the Vernier scale on any microscope stage allows reproducible movement in, for example, 1- or 2-mm steps.

3.2.2. Using a Point Counting Grid

A coherent point counting grid consists of uniformly spaced points often, although not necessarily, in a square lattice (*see* **Fig. 3A** for an example). When the grid is overlaid on an image, each point in effect samples an area corresponding to the square of the interval between points. Counting the number of points falling on the tissue component of interest (e.g., Sirius Red-stained collagen) relative to the number falling on the reference component (e.g., renal interstitium, lung parenchyma) thus yields an area fraction of the component of interest relative to the reference component, which is in turn a measure of the volume fraction. No calibration is required.

The simplest way of implementing this approach is with a video camera attached to a suitable microscope. The image is projected on to a monitor and a grid printed on to a transparency sheet is overlaid on the screen. Point counting in each field then allows efficient quantification of fibrosis as a volume fraction (**Fig. 3B**) while permitting the user to rapidly exclude tissue components

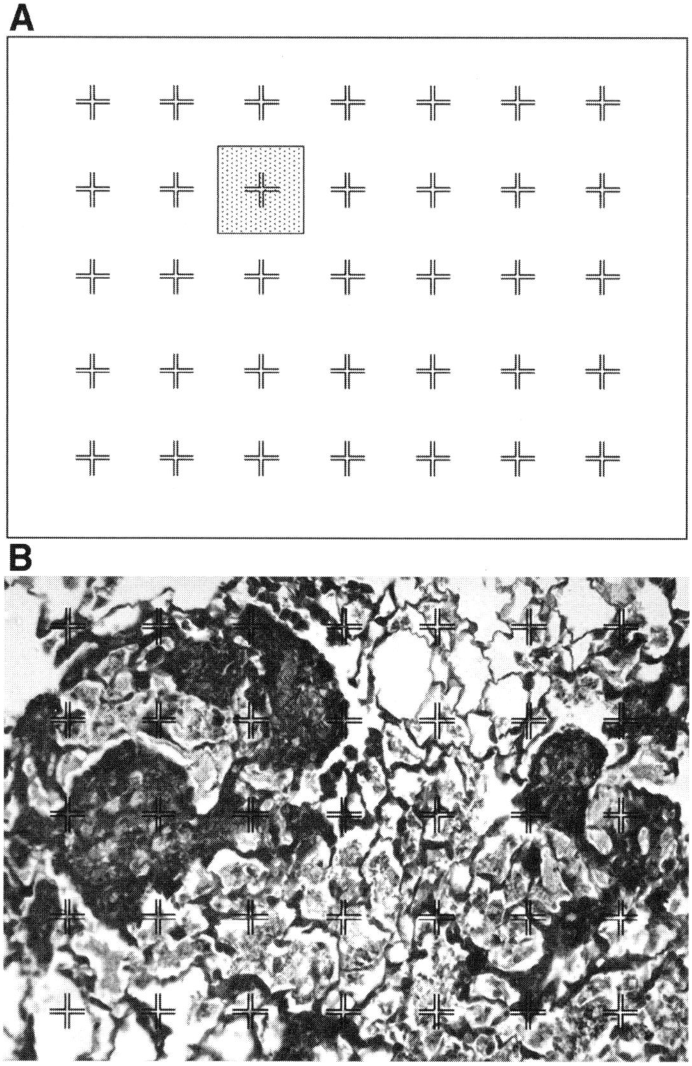

Fig. 3. Using a point counting grid. **(A)** A square lattice of points forming a coherent grid. Each point samples an area around it corresponding to the shaded square. **(B)** The grid applied to a Masson's trichrome-stained section of experimental pulmonary fibrosis induced by intratracheal administration of silica particles.

that are not relevant to the assessment. The author successfully employed this approach in an early study of experimental silicotic pulmonary fibrosis in mice to demonstrate temporal progression of lesions *(15)*. Point counting using a transparent overlay can equally effectively be performed on an image series acquired with a digital camera and is easier than superimposing a computer-generated grid. Note that valid comparison between different experimental groups requires that sample preparation is comparable. Because the number of points falling on the region of interest in the tissue section provides an assessment of the area sampled, it is also possible to use point counting in combination with counting of cellular profiles to obtain an estimate of the numerical density of a cell population within a tissue (*see* **Note 4**).

3.3. Quantifying Fibrosis Using Computer-Assisted Measurement

Interactive computer-assisted measurement is the preferred technique for quantifying length and thickness in microscopic sections. This requires appropriate calibration (*see* **Note 5**).

Various software packages are available to facilitate computer-assisted morphometry but entirely satisfactory results may be achievable with the software supplied with digital cameras intended for use for microscopy. An interactive approach to measurement allows exclusion of technically unsatisfactory fields. Measurement of length or thickness can be performed in an unbiased fashion using an appropriate approach to sampling. For example, in studies from the author's laboratory, subepithelial fibrosis in an experimental model of asthma has been quantified by computer-assisted measurement using three predetermined sampling points in each field and systematically sampling at fixed intervals *(6)*. The approach is illustrated in **Fig. 4**.

Computer-assisted morphometry is accurate and very convenient for a variety of purposes, but the validity of the measurement remains dependent on the appropriate application of technology by the operator. For example, area measurement can be performed using computer-assisted morphometry instead of point counting, but this requires all measurements to be performed on slides stained in a single batch and introduces additional variables such as light source and instrument drift, appropriate and consistent definition of thresholds, and so on. Although such measurement can potentially be automated, an interactive approach permits exclusion of nonrelevant areas or technically unsatisfactory fields *(16)*. There are even more pitfalls associated with computer-assisted morphometry of immunostained sections (*see* **Note 6**).

4. Notes

1. Although extensive accumulation of collagen is usually obvious in routine hematoxylin and eosin-stained sections, a number of staining methods permit improved demonstration of fibrillar collagen. Among the most useful staining methods are Masson's trichrome stain, Sirius Red, and Gordon and Sweet's reticulin stain *(17)*. Masson's trichrome and other trichrome stains such as picro-Mallory or Martius Scarlet Blue yield excellent reproducible staining, but require technical

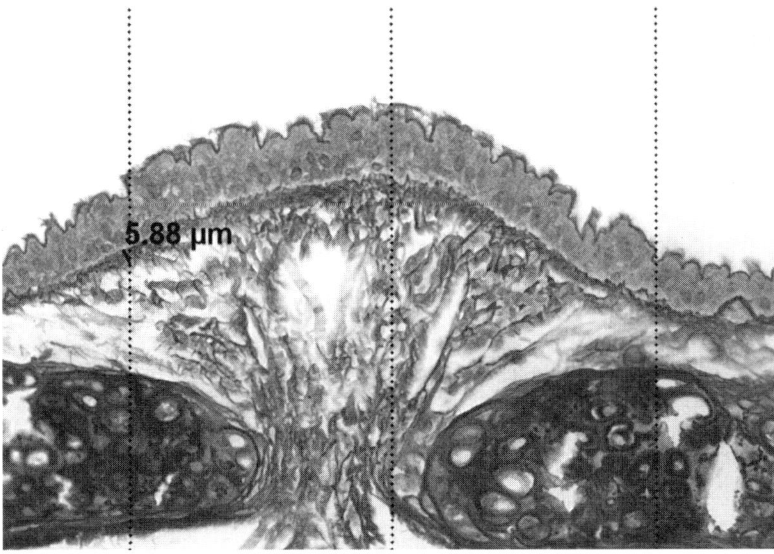

Fig. 4. Computer-assisted measurement of subepithelial fibrosis in an experimental model of chronic asthma in mice. Images were acquired using a Spot™ Cooled Color Digital camera (Diagnostic Instruments, Sterling Heights, MI). In each field, measurements were performed at three points corresponding to the intersections between the fibrotic zone and lines overlaid on the screen. The mouse was used to draw a line defining the beginning and end of the zone, at right angles to the epithelial surface, and a measurement of the thickness was obtained using the Spot software.

skill and should be performed by a specialist histology laboratory. Sirius Red is a much simpler staining method which provides comparable results (**Fig. 1A**) and its sensitivity may be enhanced by examination under polarized light (**Fig. 1B**). The birefringence of collagen fibers stained with Sirius Red is dependent on their pattern of physical aggregation. Type I collagen, which forms thick fibers, typically exhibits red or yellow birefringence, while type III collagen which forms thin (reticulin) fibers is typically green *(17)*. However, differentiation of collagen subtypes is best achieved by immunohistochemistry. A silver impregnation stain for reticulin may be a more sensitive method for demonstrating early fibrosis in tissues (**Fig 1C**).

2. If using an iron hematoxylin stain such as Weigert's hematoxylin, nuclear staining may be performed before staining with Sirius Red. However, picric acid removes staining with an alum hematoxylin such as the modified Harris' hematoxylin described here, hence nuclear staining needs to performed after Sirius Red.
3. Howard and Reed *(18)* make the case for point counting very elegantly: "...the vast majority of biological microscopy images are of low and variable contrast and often phase identification requires both light intensity information and tex-

ture and context (i.e., a human's knowledge)...Therefore, in the majority of biological applications that use conventional transmitted light microscopy, image processing and analysis are easily outclassed in terms of statistical and practical efficiency by manual point counting methods. The fact that the 'tools of the trade' required for volume fraction estimation boil down to a range of transparent point grids shouldn't mask the fact that the method is well founded mathematically and very efficient practically." A number of recently published reports demonstrate the continuing usefulness of point counting for assessment of cardiac, pulmonary and hepatic fibrosis ***(19–21)***.

4. Strictly speaking, this approach yields a profile density per unit area and is subject to error related to variations in section thickness and artefacts resulting from tissue shrinkage. Nevertheless, counting cellular profiles in parallel with point counting is rapid and efficient. The approach was used by the author to quantify immunoreactive T- and B-lymphocytes in silicotic pulmonary fibrosis ***(15)*** and is equally applicable to cells identified by any appropriate morphological technique ranging from enzyme histochemistry to *in situ* hybridization. However, manual counting of cellular profiles is only feasible if the cell type being enumerated is not excessively abundant. A nuclear counterstain is desirable to ensure that only profiles which include a nucleus within the plane of section are counted: this minimizes errors related to the plane of section ***(14)***. When very large numbers of cells are to be counted, computer-assisted enumeration may be more appropriate, or a semilogarithmic scoring system may yield sufficient information ***(22)***.
5. If a calibration slide is not readily available, accurate calibration can be achieved on images of the ruled grid of a hemocytometer chamber. In the outer squares of the grid, each 1 mm^2 region is divided at 250-μm intervals, while in the center square, subdivisions of the smaller 200-μm squares are at 50-μm intervals.
6. When quantifying intensity of immunostaining, it is important to recognize that the choice of reporter reagent and technique has a significant impact on the approach to quantification. Using immunofluoresence, the intensity of emission is directly proportional to the amount of antigen detected in the tissue section. It is therefore legitimate to perform computer-assisted measurement of the area and intensity of immunostaining in digitally captured images, and to quantify staining in terms of the product of these values. In contrast, the amount of insoluble colored reaction product generated by an enzymatically-labeled reporter reagent is not linearly related to the amount of antigen in the tissue. This is especially true for immunoperoxidase staining, because horseradish peroxidase is a suicidal enzyme. Therefore, although computer-assisted measurement of the area of staining above an operator-determined threshold is appropriate, quantifying color intensity is potentially misleading. The degree of immunoreactivity should instead be semiquantitatively assessed by grading, for example grade 0 = no staining, grade 1 = weak staining, grade 2 = moderate staining, and grade 3 = strong staining. Such data must then be analyzed using appropriate nonparametric statistical methods (e.g., a Mann-Whitney test, or a Kruskal-Wallis test followed by Dunn's multiple comparison procedure) ***(23)***. Other

caveats apply to enumeration of immunoreactive cells (or cells otherwise distinguished by some staining characteristic, e.g., using enzyme histochemistry or *in situ* hybridization) using computer-assisted morphometry, which is particularly susceptible to errors related to threshold setting.

Acknowledgment

The author thanks Mr. Gavin McKenzie for assistance with the assessment of various collagen stains and for advice about staining techniques.

References

1. Weibel, E. R. (1990) Morphometry: stereological theory and practical methods, in *Models of Lung Disease: Microscopy and Structural Methods* (Gil, J., ed.), Marcel Dekker, NY, pp. 199–252.
2. Altraja, A., Laitinen, A., Virtanen, I., et al. (1996) Expression of laminins in the airways in various types of asthmatic patients: a morphometric study. *Am. J. Respir. Cell Mol. Biol.* **15,** 482–488.
3. Lazenby, A. J., Crouch, E. C., McDonald, J. A., and Kuhn, C. (1990) Remodeling of the lung in bleomycin-induced pulmonary fibrosis in the rat. An immunohistochemical study of laminin, type IV collagen, and fibronectin. *Am. Rev. Respir. Dis.* **142,** 206–214.
4. Wilson, J. W. and Li, X. (1997) The measurement of reticular basement membrane and submucosal collagen in the asthmatic airway. *Clin. Exp. Allergy* **27,** 363–371.
5. Uh, S. T., Inoue, Y., King, T. E., Jr., Chan, E. D., Newman, L. S., and Riches, D. W. (1998) Morphometric analysis of insulin-like growth factor-I localization in lung tissues of patients with idiopathic pulmonary fibrosis. *Am. J. Respir. Crit. Care Med.* **158,** 1626–1635.
6. Kumar, R. K., Herbert, C., Thomas, P. S., et al. (2003) Inhibition of inflammation and remodeling by roflumilast and dexamethasone in murine chronic asthma. *J. Pharmacol. Exp. Ther.* **307,** 349–355.
7. Broekelmann, T. J., Limper, A. H., Colby, T. V., and McDonald, J. A. (1991) Transforming growth factor beta1 is present at sites of extracellular matrix gene expression in human pulmonary fibrosis. *Proc. Natl. Acad. Sci. USA* **88,** 6642–6646.
8. Zhang, K., Flanders, K. C., and Phan, S. H. (1995) Cellular localization of transforming growth factor-beta expression in bleomycin-induced pulmonary fibrosis. *Am. J. Pathol.* **147,** 352–361.
9. Lee, C. G., Homer, R. J., Zhu, Z., et al. (2001) Interleukin-13 induces tissue fibrosis by selectively stimulating and activating transforming growth factor beta(1). *J. Exp. Med.* **194,** 809–821.
10. Fend, F. and Raffeld, M. (2000) Laser capture microdissection in pathology. *J. Clin. Pathol.* **53,** 666–672.
11. Ornstein, D. K., Gillespie, J. W., Paweletz, C. P., et al. (2000) Proteomic analysis of laser capture microdissected human prostate cancer and in vitro prostate cell lines. *Electrophoresis* **21,** 2235–2242.

12. Specht, K., Richter, T., Muller, U., Walch, A., Werner, M., and Hofler, H. (2001) Quantitative gene expression analysis in microdissected archival formalin-fixed and paraffin-embedded tumor tissue. *Am. J. Pathol.* **158,** 419–429.
13. Junqueira, L. C. U., Bignolas, G., and Bretnani, R. R. (1979) Picrosirius staining plus polarization microscopy, a specific method for collagen detection in tissue sections. *Histochem. J.* **11,** 447–455.
14. Weibel, E. R. (1979) *Stereological Methods.* Academic Press, New York.
15. Kumar, R. K. (1989) Quantitative immunohistologic assessment of lymphocyte populations in the pulmonary inflammatory response to intratracheal silica. *Am. J. Pathol.* **135,** 605–614.
16. De Heer, E., Sijpkens, Y. W., Verkade, M., et al. (2000) Morphometry of interstitial fibrosis. *Nephrol. Dial. Transplant.* **15(Suppl 6),** 72–73.
17. Montes, G. S. (1996) Structural biology of the fibres of the collagenous and elastic systems. *Cell Biol. Int.* **20,** 15–27.
18. Howard, C. V. and Reed, M. G. (1998) Unbiased stereology, in *Three-Dimensional Measurement in Microscopy.* Bios Scientific, Oxford.
19. Dolhnikoff, M., Mauad, T., and Ludwig, M. S. (1999) Extracellular matrix and oscillatory mechanics of rat lung parenchyma in bleomycin-induced fibrosis. *Am. J. Respir. Crit. Care Med.* **160,** 1750–1757.
20. Zaitoun, A. M., Al Mardini, H., Awad, S., Ukabam, S., Makadisi, S., and Record, C. O. (2001) Quantitative assessment of fibrosis and steatosis in liver biopsies from patients with chronic hepatitis C. *J. Clin. Pathol.* **54,** 461–465.
21. Cittadini, A., Monti, M. G., Isgaard, J., et al. (2003) Aldosterone receptor blockade improves left ventricular remodeling and increases ventricular fibrillation threshold in experimental heart failure. *Cardiovasc. Res.* **58,** 555–564.
22. Tedla, N., Palladinetti, P., Kelly, M., et al. (1996) Chemokines and T lymphocyte recruitment to lymph nodes in HIV infection. *Am. J. Pathol.* **148,** 1367–1373.
23. Kumar, R. K., Thomas, P. S., Seetoo, D. Q., et al. (2002) Eotaxin expression by epithelial cells and plasma cells in chronic asthma. *Lab. Invest.* **82,** 495–504.

11

Methods for Measuring Hydroxyproline and Estimating In Vivo Rates of Collagen Synthesis and Degradation

Robin J. McAnulty

Summary

A major pathogenic feature of fibrotic diseases is the excessive and disorganized deposition of collagens. This results from changes in both synthetic and degradative pathways. The post-translational hydroxylation of proline to hydroxyproline and the relative abundance of hydroxyproline in collagens, compared with other proteins, facilitates its use as a relatively specific marker of collagen content and metabolism. This chapter describes in vivo methods for the estimation of collagen synthesis and degradation rates, as well as the proportion of newly synthesised collagen rapidly degraded intracellularly. These pathways have all been shown to play important roles in the altered deposition of collagen associated with the development of fibrosis. The methods are based on the incorporation of radiolabeled proline into collagen as hydroxyproline and its measurement in intact protein and collagen breakdown products. In addition, an accurate and highly sensitive high-performance liquid chromatography method is described for the measurement of hydroxyproline for in vivo and in vitro studies.

Key Words: Collagen; synthesis; degradation; turnover; metabolism; hydroxyproline; fractional synthesis rate.

1. Introduction

The organs and tissues of the body contain a complex extracellular matrix which maintains their structure and plays important roles in their function. The most abundant of the extracellular matrix proteins are the collagens. The content of collagens in a tissue depends on both synthetic and degradative processes. Therefore, any change in the deposition of collagens depends on an alteration in the balance of these processes. In growth and development and wound healing, these processes are tightly regulated to maintain or restore tissue architecture and function. However, in pathologies where fibrosis is a feature, there is a net increase in the deposition of extracellular matrix proteins, including collagens, which are often deposited in a disorganized manner, severely limiting tissue function. Fibrotic diseases affect many organs and tis-

From: *Methods in Molecular Medicine, Vol. 117: Fibrosis Research: Methods and Protocols*
Edited by: J. Varga, D. A. Brenner, and S. H. Phan © Humana Press Inc., Totowa, NJ

sues including, lung, liver, kidney, heart, blood vessels, gut, and skin (*see* **refs. *1–5*** for recent reviews). Increased deposition of collagen or fibrosis can result from increased synthesis, decreased degradation, or a combination of these processes. It is well known that there are major changes in both the synthetic and degradative processes during the development of fibrosis. Therefore, methods have been developed to accurately estimate rates of collagen synthesis and degradation to determine their relative importance in the pathogenesis of fibrosis ***(6–8)***.

The incorporation of proline into pre-procollagen followed by its posttranslational hydroxylation to hydroxyproline has been exploited in the assessment of collagen content and the estimation of rates of collagen synthesis and degradation. The relative abundance of hydroxyproline in collagens, compared with that of other proteins, further facilitates its use as a relatively specific marker of collagen content and metabolism.

The incorporation of radiolabeled proline into protein as hydroxyproline is therefore used to estimate rates of collagen synthesis. In addition, the appearance of radiolabeled hydroxyproline, free or in low molecular weight moieties, in tissues can be measured as an index of the proportion of procollagen which is degraded intracellularly within minutes of its synthesis. This pathway is of importance because in normal tissues, the proportion of newly synthesised procollagen degraded ranges from 10 to 90% of the total procollagen synthesised ***(6,7,9–14)***. Furthermore, the proportion of newly synthesised procollagen degraded has been shown to be regulated during normal growth and aging ***(13,15,16)***, and during various pathologic processes ***(6,9–11,14,17,18)***. Changes in this rapid degradation pathway can therefore make a significant contribution to alterations in collagen deposition. Extracellular degradation of collagens by matrix metalloproteinases also play important roles in regulating collagen content, and an estimate of this can be derived from differences between the rates of collagen synthesis and deposition ***(6,8,16,19,20)***. Alternatively, an index of this process can be obtained from measurements of unlabelled hydroxyproline, free or in low-molecular-weight moieties, in tissues compared with total tissue hydroxyproline ***(6,16)***.

2. Materials

1. L-[U-^{14}C]proline (Amersham Biosciences, CFB71).
2. Dowex 50W-X8 cation exchange resin, 200 to 400 mesh.
3. L-Proline (Sigma, P0380).
4. Phosphate-buffered saline (PBS).
5. Ethanol.
6. Hydrochloric acid (HCl).
7. 0.65-μm filters (Millipore, type DA, pore size 0.65 μm).

8. Powdered charcoal.
9. Trans-4-hydroxy-L-proline (Sigma, H5534).
10. Trans-4-hydroxy-L-proline: 1 mg/mL in 100 μ*M* HCl.
11. L-Hydroxy[2-^{14}C]proline (Amersham Biosciences, custom synthesis).
12. Phenolphthalein pH indicator solution (1% in propan-2-ol).
13. Potassium hydroxide (KOH).
14. Borate buffer: 1 *M* boric acid adjusted to pH 8.7 with 10 *M* KOH.
15. Alanine: 10% aqueous solution adjusted to pH 8.7 with 1 *M* KOH.
16. Chloramine-T: 0.25 *M* in 2-methoxyethanol, make fresh as required.
17. 3.6 *M* Sodium thiosulphate (heat gently to dissolve).
18. Potassium chloride.
19. Toluene.
20. Silicic acid: 200 to 400 mesh.
21. Glacial acetic acid.
22. Ninhydrin solution: 2.5 g ninhydrin mixed with 60 mL glacial acetic acid and 40 mL 6 *M* orthophosphoric acid, make fresh as required.
23. 2,5-diphenyloxazole (PPO).
24. Erhlichs reagent: 5 g 4-dimethylaminobenzaldehyde mixed with 90 mL ethanol and 10 mL of 12 *M* HCl, make fresh as required.
25. Trans-4-hydroxy-L-proline: 25 μ*M* in 100 μ*M* HCl.
26. Potassium tetraborate buffer: 0.4 *M* adjusted to pH 9.5 with HCl.
27. 7-chloro-4-nitrobenzo-2oxa-1,3-diazole (NBD-Cl): 36 m*M* dissolved in methanol. Store protected from light at 4°C. Stable for 1 wk.
28. Sodium acetate: 167 m*M* in 26% acetonitrile (v/v) adjusted to pH 6.4 with orthophosphoric acid.
29. Low dead volume syringe filters (Millipore, type GV, pore size 0.22 μm).
30. High-performance liquid chromatography (HPLC) buffer A: 50 m*M* sodium acetate in 8% acetonitrile adjusted to pH 6.4 with orthophosphoric acid and filtered through 0.22-μm filters.
31. HPLC buffer B: 75% aqueous acetonitrile (v/v) filtered through 0.22-μm filters.

3. Methods

3.1. Purification of Radiolabeled Proline

Commercially available preparations of L-[U-^{14}C]proline contain low levels of radiolabelled contaminants, including hydroxyproline, and must therefore be further purified prior to use.

1. Equilibrate cation exchange columns (1 cm × 50 cm packed with Dowex 50W-X8, 200–400 mesh resin) with 1.5 *M* HCl at a flow rate of 1 mL/min.
2. Load radiolabeled proline and elute with 1.5 *M* HCl at a flow rate of 1 mL/min.
3. Collect fractions of 5 mL and pool samples containing proline, identified by scintillation counting of 10-μL aliquots. Under these conditions, proline usually elutes between 180 mL and 240 mL.

4. Evaporate fractions containing proline to dryness using a centrifugal vacuum concentrator (Savant, Speed-Vac), redissolve in H_2O, and store at 4°C prior to use. Purified solutions can be stored under these conditions for at least 1 mo without any obvious major change in chemical composition.

3.2. In Vivo Incorporation of Radiolabeled Proline Into Collagen and Posttranslational Hydroxylation

1. Animals are injected either intravenously or intraperitoneally with phosphate buffered saline containing both L-[U-^{14}C]proline and unlabeled proline. For rats, the injection solution should contain 1.85 MBq radiolabeled and 1.4 mmol unlabeled proline per 100 g body weight, and for mice 300 KBq radiolabeled and 28 µmol unlabeled proline per 1 g body weight (*see* **Notes 1** and **2**).
2. Animals are killed 30 min after the injection of proline and the exact time from injection to death recorded.
3. Following exsanguination, the vasculature of the tissue of interest is perfused free of blood with ice-cold PBS and the tissue removed, weighed, and rapidly frozen in liquid nitrogen.
4. Tissues may then be stored between –40 and –80°C prior to analysis.

3.3. Preparation of Tissues for Proline- and Hydroxyproline-Specific Radioactivity Measurements

Tissues are processed as indicated in the schematic diagram (**Fig. 1**) and described in detail as follows.

1. Homogenize up to 1 g of preweighed tissue (*see* **Note 3**) in 5 mL of an aqueous solution of ice-cold 67% ethanol using a high-speed mechanical homogenizer (e.g., Ultraturrax). In addition to samples from animals injected with radiolabeled proline, three unlabeled samples are processed for use as assay blanks and to determine assay efficiencies for the recovery of proline and hydroxyproline (*see* **Subheading 3.5.1.**).
2. Wash the homogenizer head with 2.5 mL 67% ethanol and add to the tissue homogenate.
3. Leave to stand at 4°C overnight to precipitate proteins.
4. Centrifuge at 15,000*g* for 30 min at 4°C.
5. Retain the supernatant and resuspend the pellet containing protein twice more in 2.5 mL of 67% ethanol followed by centrifugation as in **step 4** above and combine supernatants from each of the washes with the initial supernatant.
6. Dry the pellet (protein-bound pool) under vacuum and hydrolyse in 2 mL 6 *M* HCl in sealed tubes for 16 h at 110°C.
7. Filter the pooled tissue supernatants (tissue free pool) through a 0.65-µm filter and evaporate to dryness using a centrifugal vacuum concentrator (Savant, Speed-Vac).
8. Dissolve the residue in 1.5 mL H_2O. Transfer two-thirds of this solution (1 mL) to a hydrolysis tube and add HCl to a final concentration of 6 *M*, seal and hydrolyze for 16 h at 110°C. Add 3.5 mL H_2O to the remaining one-third of the solu-

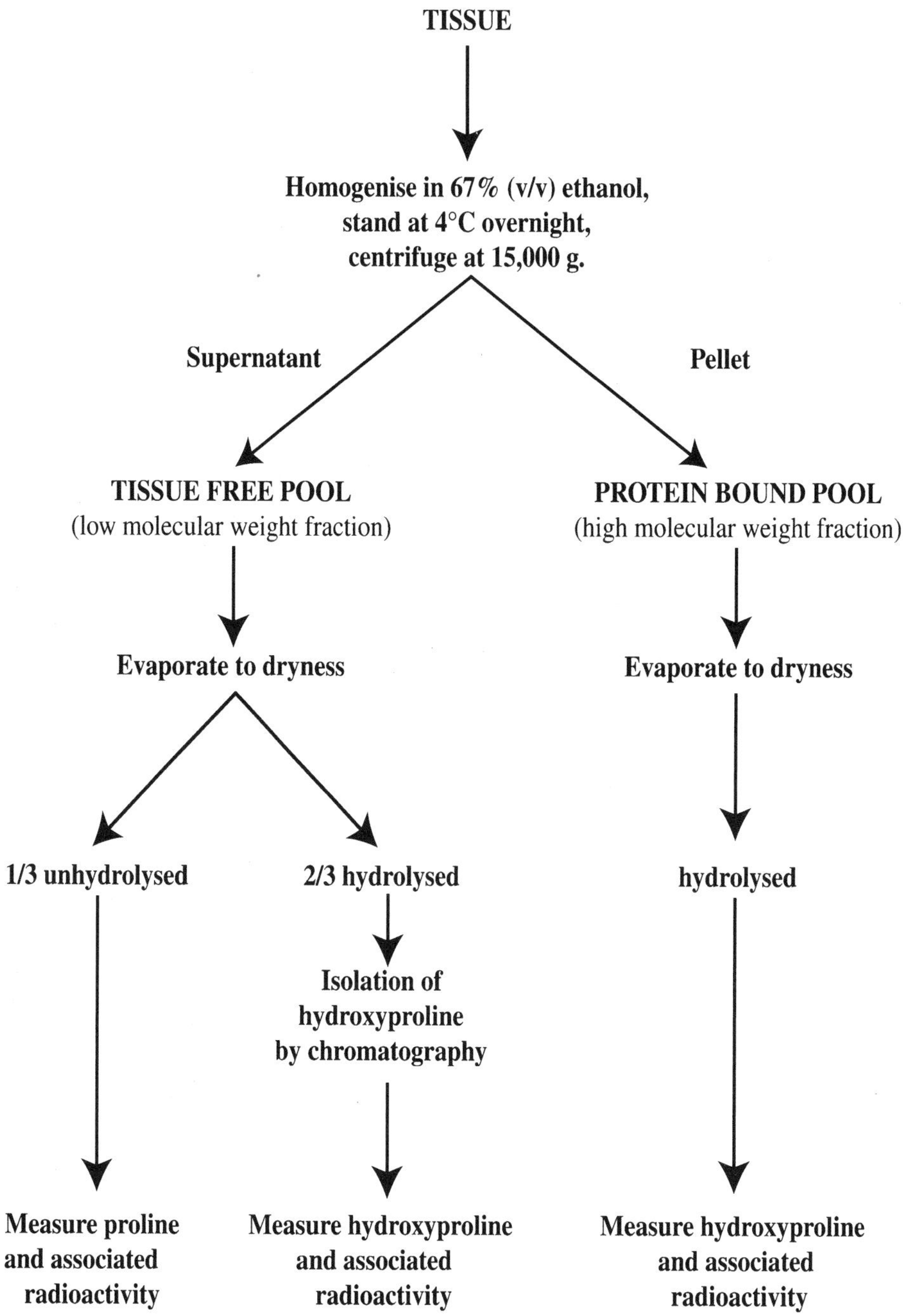

Fig. 1. Schematic diagram for the processing of tissue samples to measure collagen synthesis and degradation.

tion (0.5 mL) and transfer to assay tubes (*see* **Subheading 3.5.1.**) for measurement of tissue-free, proline-specific radioactivity.

9. To decolorize the protein-bound and tissue free pool hydrolysates, add approx 70 mg of charcoal to each sample, mix, and filter through 0.65-µm filters. Wash the filter three times with 1 mL H_2O and combine washings with filtered hydrolyzate. Transfer protein-bound pool samples to assay tubes (*see* **Subheading 3.5.1.**) and isolate tissue-free hydroxyproline by chromatography (*see* **Subheading 3.4.**).

3.4. Isolation of Tissue-Free Hydroxyproline (see Note 4)

1. Dilute the filtrates from the hydrolyzed tissue-free pool to 1.5 *M* HCl by addition of H_2O.
2. Isolate hydroxyproline by cation exchange chromatography as described in **Subheading 3.1.** (*see* **Note 5**). Collect 5-mL fractions and pool samples containing hydroxyproline identified by scintillation counting of 100-µL aliquots. Under these conditions, hydroxyproline elutes between 90 and 120 mL.
3. Evaporate fractions containing hydroxyproline to dryness using a centrifugal vacuum concentrator (Savant, Speed-Vac), redissolve in 4 mL H_2O, and transfer to assay tubes (*see* **Subheading 3.5.1.**).

3.5. Measurements of Proline, Hydroxyproline, and Their Specific Radioactivities

The amounts of proline and hydroxyproline, as well as their associated radioactivity in the tissue fractions, are measured using a method based on that of Stegemann *(21)* with a number of modifications *(7,22–27)*. The method involves the oxidation of proline and hydroxyproline to toluene-extractable products as illustrated in **Fig. 2** and described in detail as follows.

3.5.1. Oxidation of Proline and Hydroxyproline, and Extraction of Their Oxidation Products

1. Transfer samples for tissue-free, proline-specific radioactivity measurements (**Subheading 3.3.**), protein-bound (**Subheading 3.3.**), and tissue-free (**Subheading 3.4.**) hydroxyproline-specific radioactivity measurements to glass assay tubes with Teflon-lined screw caps (Pyrex, 20 mm × 200 mm).
2. Generate a standard curve for hydroxyproline with assay tubes containing 0, 5, 10, 20, 40, 60, 80, and 100 µg hydroxyproline from a stock solution of trans-4-hydroxy-L-proline (1 mg/mL in 100 µ*M* HCl).
3. In each assay, three nonradiolabeled samples are included for tissue-free pool or protein-bound pool hydrolyzates for calculation of extraction efficiencies of proline and hydroxyproline. To two of these tubes, a known amount of either L-[U-^{14}C]proline (nominally containing 60,000 dpm, approx 1 KBq) or L-hydroxy-[2-^{14}C]proline (nominally 60,000 dpm) is added (*see* **Note 6**). The remaining blank sample is used to determine background radioactivity for the assay. L-Hydroxy[2-^{14}C]proline (nominally 60,000 dpm) is also added to the tubes containing the top two concentrations of the hydroxyproline standard curve.

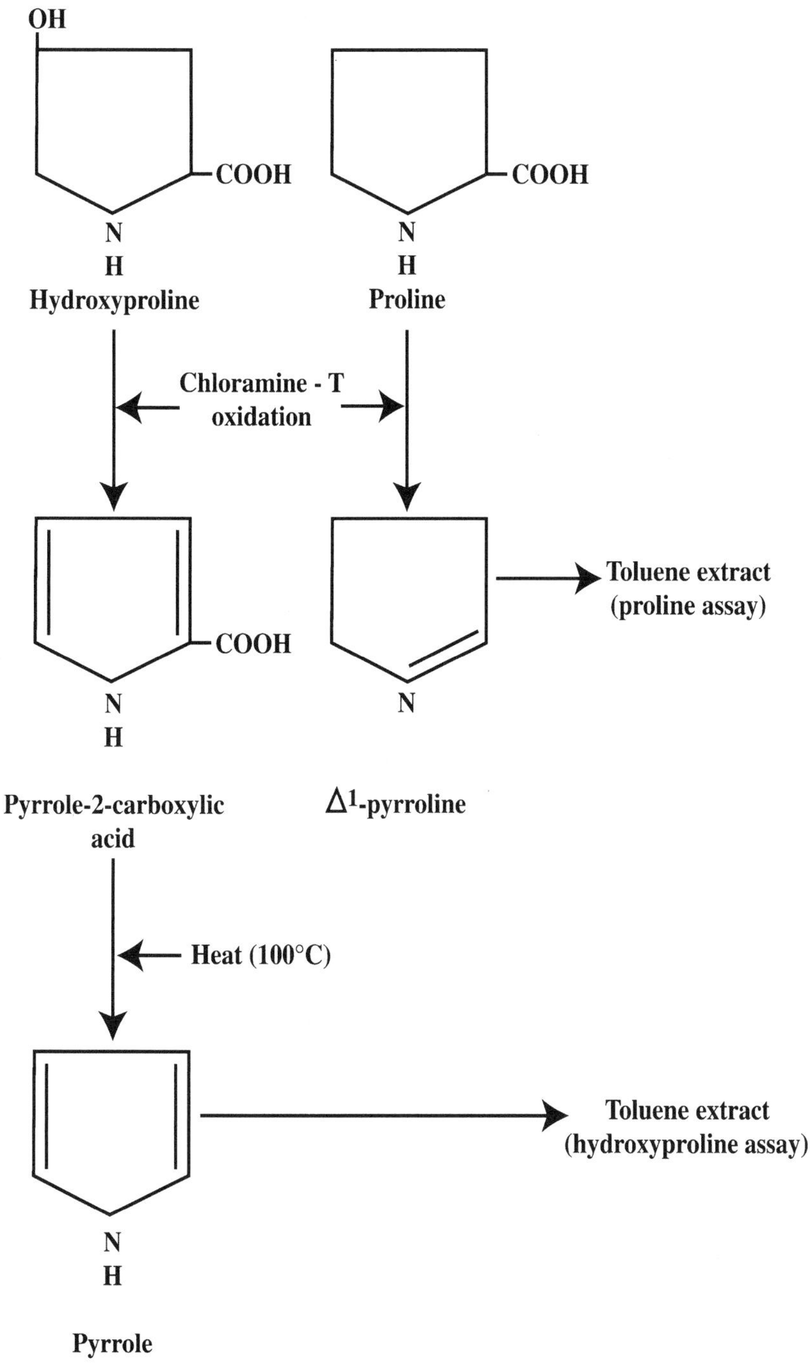

Fig. 2. Chemical reactions involved in the assay of proline and hydroxyproline.

4. Add 50 µL of phenolphthalein pH indicator solution (1% in propan-2-ol) to each tube.
5. Adjust the pH to between 8.3 and 8.9 by alternating dropwise addition of decreasing concentrations of 1 *M* KOH, 1 *M* HCl, 0.3 *M* KOH, and 0.1 *M* HCl until a pale pink color is obtained indicating the correct pH. Mix and check color. Readjust pH if necessary.
6. Equalize the volumes in the tubes with H_2O.
7. Adjust to pH 8.7 by addition of 2 mL borate buffer.
8. Add 1 mL alanine solution and mix.
9. Timed chloramine-T oxidation reaction:
   a. Treat samples in groups of four.
   b. Over a 60-s interval, add 2 mL chloramine-T solution to each of four samples in the group and vortex each tube vigorously.
   c. At the end of 60 s, repeat process with next set of samples and continue in 60-s cycles until all samples are processed.
   d. After 20 min, stop the reaction by addition of 6 mL 3.6 *M* sodium thiosulfate to each of four samples over 60 s and vortex each tube vigorously.
   e. Repeat until oxidation reaction is stopped in all samples.
10. Saturate each sample with KCl.
11. Add 10 mL toluene.
12. Cap tightly and shake vigorously for 10 min on a horizontal shaker.
13. Allow the aqueous and solvent phases to separate.
14. Remove the upper solvent phase taking care not to remove any of the aqueous phase and retain for measurement of the oxidation product of proline, Δ^1 pyrroline (*see* **Subheading 3.5.2.**). Tubes containing the unhydrolyzed tissue-free pool samples require no further processing.
15. For hydrolyzed tissue-free pool and protein-bound pool samples, carry out three further extractions with toluene, discarding the toluene extract each time to reduce the amount of Δ^1 pyrroline remaining in the aqueous phase ***(23,24)***.
16. Cap the tubes tightly and heat at 100°C for 30 min to convert the oxidation product of hydroxyproline, pyrrole-2-carboxylic acid, to pyrrole.
17. After 30 min, cool the samples rapidly by plunging in to ice.
18. Resaturate with KCl if necessary.
19. Add 12.5 mL toluene to each tube, cap tightly, and shake vigorously for 10 min on a horizontal shaker.
20. Allow phases to separate, transfer the toluene extracts to fresh tubes, and shake twice with 800 mg of silicic acid to remove any remaining Δ^1 pyrroline and retain toluene extract for measurement of hydroxyproline (*see* **Subheading 3.5.3.**).

3.5.2. Assay of Proline Extract

3.5.2.1. Colorimetric Assay

Proline is assayed according to the method of Troll and Lindsley ***(28)***.

1. Take 1 mL of the first toluene extract (**Subheading 3.5.1., step 14**) from the unhydrolyzed tissue-free pool samples and place in screw capped glass tubes (*see* **Note 7**).

2. Prepare standards containing 0 to 0.1 μmol L-proline in 1 mL H_2O (*see* **Note 8**).
3. Add 2 mL H_2O to standards and 3 mL to samples.
4. Add 3 mL glacial acetic acid and 3ml ninhydrin solution to each tube.
5. Cap the tubes and heat at 100°C for 60 min.
6. Add toluene to give a final volume of 3.5 mL and extract the chromophore into toluene by shaking.
7. Separate the aqueous and solvent phases by centrifugation (600*g* for 10 min) (*see* **Note 9**).
8. Measure the absorbance of the solvent phase at 515 nm.

3.5.2.2. Radioactivity Determination

1. Transfer 8 mL of the toluene extracts (**Subheading 3.5.1., step 14**) from unhydrolyzed tissue-free pool samples and all blank and isotopically "spiked" samples (*see* **Subheading 3.5.1., step 3**) to 20-mL scintillation vials.
2. Add 4 mL of toluene containing 1.2% PPO.
3. Measure radioactivity in a scintillation counter with correction for counting efficiency and quenching.

3.5.3. Assay of Hydroxyproline Extract

The assay of pyrrole is based on its ability to form a chromophore with 4-dimethylaminobenzaldehyde *(22)*.

3.5.3.1. Colorimetric Assay

1. Take aliquots of the second toluene extract (**Subheading 3.5.1., step 20**), 100 μL protein-bound pool hydrolyzate, 1 mL hydrolyzed tissue-free pool, 1 mL hydroxyproline standards (*see* **Note 7**).
2. Make volume up to 1 mL with toluene.
3. Add 5 mL Ehrlichs reagent, mix, and leave at room temperature for 30 min to allow chromophore to develop.
4. Measure absorbance at 560 nm.

3.5.3.2. Radioactivity Determination

1. Transfer 10 mL of toluene extracts (**Subheading 3.5.1., step 20**) to 20-mL scintillation vials.
2. Add 2 mL of toluene containing 2.4% PPO.
3. Measure radioactivity in a scintillation counter with correction for counting efficiency and quenching.

3.6. Calculations

3.6.1. Proline

Tissue-free proline can be calculated from the following equation:

$$\text{Proline } \mu(\text{mol}) = \text{Sample absorbance/Absorbance for 1 } \mu\text{mol proline}$$

$$\times \text{ Volume of toluene extract/Volume of toluene extract assayed}$$

$$\times \text{ 100/Sample proline extraction efficiency}$$

$$\times 3$$

The absorbance for 1 μmol of proline can be obtained from the standard curve generated for each assay. In our laboratory, for 25 consecutive assays, the absorbance/μmol ranged from 3.81 to 4.50 (mean 4.20 ± 0.04 SEM). The sample proline extraction efficiency is calculated from the assay of blank samples spiked with known amounts of radiolabeled proline (**Subheading 3.5.1.**). In our laboratory, these routinely give extraction efficiencies of between 50% and 55% for tissue-free pool samples. Values are multiplied by three to take account of the splitting of the sample into hydrolyzed and unhydrolyzed fractions.

Radioactivity in proline can be calculated from the following equation:

$$\text{Proline (dpm)} = (\text{Sample dpm} - \text{Blank dpm})$$

$$\times \text{ Volume of toluene extract/Volume of toluene extract counted}$$

$$\times \text{ 100/Sample proline extraction efficiency}$$

$$\times \text{ Correction for isotope loss}$$

$$\times 3$$

During the assay procedure, the carboxyl carbon is lost during the conversion of proline to Δ^1-pyrroline, hence the loss of one of the five radiolabeled carbon atoms. The correction factor for isotope loss is therefore 1.25.

The proline-specific radioactivity is calculated from the ratio of radioactivity to amount of proline and expressed as dpm/μmol.

3.6.2. Hydroxyproline

Free- and protein-bound hydroxyproline (hyp) can be calculated from the following equation:

$$\text{Hydroxyproline } (\mu\text{g}) = \text{Sample absorbance/Absorbance for 1 } \mu\text{g hyp}$$

$$\times \text{ Volume of hyp standard assayed/Volume of sample assayed}$$

$$\times \text{ Standard hyp extraction efficiency/Sample hyp extraction efficiency}$$

The absorbance for 1 μg of hydroxyproline is calculated from a standard curve constructed from standard solutions of hydroxyproline, assayed in an identical manner to that for samples, in each assay (*see* **Subheading 3.5.1.2.**) The absorbance/μg ranged from 0.0029 to 0.0043 with a mean of 0.0037 ± 0.0004 SEM for 10 consecutive assays in our laboratory. Hydroxyproline is extracted with varying efficiencies in standards and different biological samples. Therefore, extraction efficiencies are estimated in each assay and for each type of sample (*see* **Subheading 3.5.1.3.**) by addition of known amounts of hydroxy[2-^{14}C]proline to blank samples and standards and calculation of the percentage recovery. In our laboratory, in 10 consecutive assays the extraction efficiency of hydroxyproline from tissue protein-bound hydrolyzates was 20.9 ± 1.3%, and from hydroxyproline standards was 37.0 ± 1.6%. Tissue-free hydroxyproline extraction efficiencies are similar to those for hydroxyproline standards. In addition, tissue-free hydroxyproline values must be multiplied by 3/2 to take account of the splitting of the sample into hydrolyzed and unhydrolyzed fractions.

The radioactivity in hydroxyproline is calculated according to the following equation:

$$
\begin{aligned}
&\text{Hydroxyproline (dpm)} = (\text{Sample dpm} - \text{Blank dpm}) \\
&\times \text{Volume of toluene extract/Volume of toluene extract counted} \\
&- \text{Carryover of proline oxidation product} \\
&\times 100/\text{Sample hydroxyproline extraction efficiency} \\
&\times \text{Correction for isotope loss}
\end{aligned}
$$

In the hydroxyproline assay, it is necessary to correct for carryover of the proline oxidation product Δ^1-pyrroline into the pyrrole extract (*see* **Fig. 2**). This is measured in blank protein-bound pool samples spiked with known amounts of radiolabeled proline. Typical carryover ranges between 0.14% and 0.58%. Hydroxyproline extraction efficiencies are calculated from blank samples containing known amounts of hydroxy[2-^{14}C]proline (*see* **Subheading 3.5.1., step 3**). Values also have to be corrected for isotope loss during the assay. For tissues labeled with L-[U-^{14}]proline, values are multiplied by 1.25 as a result of the loss of the carboxyl carbon atom during the conversion of pyrrole-2-carboxylic acid to pyrrole (*see* **Fig. 2**) (*see* **Note 10**). In addition, tissue-free hydroxyproline values must be multiplied by 3/2 to take account of the splitting of the sample into hydrolyzed and unhydrolyzed fractions.

Hydroxyproline-specific radioactivities are calculated from the ratio of radioactivity to molar amount of hydroxyproline and expressed as dpm/μmol.

Hydroxyproline (μmol) are calculated assuming a molecular weight for hydroxyproline of 131.1.

3.7. Estimates of Collagen Synthesis and Degradation

3.7.1. Collagen Fractional Synthesis Rate

The fractional rate of collagen synthesis is estimated as previously described ***(26)*** using the general equation:

$$\text{Fractional synthesis rate (\%/d)} = \text{Protein specific radioactivity} / \text{Estimate of precursor pool specific radioactivity} \times 100/\text{Time}$$

For collagen, the protein-specific radioactivity represents the total of tissue-free and protein-bound hydroxyproline-specific radioactivity and the unhydrolyzed tissue-free, proline-specific radioactivity represents the estimate of the precursor amino acid pool-specific radioactivity from which collagen is synthesized. Time is the period over which radiolabeled proline is being incorporated into protein measured in days, in this case the time from injection of the animal until death (*see* **Subheading 3.2.**).

3.7.2. Collagen Fractional Degradation Rate

Fractional rates of collagen degradation can be derived from the difference between the synthesis rate and the rate of change in protein content/growth rate ***(6,8)***. To obtain growth rates, collagen content of a defined organ or tissue must be measured over a period of time, for example during the growth of the animal or during the development of fibrosis. Collagen growth rates are determined at each time from the mean of rates of collagen growth, obtained using data from the time-points before and after the time at which the measurement is being made. If there is no significant change in collagen content between time-points, the growth rate is assumed to be zero. Fractional growth rates are then calculated from the mean collagen growth rate (mg/d) as a fraction of the collagen content (mg) at that time and expressed as a percentage ***(6,8)***.

3.7.3. Estimation of the Proportion of Newly Synthesized Procollagens Degraded

The proportion of procollagen molecules degraded rapidly after their synthesis can be estimated from the relative amounts of radioactivity associated with hydroxyproline in the tissue-free and protein-bound pools according to the equation:

Degradation of newly synthesised procollagens (%) = Radioactive hyp in tissue free pool (dpm)/Total radioactive hyp in tissue (dpm)

$$\times 100/1$$

3.7.4. Index of Degradation of "Mature" Collagen

An index of the degradation of "mature" collagens can be obtained by a similar calculation to that used for calculating degradation of newly synthesised procollagens (**Subheading 3.7.3.**), except molar amounts of free and total hydroxyproline are used, instead of radioactivity, and expressed as a ratio ***(6,8,16,19,20,29)***.

3.8. Alternative Method for Measuring Hydroxyproline by HPLC

Hydroxyproline can also be measured by 4-chloro-7-nitrobenz-2-oxa-1,3-diazole (NBD-Cl) derivatization of hydrolyzates, isolation by reverse-phase high-pressure liquid chromatography, and post column detection of the chromophore or radioactivity associated with hydroxyproline (*see* **Note 11**). NBD-Cl has several advantages compared with other derivatizing agents utilized to measure hydroxyproline. It reacts at an order of magnitude faster and displays a different absorbtion spectrum with secondary amino acids, proline and hydroxyproline, than with primary amino acids. These properties allow optimization of the reaction, separation, and detection conditions increasing rate of analysis and assay sensitivity ***(30,31)***. This highly sensitive method is suitable for measuring hydroxyproline from in vitro cell culture studies ***(31–33)*** and for measuring tissue hydroxproline levels ***(34)***.

3.8.1. Amino Acid Derivatization

1. Hydrolyze sample in 2 mL 6 *M* HCl at 110°C for 16 h. Samples may include, precipitated protein from cell cultures (*see* **Note 12**), tissues (as described in **Subheading 3.3., steps 1–6**), or 10 to 100 mg tissue for measurement of total tissue hydroxyproline (*see* **Note 13**).
2. Add 30 mg charcoal, mix, and filter (Millipore, 0.65 µm).
3. Dilute filtered sample hydrolyzate with H_2O, as appropriate, to ensure that 100 µL contains less than 250 pmol hydroxyproline.
4. Place a 100-µL aliquot of the diluted hydrolyzate in a 1.5-mL microcentrifuge tube and evaporate to dryness in a centrifugal vacuum concentrator (Savant, Speed-Vac).
5. Dissolve residue in 100 µL H_2O.
6. Place 100 µL of standard hydroxyproline (25 µ*M* *trans*-4-hydroxy-L-proline) in a 1.5-mL microcentrifuge tube.
7. Add 100 µL potassium tetraborate (0.4 *M*, pH 9.5) to samples and standards.

8. Add 100 µL NBD-Cl (36 m*M* in methanol).
9. Protect tubes from light and incubate at 37°C for 20 min.
10. Stop reaction by addition of 50 µL of 1.5 *M* HCl.
11. Add 150 µL of 167 m*M* sodium acetate, pH 6.4, in 26% acetonitrile (v/v).
12. Filter through a low dead volume syringe filter (Millipore, type GV, pore size 0.22 µm) and purge with air to remove any trapped sample from the filter.
13. Load 100 µL of derivatized sample onto HPLC column as described in **Subheading 3.8.2.** (*see* **Note 14**).

3.8.2. Chromatography

NBD-hydroxyproline is isolated using a reverse-phase cartridge column (LiChroCART LiChrospher 250 mm × 4 mm, 5 µm particle size, 100 RP-18) protected by a directly coupled precolumn (LiChrosorb, 4 mm × 4 mm, 5µm, RP-18) maintained at 40°C and a flow rate of 1 mL/min. NBD-amino acids are separated and eluted with an acetonitrile gradient. Post-olumn detection of the yellow/orange chromophore is achieved by continuous monitoring of the column eluent at 495 nm and the signal processed by computer integration. NBD-hydroxyproline elutes at approx 5.5 min and radiolabeled NBD-hydroxyproline can be detected by collecting fractions over 15-s periods (0.25 mL) between 3.5 and 7.5 min and counting on a scintillation counter or by using an in-line, flow-through scintillation counter. Hydroxyproline content is determined by comparison of the peak areas of samples wtih those generated from standard solutions derivatized and separated under identical conditions on the same day.

1. Equilibrate column with 100% buffer A (50 m*M* sodium acetate in 8% aqueous acetonitrile, pH 6.4) for 40 min prior to running samples.
2. Inject 100 µL of filtered derivatized sample (**Subheading 3.8.1.**) onto the column.
3. Increase the proportion of buffer B (75% acetonitrile, 25% H_2O) from 0% to 5% between 0 and 5 min.
4. Increase buffer B from 5 to 80% between 5 and 6 min.
5. Decrease buffer B from 80 to 0% between 12 and 12.5 min (*see* **Note 15**).
6. Maintain in 100% buffer A between 12.5 and 25 min to re-equilibrate the column prior to injection of the next sample.

3.8.3. Calculations

Because 100 µL of the 500 µL derivatized sample is loaded on to the column, the peak area for standard hydroxyproline represents 50 pmol. Therefore the amount of hydroxyproline in test samples loaded onto the HPLC column can be calculated as follows:

Hyp in test sample (pmol) = peak area test sample × peak area standard hyp/50

This value is multiplied by 5 to obtain the amount of hydroxyproline (pmol) present in the 100 µL of derivatized sample hydrolyzate (**Subheading 3.8.1., step 5**). Correction for any dilution (**Subheading 3.8.1., step 3**), and volume of hydrolyzate (**Subheading 3.8.1., step 1**) allows calculation of total hydroxyproline in the original sample. It is not necessary to correct for the efficiency of derivatization, as the efficiency is generally 95% or greater and is similar in samples and standards.

4. Notes

1. The methods for calculating rates of collagen synthesis assume that the specific radioactivity of the precursor pool of amino acids for protein synthesis attains a plateau value rapidly after injection of the labeled precursor, and that this plateau is maintained over the period of measurement. This is achieved by injecting large amounts of unlabeled proline to "flood" the natural pools of free proline in the tissue from which proteins are synthesized *(7,26)*. As a result of varying rates of metabolism between species, it is necessary to vary the amount of radiolabeled and unlabeled proline accordingly *(7,8,26)*. The methods also assume that incorporation of the labeled precursor into protein occurs in a linear manner with respect to time *(7,26)*. In addition, estimation of the proportion of newly synthesized procollagens degraded rapidly after synthesis assumes that the appearance of hydroxy-^{14}C-proline occurs rapidly and in a linear manner with respect to time *(7)*. Hydroxy-^{14}C-proline-free and in low-molecular-weight moieties has been shown to appear in a linear manner with respect to time; however, a plateau is attained after a period of time owing to equilibration of the rate of appearance with the rate of loss from the tissue. The parameters for measuring fractional rates of collagen synthesis have been previously validated for various tissues in mice *(8)*, rats *(7,13)*, rabbits *(6,26)*, and chickens *(15)*. The methods for measuring collagen degradation have been most extensively validated in rats *(7,13,19,20)* and rabbits *(6)*, but only partial validation has been carried out for mice *(8)*. Therefore, further validation would be required for the use of these methods for different incorporation times, tissues, and species.
2. The rate of proline metabolism, collagen content, rates of collagen metabolism, and rate of loss of free hydroxyproline vary between tissues and species. It is therefore important to conduct pilot experiments to ensure that for the tissue of interest, tissue-free proline-specific radioactivity is close to that of the injected solution and that sufficient levels of radiolabeled hydroxyproline are generated in all the fractions for accurate measurement. The amounts of radiolabeled and unlabeled proline and incorporation times indicated under **Subheading 3.2.** should be appropriate for studies of lung, heart, aorta, skin, skeletal muscle, and liver in rats *(7,13,16,19,20,35)* and for lung in mice *(8)*. They also represent good starting doses for the assessment of other tissues in these species. As a general rule, study of smaller tissues or tissues with lower concentrations of collagen will require an increase in the dose of radiolabeled proline and *vice versa*. Smaller

species tend to have higher rates of proline metabolism and will hence require increases in both radiolabeled and unlabeled proline to maintain the tissue-free, proline-specific radioactivity at a level close to that of the injected solution. If the tissue-free, proline-specific radioactivity is not similar to that of the injected solution (i.e., less than 90%), check the free proline concentration of injected animal tissues and, if less than 10 times that for uninjected animals, increase the amount of unlabeled proline injected. However, in some tissues, free proline concentrations may be more than 10 times those in the uninjected animal tissues but have specific radioactivities less than 90% of that of the injected solution. This often occurs in tissues such as heart and skeletal muscle; however, good estimates of collagen synthesis rates may still be obtained providing that the tissue-free proline-specific radioactivity remains similar over the incorporation period and that incorporation of radiolabeled proline into hydroxyproline is linear over this period *(7)*.

3. Tissues larger than 1 g can be crushed to a powder under liquid nitrogen using a pestle and mortar and up to 1 g of preweighed tissue used for assay.
4. To calculate the proportion of newly synthesized procollagen degraded, measurement of radioactive hydroxyproline, free or in low-molecular-weight peptides, is required. The proportion of hydroxyproline compared with proline in these fractions is very small, and extraction procedures for oxidation products of proline and hydroxyproline are not 100% efficient (**Subheading 3.5.**). This leads to carryover of the oxidation product of proline, Δ^1 pyrroline, into the oxidized hydroxyproline extract. Multiple toluene extractions of Δ^1 pyrroline does not reduce this carryover to a sufficient extent to allow accurate measurement of hydroxyproline. Therefore, to avoid potentially large errors, prior isolation of hydroxyproline by column chromatography is required.
5. Separate columns should be used for purification of proline and isolation of hydroxyproline, as large amounts of proline relative to those in analytical samples get trapped on the purification column.
6. L-Hydroxy-[2-^{14}C]proline can be obtained from Amersham Biosciences by custom synthesis.
7. The volume of toluene extract assayed may need to be varied depending on the tissue being studied to ensure values fall within the limits of the standard curves.
8. Use of proline for the standard curve is valid, because Δ^1 pyrroline and proline react stoichiometrically with ninhydrin to produce a chromophore with an identical extinction coefficient at 515 nm *(27)*.
9. Occasionally, the solvent phase remains cloudy as a result of droplets of the aqueous phase being trapped in the solvent. This can be overcome by the addition of 50 µL of ethanol.
10. Use of alternative isotopes of proline to L-[U-^{14}C]proline is possible, but requires careful validation of the correction for isotope loss. This is particularly important for tritiated proline, where losses may be a result of effects other than chemical reactions in the assay, including variation in the proportion of hydrogens that are tritiated at the designated site, variable loss of isotope during tissue processing,

and differential metabolism of radiolabeled and unlabeled compounds in vivo *(7,27)*.

11. When using this method to measure tissue hydroxyproline-specific radioactivity, it may be necessary to do two HPLC column runs. One with sample loading to analyze the molar amount of hydroxyproline, and one with a much higher loading to accurately measure the radioactivity associated with hydroxyproline.
12. To aid recovery of proteins from cell culture studies with small numbers of cells, ethanol-precipitated proteins can be collected on acid-resistant filters (Millipore, type HV, pore size 0.45µm) using a multiport vacuum filtration unit (Millipore) as previously described ***(33)***. The filter together with adherent protein can then be transferred directly to the hydrolysis tube with minimal losses.
13. Because most tissues contain less than 3% hydroxyproline, which is free or in small peptides, unless measurement of hydroxyproline in collagen breakdown products is required tissue collagen content can be estimated without prior precipitation of protein.
14. NBD-Cl and NBD-amino acids are light-sensitive at room temperature, with rapid loss of the chromophore. However, stability of the product is greatly increased at 4°C. Therefore, it is recommended that a cooled autosampler with darkened sample vials be used in conjunction with the HPLC system, allowing batch derivatization and automated analysis.
15. This gradient profile is designed to optimize isolation of hydroxyproline while minimizing time between sample runs. However, if desired, the profile can be altered to isolate and quantify other amino acids including proline.

References

1. Manabe, I., Shindo, T., and Nagai, R. (2002) Gene expression in fibroblasts and fibrosis: involvement in cardiac hypertrophy. *Circ. Res.* **91,** 1103–1113.
2. Simms, R. W. and Korn, J. H. (2002) Cytokine directed therapy in scleroderma: rationale, current status, and the future. *Curr. Opin. Rheumatol.* **14,** 717–722.
3. Bedossa, P. and Paradis, V. (2003) Liver extracellular matrix in health and disease. *J. Pathol.* **200,** 504–515.
4. Desmouliere, A., Darby, I. A., and Gabbiani, G. (2003) Normal and pathologic soft tissue remodeling: role of the myofibroblast, with special emphasis on liver and kidney fibrosis. *Lab. Invest.* **83,** 1689–1707.
5. White, E. S., Lazar, M. H., and Thannickal, V. J. (2003) Pathogenetic mechanisms in usual interstitial pneumonia/idiopathic pulmonary fibrosis. *J. Pathol.* **201,** 343–354.
6. Laurent, G. J. and McAnulty, R. J. (1983) Protein metabolism during bleomycin-induced pulmonary fibrosis in rabbits: in vivo evidence for collagen accumulation because of increased synthesis and decreased degradation of the newly synthesised collagen. *Am. Rev. Respir. Dis.* **128,** 82–88.
7. McAnulty, R. J. and Laurent, G. J. (1987) Collagen synthesis and degradation in vivo. Evidence for rapid rates of collagen turnover with extensive degradation of newly synthesised collagen in tissues of the adult rat. *Collagen Rel. Res.* **7,** 93–104.

8. McAnulty, R. J., Moores, S. R., Talbot, R. J., Bishop J. E., Mays, P. K., and Laurent, G. J. (1991) Long-term changes in mouse lung following inhalation of a fibrosis-inducing dose of $^{239}PuO_2$: changes in collagen synthesis and degradation rates. *Int. J. Radiat. Biol.* **59,** 229–238.
9. Schneir, M. and Golub, L. (1981) The effect of streptozotocin-induced diabetes on collagen catabolism, in *Streptozotocin: Fundamentals and Therapy.* (Agarwal, M. K., ed.), Elsevier/North-Holland Biomedical Press, Amsterdam: pp. 161–182.
10. Schneir, M., Ramamurthy, N. S., and Golub, L. (1984) Extensive degradation of recently synthesised collagen in gingiva of normal and streptozotocin-induced diabetic rats. *J. Dent. Res.* **63,** 23–27.
11. Schneir, M., Ramamurthy, N. S., and Golub, L. (1985) Dietary ascorbic acid normalizes diabetes-induced underhydroxylation of nascent type I collagen molecules. *Collagen Rel. Res.* **5,** 415–422.
12. Turner, J. E., Oliver, M. H., Guerreiro, D., and Laurent, G. J. (1986) Collagen metabolism during right ventricular hypertrophy following induced lung injury. *Am. J. Physiol.* **251,** H915–H919.
13. Mays, P. K., McAnulty, R. J., Campa, J. S., and Laurent, G. J. (1991) Age-related changes in collagen synthesis and degradation in rat tissues: importance of degradation of newly synthesised collagen in regulating collagen production. *Biochem. J.* **276,** 307–313.
14. Bishop, J. E., Rhodes, S., Laurent, G. J., Low, R. B., and Stirewalt, W. S. (1994) Increased collagen synthesis and decreased collagen degradation in right ventricular hypertrophy induced by pressure overload. *Cardiovasc. Res.* **28,** 1581–1585.
15. Laurent, G. J., McAnulty, R. J., and Gibson, J. (1985) Changes in collagen synthesis and degradation during skeletal muscle growth. *Am. J. Physiol. Cell Physiol.* **249,** C352–C355.
16. McAnulty, R. J., Staple, L. H., Guerreiro, D., and Laurent, G. J. (1988) Extensive changes in collagen synthesis and degradation during compensatory lung growth. *Am. J. Physiol. Cell Physiol.* **255,** C754–C759.
17. Pickrell, J. A., Hahn, F. F., Rebar, A. H., Horoda, R. A., and Henderson, R. F. (1987) Changes in collagen metabolism and proteinolysis after repeated inhalation exposure to ozone. *Exp. Mol. Pathol.* **46,** 159–167.
18. Nirmala, C., Anand, S., and Puvanakrishnan, R. (1999) Curcumin treatment modulates collagen metabolism in isoproterenol induced myocardial necrosis in rats. *Mol. Cell. Biochem.* **197,** 31–37.
19. Mays, P. K., McAnulty, R. J., and Laurent, G. J. (1989) Age-related changes in lung collagen metabolism: a role for degradation in regulating lung collagen production. *Am. Rev. Respir. Dis.* **140,** 410–416.
20. Mays, P. K., McAnulty, R. J., and Laurent, G. J. (1991) Age-related changes in total protein and collagen metabolism in rat liver. *Hepatology* **14,** 1224–1229.
21. Stegemann, H. (1958) Mikrobestimmung von hydroxyproline mit chloramin-T und p-dimethylaminobenzaldehyd. Hoppe-Seyler's Z. *Physiol. Chem.* **311,** 41–45.
22. Prockop, D. J. and Udenfriend, S. (1960) A specific method for the analysis of hydroxyproline in tissues and urine. *Anal. Biochem.* **1,** 228–239.

23. Prockop, D. J., Udenfriend, S., and Lindstedt, S. (1961) A simple technique for measuring the specific activity of labelled hydroxyproline in biological materials. *J. Biol. Chem.* **236,** 1395–1398.
24. Peterkofsky, B. and Prockop, D. J. (1962) A method for the simultaneous measurement of radioactivity of proline-C^{14} and hydroxyproline-C^{14} in biological materials. *Anal. Biochem.* **4,** 400–406.
25. Woessner, J. F. (1976) Measurement of the specific activities of proline and hydroxyproline in connective tissues, in *The Methodology of Connective Tissue Research* (Hall, D. A., ed.), Academic, London: pp. 247–251.
26. Laurent, G. J. (1982) Rates of collagen synthesis in lung, skin and muscle obtained *in vivo* by a simplified method using [^{3}H]proline. *Biochem. J.* **206,** 535–544.
27. Laurent, G. J., McAnulty, R. J., and Oliver, M. H. (1982) Anomalous tritium loss in the measurement of tissue hydroxyl-[5-^{3}H]-proline specific activity following chloramine T oxidation. *Anal. Biochem.* **123,** 223–228.
28. Troll, W. and Lindsley, J. (1955) A photometric method for the determination of proline. *J. Biol. Chem.* **215,** 655–660.
29. Woessner, J. F. (1970) Collagen remodelling in chick skin embryogenesis, in *Chemistry and Molecular Biology of the Intracellular Matrix* (Balazs, E. A., ed.), Academic, London: pp. 1663–1669.
30. Lindblad, W. J. and Diegelmann, R. F. (1984) Quantitation of hydroxyproline isomers in acid hydrolysates by high-performance liquid chromatography. *Anal. Biochem.* **138,** 390–395.
31. Campa, J. S., McAnulty, R. J., and Laurent, G. J. (1990) Application of high-pressure liquid chromatography to studies of collagen production by isolated cells in culture. *Anal. Biochem.* **186,** 257–263.
32. McAnulty, R. J., Campa, J. S., Cambrey, A. D., and Laurent, G. J. (1991) The effect of transforming growth factor β on rates of procollagen synthesis and degradation in vitro. *Biochim. Biophys. Acta.* **1091,** 231–235.
33. McAnulty, R. J., Chambers, R. C., and Laurent, G. J. (1995) Regulation of fibroblast procollagen production: transforming growth factor-β_1 induces prostaglandin E_2 but not procollagen synthesis via a pertussis toxin-sensitive G-protein. *Biochem. J.* **307,** 63–68.
34. Mutsaers, S. E., Foster, M. L., Chambers, R. C., Laurent, G. J., and McAnulty, R. J. (1998) Increased endothelin-1 and its localization during the development of bleomycin-induced pulmonary fibrosis in rats. *Am. J. Respir. Cell Mol. Biol.* **18,** 611–619.
35. Shivakumar, K. and Prakash Kumar, B. (1997) Magnesium deficiency enhances oxidative stress and collagen synthesis in vivo in the aorta of rats. *Int. J. Biochem. Cell Biol.* **29,** 1273–1278.

12

Approaches to Evaluation of Fibrogenic Pathways in Surgical Lung Biopsy Specimens

Cory M. Hogaboam, Kristin J. Carpenter, Holly Evanoff, and Steven L. Kunkel

Summary

Idiopathic interstitial pneumonias (IIPs) are a heterogeneous group of pulmonary fibrotic disorders consisting of several clinicopathologic entities with differing histopathologic patterns, clinical course, response to therapy, and prognosis *(1–3)*. It is now recognized that accurate diagnosis is required in IIP, particularly in distinguishing various clinicopathologic entities of this disease from usual interstitial pneumonia, the most common histological pattern in IIP. Although no longer considered the "gold standard" for diagnosis *(2)*, surgical lung biopsies (SLBs) have provided clinicians and researchers with important clues as to the identity of soluble mediators that may account for the subtype differences in IIP. Given that the expression of chemokine ligands and chemokine receptors appear to be markedly altered during the development of pulmonary fibrosis in IIP *(4)*, we have focused on the characterization of these mediators in IIP and non-IIP SLBs and in primary human fibroblast lines grown from these biopsies. Herein, we describe laboratory techniques routinely employed to detect these important profibrotic factors and their corresponding receptors in SLBs and in primary human fibroblast lines.

Key Words: Pulmonary fibrosis; interstitial pneumonia; fibroblasts; chemokines; chemokine receptors.

1. Introduction

1.1. *Idiopathic Interstitial Pneumonias*

Chronic pulmonary fibrosis of known and idiopathic origin presents extraordinary clinical challenges for which treatment options show limited effectiveness *(5)* or toxicity *(6,7)*, and the median survival rate following diagnosis has changed little *(8,9)*. Known profibrotic stimuli include radiation, inhaled mineral and organic particles, gaseous oxidants, pharmaceuticals, and infectious organisms *(10)*, whereas debate persists regarding the identity of etiological

From: *Methods in Molecular Medicine, Vol. 117: Fibrosis Research: Methods and Protocols*
Edited by: J. Varga, D. A. Brenner, and S. H. Phan © Humana Press Inc., Totowa, NJ

factors that initiate the clinicopathological entities of idiopathic interstitial pneumonias (IIPs) ***(11,12)***. IIP are a diverse group of disorders involving the distal pulmonary parenchyma, which share numerous features but are felt to be sufficiently different to justify designation as separate disorders ***(13)***. Their pathogenesis remains unclear, but is thought to center around an injury (or multiple injuries) to the lung followed by attempts to heal this injury. Fibroblastic foci, small aggregates of actively proliferating fibroblasts, are believed to represent the organization of prior foci of injury and indicate that fibrosis is active and ongoing. Recent studies have renewed interest in categorizing patients with IIP according to histological features ***(3,13,14)***. Patients previously diagnosed with IIP are now divided into numerous categories including usual interstitial pneumonia (UIP), nonspecific interstitial pneumonia (NSIP), and others. The presence of fibroblastic foci in UIP lung biopsies is a key histological feature in the differential diagnosis ***(13)***. Patients with NSIP have a better prognosis and response to immunosuppressive therapy than those with UIP ***(7,15–17)***. In addition, those patients with a predominantly cellular form of NSIP (NSIP-cellular) appear to have the best prognosis compared with those demonstrating a predominantly fibrotic form of NSIP (NSIP-fibrotic) ***(13,17)***.

1.2. The Dynamic Pulmonary Fibroblast

Little controversy surrounds the fact that the pulmonary fibroblast is the major instigator and/or effector of these diseases ***(18)***. The relative importance of the pulmonary fibroblast during chronic IIP is highlighted by growing evidence that inflammatory cells are often conspicuously absent in certain types of IIP, and these patients typically respond poorly to potent anti-inflammatory therapy ***(6,7,17,19,20)***. This paradox coincides with a number of experimental findings demonstrating that inflammation is necessary but is only one component of many required to induce and maintain chronic fibrosis ***(21)***. In keeping with an evolving hypothesis that IIP is an abnormal wound healing disease ***(19)***, the pulmonary fibroblast represents a major target in the treatment of these diseases.

1.3. Chemokines

Chemokines are small (approx 8–14 kDa), soluble, and membrane-bound proteins that have been subdivided into four major families based on the juxtaposition of cysteine residues in the proteins N-terminus. Nearly 50 human chemokines have now been identified, necessitating the need for a new classification system recently proposed by Zlotnik and Yoshie ***(22)***. Accordingly, the four families include 28 CC ligands (CCL), 15 CXCL, 2 XCL, and 1 CX3CL. The human CCL chemokine family is comprised of the macrophage inflammatory proteins (i.e., MIP-1α/CCL3), the monocyte chemoattractant proteins (i.e., MCP-1/CCL2), eotaxin/CCL11, and I-309/CCL1 *(22)*. These chemokines predominately affect the directional movement of mononuclear cells (i.e., T-cells, monocytes, and macrophages). An additional subgroup of CCLs, includes CCL19 and CCL21, which have been shown to direct lymphocyte and dendritic cell trafficking to and from lymphoid tissues during immune surveillance *(23)*. The CXC chemokines comprise the second major family of chemokines, which were originally described as neutrophil chemotactic and activating factors. Examples include interleukin (IL)-8/CXCL8), interferon inducible protein (IP)-10/CXCL10), and monokine-induced by interferon γ (MIG/CXCL9). Two other smaller families of chemokines have also been identified through bioinformatics analysis and include the C (lymphotactin/XCL1) and CX3C (fractalkine/CX3CL1) chemokines. Lymphotactin/XCL is a potent chemoattractant for T- and natural-killer (NK) cells *(24,25)*, whereas fractalkine/CX3CL is a membrane-bound chemokine that firmly adheres mononuclear cells to the endothelium *(26)*. The pace of chemokine discovery has slowed considerably over the past few years, leading some to suggest that the list of human chemotactic chemokines has neared completion *(22)*.

1.4. Chemokines and Pulmonary Fibrosis

Chemokines affect both the initiation and maintenance of the inflammatory response and contribute to the abnormal tissue repair process in IIP. CXCL8 is markedly increased in IIP *(27–29)* and appears to be an important factor in the recruitment of neutrophils and the development of neutrophilic alveolitis ***(30–32)***. In addition, CXCL8 and ENA-78/CXCL5 promote neovascularization during IIP ***(33,34)***. Stronger evidence exists that the CC chemokines have major roles in fibrosing interstitial diseases. For example, CCL2 has been shown to be markedly elevated at early and late stages in interstitial lung diseases ***(29,35–40)***. CCL2 is a potent chemoattractant for T-cells ***(41)*** and monocytes ***(42)***, both prominent cells in interstitial lung diseases ***(43,44)***. Alveolar macrophages, epithelial cells, smooth muscle cells, and pulmonary fibroblasts isolated from IIP patients exhibit enhanced CCL2 generation ***(35)***. Although all of these studies have given us "snapshots" of the various chemokines that may contribute to the pathology of IIP, our understanding of the sequence of events that leads to changes in chemokine synthesis is limited. The exact nature of the effects of these mediators in IIP is also unknown.

1.5. Chemokine Receptors and Experimental Pulmonary Fibrosis

There is at present no literature pertaining to the expression of chemokine receptors in IIP, particularly in different histopathological groups. Reports regarding the role of chemokine receptors during experimental lung fibrosis have been scarce despite the availability of specific antibodies and chemokine receptor knockout mice. CCR1-positive cells that accumulate in interstitial inflammatory sites are major contributors to the fibrotic response during bleomycin-induced lung injury *(45)*. Bleomycin-challenged mice treated with anti-CCR1 antibody exhibit a significantly reduced accumulation of inflammatory cells and collagen deposition and a dramatic improvement of survival. We have recently examined the role of CCR1 in a model of allergic airway remodeling normally associated with subepithelial fibrosis, and noted that mice lacking CCR1 as a result of gene knockout failed to develop this fibrotic response *(46)*. CCR2, but not CCR5 *(47)*, is involved in the development of experimental pulmonary fibrosis owing to fluorescein isothiocyanate (FITC) *(47)* and bleomycin *(48)*. At 26 wk after radiation exposure, CCR1, CCR2, CCR5, and CCR6 were elevated in fibrosis-sensitive mice, whereas SDF-1α/CXCL12 and CCR1 were elevated in fibrosis-resistant mice *(4)*. More recently, Hashimoto and colleagues *(49)* showed that bone marrow-derived lung fibroblasts expressed the chemokine receptors CXCR4 and CCR7 and responded chemotactically to their cognate ligands (i.e., CXCL12 and secondary lymphoid chemokine/CCL21, respectively). Together, these studies provide compelling evidence that those chemokine receptor-positive cells in the lung play significant roles in the pathogenesis of pulmonary fibrosis in mice.

1.6. Chemokine Receptors in IIP

1.6.1. Surgical Lung Biopsies

Given these promising data from the published experimental studies, detailed examination of specific chemokine receptors in clinical IIP is warranted. During an immunohistochemical screening of whole lung sections from IIP and non-IIP surgical lung biopsies (SLBs) for the expression of chemokine receptors, we were surprised to find the prominent expression of CXCR4 in IIP SLBs (**Fig. 1**). Prominent CXCR4 expression was observed in SLBs from UIP, NSIP-fibrotic, and respiratory bronchiolitis-associated interstitial lung disease (RBILD) patients. Although we observed intense CXCR4 expression in macrophages in all of these patient groups and in non-IIP SLBs, the pattern of CXCR4 expression suggested to us that this chemokine receptor was not exclusively associated with immune cells. A similar pattern of expression was observed when we examined CCR7; however, this chemokine receptor appeared to be limited to nonhematopoietic cells found in distinct foci present in IIP SLBs (not shown). These observations were surprising in light of previous observations that both CC chemokine receptors are solely expressed on cells of hematopoietic origin, namely lymphocytes *(50)*. However, beyond their role in immune cell trafficking, there is a growing body of recent data suggesting that these chemokine receptors are present on cells of nonhematopoietic

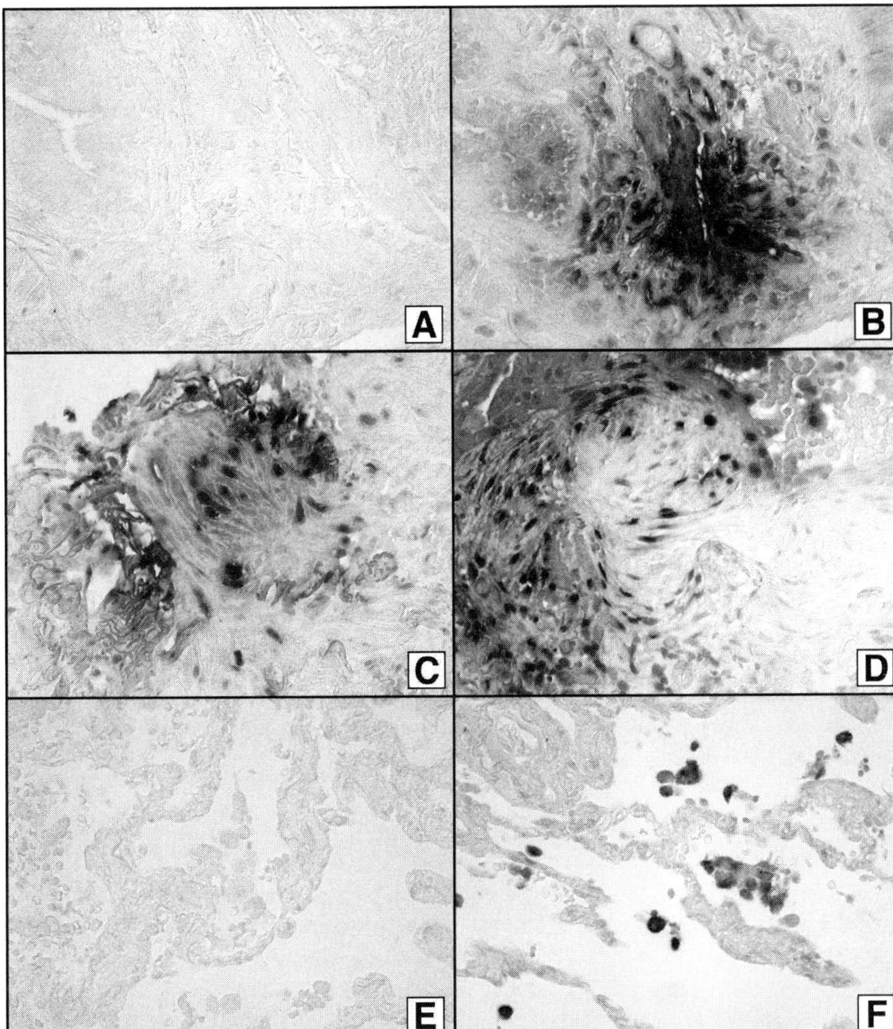

Fig. 1. Immunohistochemical localization of CXCR4 in fistological sections from usual interstitial pneumonia (UIP) (**A–D**) and RBILD (**E** and **F**) surgical lung biopsies (SLBs). Focal expression CXCR4 was observed in UIP SLBs (**B**). Fibroblastic foci also contained cells that stained strongly for CXCR4 (**C** and **D**). The appropriate negative staining for each lung is shown in (**A**) and (**E**). Original magnification for all panels was 400×.

origin. Breast cells do not constitutively express this chemokine receptors; however, the expression of CCR7 and CXCR4 on breast cancer cells explained, in part, the metastatic properties of breast tumors ***(51)***.

1.6.2. Primary Human Fibroblast Lines

Using immunohistochemical techniques, a number of interesting observations were made regarding putative cytokines that regulate the expression of CCR7 on IIP primary fibroblast lines. UIP and NSIP-fibrotic fibroblast lines exhibit strong constitutive expression of CCR7, whereas fibroblast lines from non-IIP patients do not exhibit any CCR7. The addition of TNF-α to all IIP, but not non-IIP, fibroblast lines examined to date markedly upregulated the protein expression of CCR7. In contrast, the presence of IL-10 in cultures of human fibroblasts inhibited the constitutive and the TNF-α-induced expression of CCR7 on IIP fibroblasts. Examples of the CCR7 expression we detected on a RBILD fibroblast line are shown in **Fig. 2**.

2. Materials

2.1. Tissue Culture

1. Dulbeco's modified Eagle's medium (DMEM)
2. 2% (v/v) Antibiotic-antimycotic
3. Hypotonic buffer: 150 m*M* NH_4Cl, 10 m*M* $NaHCO_3$, 1 m*M* ethylenediaminetetraacetic acid (EDTA).
4. 0.25% Porcine trypsin (containing 0.02% EDTA-2Na, without calcium and magnesium).
5. Tissue culture plates (two-well LAB-TEK® chamber culture slides, 6-, 12-, or 24-well plates).
6. 37°C humidified CO_2 incubator.

2.2. Immunochemistry

1. 4% Paraformaldehyde.
2. L-Lysine-coated slides.
3. Xylene.
4. Ethanol (EtOH: 50, 70, 90, 100%).
5. Citric acid buffer: 3.84 g anhydrous citrate in 2 L distilled water, pH 6.0.
6. 1X Phosphate-buffered saline (PBS).
7. Buffer used for washes and primary antibody dilution: 1X PBS, 0.1% saponin, 5% nonfat powdered milk (1 L 1X PBS, 1 g saponin, 50 g nonfat powdered milk).
8. Primary antibody.
9. Biotinylated secondary antibody.
10. R&D Systems horse radish peroxidase-3-amino-9-ehtylcarbazole (AEC) anti-rabbit staining kit (vat.no. CTS006). Each kit includes Peroxidase Blocking Reagent®, Serum Blocking Reagent®, Avidin Blocking Reagent®, Biotin Blocking Reagent®, AEC Chromagen®, and HSS-HRP®.
11. Aqueous mounting medium.
12. Aluminum foil.
13. Refrigerator.

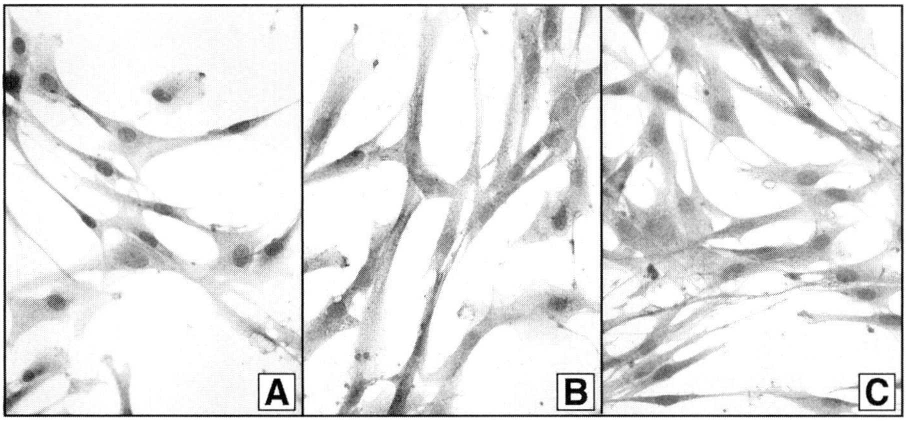

Fig. 2. Immunohistochemical localization of CCR7 on a primary fibroblast grown from a respiratory bronchioloitis-associated interstitial lung disease patient. Shown in (**A**) are fibroblasts that were left untreated for 24 h prior to immunostaining. Weak constitutive expression of CCR7 was observed on these fibroblasts (**A**). However, as shown in (**B**), the presence of 10 ng/mL of tumor necrosis factor-α for 24 h markedly upregulated CCR7 expression. The addition of interleukin-10 (at 10 ng/mL) inhibited the constitutive expression of CCR7 (**C**).

3. Methods

3.1. Lung Fibroblast Culture

Lung fibroblasts were cultured from SLBs and transbronchial biopsies (TBBs) as previously described in detail ***(52,53)***. Briefly, SLBs were delivered on ice from the operating room within 1 h after resection and transferred to DMEM containing 15% fetal bovine serum (FBS) and 2% (v/v) antibiotic-antimycotic (DMEM-15 growth medium). SLBs were mechanically separated into single cell preparations, and contaminating red blood cells lysed with hypotonic buffer for 2 min at 4°C were added to 175-mL tissue culture flasks. Pulmonary fibroblasts were grown from TBBs using an explant technique previously employed in the laboratory ***(54,55)***. Briefly, the transbronchial biopsy was cut into the base of a 60-mm tissue culture plate in a checkerboard pattern. All fibroblasts were grown at 37°C in a humidified CO_2 incubator and fed DMEM-15 growth medium three times weekly. Approximately 35 d after the addition of the dispersed cells from the SLBs and the explanting of the transbronchial biopsy, adherent cells were dispersed using 0.25% porcine trypsin. After a minimum of four passages, homogenous populations of fibroblasts were transferred to tissue culture plates for experiments. Prior to use in any experiment, lung fibroblasts were transferred to two-well LAB-TEK chamber culture slides. These cells were characterized by the following immunohistochemical staining: (1) absence of nonspecific esterase, (2) absence of Factor VIII, (3) absence of cytokeratin, (4) absence of α-smooth muscle actin, (5) absence of desmin, (6) absence of tenascin, (7) presence of vimentin, (8) presence of laminin, (9) presence of fibronectin, and (10) presence of β-actin. After the fourth passage, fibroblasts from each SLBs and transbronchial biopsy were archived in liquid nitrogen.

3.2. Immunohistochemistry

SLBs were fixed in 4% paraformaldehyde for a minimum of 12 h. Fixed samples were subsequently embedded in paraffin, thin-sectioned, and placed on L-lysine-coated slides. Slides were deparaffinized by sequential treatment:

Deparaffinization and rehydration of sections:

1. Xylene 1 min
2. Xylene 1 min
3. 100% EtOH 1 min
4. 100% EtOH 1 min
5. 90% EtOH 1 min
6. 70% EtOH 1 min
7. 50% EtOH 1 min
8. Distilled water 1 min

Microwave antigen retrieval:

1. Place slides in plastic slide holders.
2. Place holders in pressure cookers and fill to frosted mark on slides with citric acid buffer (approx 1.5 L).
3. Put rubber gasket in place, lock lid, and place rubber plug over the vent hole.
4. Microwave on full power until the yellow stem on the pressure cooker has popped. Continue to microwave for 1 min after stem has popped. This should take 10 to 12 min.
5. Remove cooker carefully. After 10 min, remove rubber plug to release steam. Let sit for 10 to 20 min at room temperature. Remove the top from the pressure cooker and allow cooling an additional 10 to 15 min at room temperature.

3.3. Immunohistochemistry Protocol

1. Rinse slides in 1X PBS and circle sections with hydrophobic slide marker.
2. Cover sample with 1 to 3 drops Peroxidase Blocking Reagent. Incubate at room temperature for 15 to 20 min.
3. Rinse sample with 1X PBS. Wash gently in milk buffer for 5 min.
4. Incubate slides with 1 to 3 drops of Serum Blocking Reagent for 15 min at 37°C.
5. Blot excess Serum Block from slides. **Do not** rinse with buffer.
6. Incubate slides with 1 to 3 drops of Avidin Blocking Reagent for 15 min at 37°C.

7. Rinse slides with 1X PBS and blot excess buffer.
8. Incubate slides with 1 to 3 drops of Biotin Blocking Reagent for 15 min at 37°C.
9. Rinse slides with 1X PBS and blot excess buffer.
10. Incubate sample with Primary Antibody and respective control IgG for 1 h.
    - Primary antibody at appropriate dilution, i.e., 1/100.
    - Isotype Control: i.e., rabbit IgG.
11. Rinse samples with 1X PBS. Wash slides in milk buffer three times for 20 min. Blot dry.
12. Incubate with 1 to 3 drops of Biotinylated Secondary Antibody for 30 min at 37°C.
    - Secondary antibody and staining kit: R&D Systems HRP-AEC anti-rabbit staining kit (cat. no. CTS006).
13. Rinse with 1X PBS. Wash in milk buffer three times for 20 min. Blot dry.
14. Incubate with 1 to 3 drops HSS-HRP for 30 min (37°C).
15. Rinse with 1X PBS. Wash in buffer three times for 2 min. Blot dry.
16. Calculate volume AEC Chromagen required for all slides (approx 100 μL per slide). One drop chromagen solution/2 m: chromagen buffer. Mix immediately prior to use.
17. Incubate slides in 100 μL AEC Chromagen solution for 2 to 20 min monitoring intensity of staining using microscope to ensure proper intensity.
18. Rinse with tap water.
19. Counter stain with hematoxylin for 20 to 30 s, rinse with tap water until it runs clear. Mount with aqueous mounting medium.
20. Cover slides with aluminum foil and store at 4°C until images have been captured.

4. Notes

1. When isolating primary culture cells, it is imperative to keep all tissue samples in a sterile environment from the moment the tissue is removed.
2. If freezing down primary cultures, do so only when the cells are undergoing vigorous proliferation, around passage 4 to 5. These cells, 0.5 to 1.0 million/ample, should be frozen, which should make it easier to bring back the frozen cells, kept in liquid nitrogen, after extended periods of time.
3. When culturing the cells for immunohistochemistry, grow the cells at a concentration that will allow the cells to spread out without growing on top of each other.
4. Remember to not vigorously wash cells when staining. It is better to blot off excess fluid. This is especially true when removing blocking antibody from the slides, as these slides should be blotted, not washed.
5. It is best to electronically capture the images as soon as possible after staining. The use of computer-captured images will allow a quick and convenient means to store and archive images for later use.

Acknowledgments

The authors thank Robin Kunkel for technical expertise. These studies were supported in part by NIH grants HL031237, HL31963, and HL32576.

References

1. Green, F. H. (2002) Overview of pulmonary fibrosis. *Chest* **122,** 334S–339S.
2. (2002) American Thoracic Society, European Respiratory Society (ATS/ERS) international multidisciplinary consensus classification of idiopathic interstitial pneumonias. *Am. J. Respir. Crit. Care Med.* **165,** 277–304.
3. Katzenstein, A. and Myers, J. (1998) Idiopathic pulmonary fibrosis. Clinical relevance of pathologic classification. *Am. J. Respir. Crit. Care Med.* **157,** 1301–1315.
4. Johnston, C. J., Williams, J. P., Okunieff, P., and Finkelstein, J. N. (2002) Radiation-induced pulmonary fibrosis: examination of chemokine and chemokine receptor families. *Radiat. Res.* **157,** 256–265.
5. Douglas, W., Ryu, J., and Schroeder, D. (2000) Idiopathic pulmonary fibrosis. Impact of oxygen and colchicine, prednisone, or no therapy on survival. *Am. J. Respir. Crit. Care Med.* **161,** 1172–1178.
6. Flaherty, K. R., Toews, G. B., Lynch, J. P., 3rd, et al. (2001) Steroids in idiopathic pulmonary fibrosis: a prospective assessment of adverse reactions, response to therapy, and survival. *Am. J. Med.* **110,** 278–282.
7. Hampton, J., Martinez, F., Orens, J., Toews, G., and Lynch III, J. (1994) Corticosteroids in idiopathic pulmonary fibrosis (IPF): Toxicity may outweigh benefits. *Am. J. Respir. Crit. Care Med.* **149,** A878.
8. Ryu, J. H., Colby, T. V., and Hartman, T. E. (1998) Idiopathic pulmonary fibrosis: current concepts. *Mayo Clin. Proc.* **73,** 1085–1101.
9. Lasky, J. A. and Brody, A. R. (2000) Interstitial fibrosis and growth factors. *Environ. Health Perspect.* **108(Suppl 4),** 751–762.
10. Kuwano, K., Hagimoto, N., and Hara, N. (2001) Molecular mechanisms of pulmonary fibrosis and current treatment. *Curr. Mol. Med.* **1,** 551–573.
11. du Bois, R. M. and Wells, A. U. (2001) Cryptogenic fibrosing alveolitis/idiopathic pulmonary fibrosis. *Eur. Respir. J. Suppl.* **32,** 43s–55s.
12. Turner-Warwick, M. (1998) In search of a cause of cryptogenic fibrosing alveolitis (CFA): one initiating factor or many? *Thorax* **53(Suppl 2),** S3–9.
13. Travis, W., Matsui, K., Moss, J., and Ferrans, V. (2000) Idiopathic nonspecific intersititial pneumonia: Prognostic signficance of cellular and fibrosing patterns. *Am. J. Surg. Path.* **24,** 19–33.
14. Myers, J. L. (1998) NSIP, UIP, and the ABCs of idiopathic interstitial pneumonias. *Eur. Respir. J.* **12,** 1003–1004.
15. Nagai, S., Kitaichi, M., Itoh, H., Nishimura, K., and Colby, T. (1998) Idiopathic nonspecific interstitial pneumonia/fibrosis: Comparison with idiopathic pulmonary fibrosis and BOOP. *Eur. Respir. J.* **12,** 1010–1019.
16. Daniil, Z., Gilchrist, F., Nicholson, A., Hansell, D., Harris, J., Colby, T., and duBois, R. (1999) A histologic pattern of nonspecific interstitial pneumonia is associated with a better prognosis than usual interstitial pneumonia in patients with cryptogenic fibrosing alveolitis. *Am. J. Respir. Crit. Care Med.* **160,** 899–905.
17. Flaherty, K. R., Toews, G. B., Travis, W. D., et al. (2002) Clinical significance of histological classification of idiopathic interstitial pneumonia. *Eur. Respir. J.* **19,** 275–283.

18. Hogaboam, C. M., Steinhauser, M. L., Chensue, S. W., and Kunkel, S. L. (1998) Novel roles for chemokines and fibroblasts in interstitial fibrosis. *Kidney Int.* **54,** 2152–2159.
19. Selman, M. and Pardo, A. (2002) Idiopathic pulmonary fibrosis: an epithelial/fibroblastic cross-talk disorder. *Respir. Res.* **3,** 3.
20. Lynch, J. P., 3rd, White, E., and Flaherty, K. (2001) Corticosteroids in idiopathic pulmonary fibrosis. *Curr. Opin. Pulm. Med.* **7,** 298–308.
21. Gauldie, J., Kolb, M., and Sime, P. J. (2002) A new direction in the pathogenesis of idiopathic pulmonary fibrosis? *Respir. Res.* **3,** 1.
22. Zlotnik, A. and Yoshie, O. (2000) Chemokines: a new classification system and their role in immunity. *Immunity* **12,** 121–127.
23. Sallusto, F., Palermo, B., Lenig, D., et al. (1999) Distinct patterns and kinetics of chemokine production regulate dendritic cell function. *Eur. J. Immunol.* **29,** 1617–1625.
24. Bianchi, G., Sozzani, S., Zlotnick, A., Mantovani, A., and Allavena, P. (1996) Migratory response of human NK cells to lymphotactin. *Eur. J. Immunol.* **26,** 3238.
25. Kelner, G. S., Kennedy, J., Bacon, K. B., et al. (1994) Lymphotactin: a cytokine that represents a new class of chemokine. *Science* **266,** 1395.
26. Kanazawa, N., Nakamura, T., Tashiro, K., et al. (1999) Fractalkine and macrophage-derived chemokine: T cell-attracting chemokines expressed in T cell area dendritic cells. *Eur. J. Immunol.* **29,** 1925–1932.
27. Ziegenhagen, M. W., Schrum, S., Zissel, G., Zipfel, P. F., Schlaak, M., and Muller-Quernheim, J. (1998) Increased expression of proinflammatory chemokines in bronchoalveolar lavage cells of patients with progressing idiopathic pulmonary fibrosis and sarcoidosis. *J. Investig. Med.* **46,** 223–231.
28. Ogushi, F., Tani, K., Maniwa, K., Ichikawa, W., Tada, H., Kawano, T., and Sone, S. (1997) Interleukin-8 in bronchoalveolar lavage fluid of patients with diffuse panbronchiolitis or idiopathic pulmonary fibrosis. *J. Med. Invest.* **44,** 53–58.
29. Car, B. D., Meloni, F., Luisetti, M., Semenzato, G., Gialdroni-Grassi, G., and Walz, A. (1994) Elevated IL-8 and MCP-1 in the bronchoalveolar lavage fluid of patients with idiopathic pulmonary fibrosis and pulmonary sarcoidosis. *Am. J. Respir. Crit. Care Med.* **149,** 655–659.
30. Lynch, J. P., 3rd, Standiford, T. J., Rolfe, M. W., Kunkel, S. L., and Strieter, R. M. (1992) Neutrophilic alveolitis in idiopathic pulmonary fibrosis. The role of interleukin-8. *Am. Rev. Respir. Dis.* **145,** 1433–1439.
31. Nakamura, H., Fujishima, S., Waki, Y., et al. (1995) Priming of alveolar macrophages for interleukin-8 production in patients with idiopathic pulmonary fibrosis. *Am. J. Respir. Crit. Care Med.* **152,** 1579–1586.
32. Carre, P. C., Mortenson, R. L., King, T. E., Jr., Noble, P. W., Sable, C. L., and Riches, D. W. (1991) Increased expression of the interleukin-8 gene by alveolar macrophages in idiopathic pulmonary fibrosis. A potential mechanism for the recruitment and activation of neutrophils in lung fibrosis. *J. Clin. Invest.* **88,** 1802–1910.
33. Keane, M. P., Arenberg, D. A., Lynch, J. P., 3rd, et al. (1997) The CXC chemokines, IL-8 and IP-10, regulate angiogenic activity in idiopathic pulmonary fibrosis. *J. Immunol.* **159,** 1437–1443.

34. Keane, M. P., Belperio, J. A., Burdick, M. D., Lynch, J. P., Fishbein, M. C., and Strieter, R. M. (2001) ENA-78 is an important angiogenic factor in idiopathic pulmonary fibrosis. *Am. J. Respir. Crit. Care Med.* **164,** 2239–2242.
35. Standiford, T. J., Rolfe, M. R., Kunkel, S. L., et al. (1993) Altered production and regulation of monocyte chemoattractant protein-1 from pulmonary fibroblasts isolated from patients with idiopathic pulmonary fibrosis. *Chest* **103,** 121S.
36. Adams, E. M., Kirkley, J., Eidelman, G., Dohlman, J., and Plotz, P. H. (1997) The predominance of beta (CC) chemokine transcripts in idiopathic inflammatory muscle diseases. *Proc. Assoc. Am. Phys.* **109,** 275–285.
37. Antoniades, H. N., Neville-Golden, J., Galanopoulos, T., Kradin, R. L., Valente, A. J., and Graves, D. T. (1992) Expression of monocyte chemoattractant protein 1 mRNA in human idiopathic pulmonary fibrosis. *Proc. Natl. Acad. Sci. USA* **89,** 5371–5375.
38. Iyonaga, K., Takeya, M., Saita, N., Sakamoto, O., Yoshimura, T., Ando, M., and Takahashi, K. (1994) Monocyte chemoattractant protein-1 in idiopathic pulmonary fibrosis and other interstitial lung diseases. *Hum. Pathol.* **25,** 455–463.
39. Boitelle, A., Gosset, P., Copin, M. C., et al. (1997) MCP-1 secretion in lung from nonsmoking patients with coal worker's pneumoconiosis. *Eur. Respir. J.* **10,** 557–562.
40. Suga, M., Iyonaga, K., Ichiyasu, H., Saita, N., Yamasaki, H., and Ando, M. (1999) Clinical significance of MCP-1 levels in BALF and serum in patients with interstitial lung diseases. *Eur. Respir. J.* **14,** 376–382.
41. Taub, D. D., Conlon, K., Lloyd, A. R., Oppenheim, J. J., and Kelvin, D. J. (1993) Preferential migration of activated CD4+ and CD8+ T cells in response to MIP-1 alpha and MIP-1 beta. *Science* **260,** 355–358.
42. Rollins, B. J., Yoshimura, T., Leonard, E. J., and Pober, J. S. (1990) Cytokine-activated human endothelial cells synthesize and secrete a monocyte chemoattractant, MCP-1/JE. *Am. J. Pathol.* **136,** 1229–1233.
43. Vath, R. R., Alexander, C. B., and Fulmer, J. D. (1982) The lymphocytic infiltrative lung diseases. *Clin. Chest Med.* **3,** 619–634.
44. Weissler, J. C. (1989) Idiopathic pulmonary fibrosis: cellular and molecular pathogenesis. *Am. J. Med. Sci.* **297,** 91–104.
45. Tokuda, A., Itakura, M., Onai, N., Kimura, H., Kuriyama, T., and Matsushima, K. (2000) Pivotal role of CCR1-positive leukocytes in bleomycin-induced lung fibrosis in mice. *J. Immunol.* **164,** 2745–2751.
46. Blease, K., Mehrad, B., Standiford, T. J., et al. (2000) Airway remodeling is absent in CCR1-/- mice during chronic fungal allergic airway disease. *J. Immunol.* **165,** 1564–1572.
47. Moore, B. B., Paine, R., 3rd, Christensen, P. J., et al. (2001) Protection from pulmonary fibrosis in the absence of CCR2 signaling. *J. Immunol.* **167,** 4368–4377.
48. Gharaee-Kermani, M., McCullumsmith, R. E., Charo, I. F., Kunkel, S. L., and Phan, S. H. (2003) CC-chemokine receptor 2 required for bleomycin-induced pulmonary fibrosis. *Cytokine* **24,** 266–276.
49. Hashimoto, N., Jin, H., Liu, T., Chensue, S. W., and Phan, S. H. (2004) Bone marrow-derived progenitor cells in pulmonary fibrosis. *J. Clin. Invest.* **113,** 243–252.

50. Kim, C. H. and Broxmeyer, H. E. (1999) SLC/exodus2/6Ckine/TCA4 induces chemotaxis of hematopoietic progenitor cells: differential activity of ligands of CCR7, CXCR3, or CXCR4 in chemotaxis vs. suppression of progenitor proliferation. *J. Leukoc. Biol.* **66,** 455–461.
51. Muller, A., Homey, B., Soto, H., et al. (2001) Involvement of chemokine receptors in breast cancer metastasis. *Nature* **410,** 50–56.
52. Hogaboam, C. M., Bone-Larson, C. L., Lipinski, S., et al. (1999) Differential monocyte chemoattractant protein-1 and chemokine receptor 2 expression by murine lung fibroblasts derived from Th1- and Th2-type pulmonary granuloma models. *J. Immunol.* **163,** 2193–2201.
53. Hogaboam, C. M., Gallinat, C. S., Bone-Larson, C., et al. (1998) Collagen deposition in a non-fibrotic lung granuloma model after nitric oxide inhibition. *Am. J. Pathol.* **153,** 1861–1872.
54. Hogaboam, C. M., Snider, D. P., and Collins, S. M. (1997) Cytokine modulation of T-lymphocyte activation by intestinal smooth muscle cells. *Gastroenterology* **112,** 1986–1995.
55. Hogaboam, C. M., Snider, D. P., and Collins, S. M. (1996) Activation of T lymphocytes by syngeneic murine intestinal smooth muscle cells. *Gastroenterology* **110,** 1456–1466.

13

Animal Models for Adult Dermal Wound Healing

Mary Birch, Annette Tomlinson, and Mark W. J. Ferguson

Summary

Wound healing in adult mammals proceeds by a series of overlapping highly coordinated events. Dermal wound repair commences with the arrest of hemorrhage followed by an inflammatory response, re-epithelialization of the wound, and formation of granulation tissue within the wound space, culminating in the production of a scar *(1,2)*. In order to study the processes involved in the repair of wounded tissue, we have developed a rodent model utilizing full thickness incisional and excisional dermal wounds, which allow for macroscopic observations and also provide tissue for the histological and immunocytochemical analysis of acute wounds and scarring.

Key Words: Fetal wound; adult wound; incisional wound; excisional wound; re-epithelialization; inflammation; extracellular matrix; collagen; CD34; TGF-β; scar.

1. Introduction

During the healing process of a mammalian adult wound, a variety of cell types migrate into the wound space from the surrounding tissues and vasculature to effect repair of the damaged tissue. This process proceeds by a series of overlapping highly coordinated events. Involvement of neutrophils, monocytes/macrophages, and lymphocytes in the inflammatory response is well documented *(3,4)*. Migration and proliferation of keratinocytes and endothelial cells promotes re-epithelialization and new blood vessel development, while fibroblasts produce extracellular matrix (ECM). Connective tissue fibroblasts participate in the reparative phase of wound healing by producing ECM proteins such as collagen and forming a connective tissue scar. In normal skin, fibroblasts are quiescent and sparsely distributed throughout the ECM. In damaged tissue, fibroblasts enter and proliferate within the wound space and have been proposed to arise from the recruitment and migration of cells from adjacent connective tissue *(1)*.

From: *Methods in Molecular Medicine, Vol. 117: Fibrosis Research: Methods and Protocols*
Edited by: J. Varga, D. A. Brenner, and S. H. Phan © Humana Press Inc., Totowa, NJ

Tissue repair begins immediately after injury with the deposition of a fibrin clot at the site of injury to prevent hemorrhage from injured blood vessels. Circulating platelets are normally discoid objects, but at the site of injury they spread into flatter shapes to plug leaks in injured blood vessels ***(1,2)***. Platelet aggregation and activation at the site of injury results in the release of inflammatory mediators including platelet-derived growth factor (PDGF), transforming growth factor (TGF)-α and -β, fibroblast growth factor (FGF), epidermal growth factor (EGF), and insulin-like growth factor (IGF) ***(5)***. These growth factors, in conjunction with chemokines, act as chemotactic signals attracting inflammatory cells, such as neutrophils and monocytes, into the wound site. A provisional fibronectin ECM is laid down within the wound space allowing cells to migrate into the wound area. An increase in vascular permeability allows cells to adhere to and pass through the capillary walls into the wound area.

Neutrophils initially predominate at the wound site in rodent dermal incisional wounds, peaking at 24 to 48 h after wounding. Macrophages start to accumulate by the recruitment from the circulating pool of peripheral blood monocytes, reaching maximum numbers 3 to 5 d postwounding ***(1,2)***. The primary function of the neutrophils and macrophages is to phagocytose pathogenic microorganisms and necrotic debris.

Lymphocytes are also recruited and function as antigen-presenting cells (APCs) and produce antibodies to facilitate the immune response to injury. The inflammatory response lasts approx 14 d and is essential for initiating repair and restoring the structural integrity of the tissue ***(1,2)***. Connective tissue fibroblasts participate in the reparative phase of wound healing by producing ECM proteins such as collagen and forming a connective tissue scar. The differentiation of fibroblasts into myofibroblasts effects wound contraction.

Migration of keratinocytes from the wound margins across the healing surface begins the re-epithelialization of the wound area. Granulation tissue is formed in the wound space by the migrating and proliferating fibroblasts, endothelial cells, and angioblasts. These processes lead to the formation of blood vessels by angiogenesis and *de novo* vascularization. The deposition of ECM molecules such as collagen results in the formation of the neodermis.

During the second week of healing in rodents, some fibroblasts assume a myofibroblast phenotype and produce contractile fibres. Tissue compaction and contraction of the wound then begins ***(1,2)***. During the transition from a provisional matrix to scar, collagen remodeling is mediated by a variety of growth factors and cytokines including TGF-β1, PDGF, EGF, FGF, interleukin (IL)-1, and tumor necrosis factor (TNF)-α ***(5)***. The ECM changes from an excess of type II to mainly type I collagen ***(2,5)***. The resolution of scar formation, usually within 6 to 12 mo of wounding, occurs when the high level of collagen synthesis returns to normal tissue levels ***(1,2)***.

Throughout this sequence of overlapping events, there are many different cell types that migrate into the wound from the surrounding tissue and the peripheral blood to effect repair of the damaged tissue. Recently, new cell types have been identified in the wound space and are involved in the processes of wound repair. A novel population of blood-borne cells with fibroblast-like properties has been recently described. These cells termed "fibrocytes" were first identified in the aspirated cells from a wound chamber, implanted subcutaneously for 2 d in a mouse *(7)*. In culture, these cells had an adherent, spindle-shaped morphology. The fibrocyte stains strongly for the fibroblast markers collagen I and vimentin, and negative for nonspecific esterases, indicating that these cells are not derived from adherent peripheral blood monocytes, which are also found in wound chambers.

During tissue maturation, significant apoptosis of blood vessels, inflammatory cells, and myofibroblasts reduces the cellularity and vascularity of the wound area, which over a period of many months brings about the formation of a mature scar. This scar can have variable "function," characterized by the pattern of matrix deposition.

The embryonic response to injury is fundamentally different from that of an adult in that tissue is regenerated and healing occurs without scar formation *(8)*. With increasing fetal age, there is a transition to a scarring phenotype. Rates of healing in the elderly are associated with alterations in inflammation, cytokine and growth factor levels, and changes in adhesion molecule expression; however, scar quality is improved ***(9,10)***.

A change in the ordered response of healing in typical acute injuries, which result in mature scar formation, results in a chronic nonhealing wound ***(11,12)***. At the other end of the healing spectrum, excessive scarring, e.g., keloids and hypertrophic scars, can occur.

At present, there is an absence of in vivo models of chronic nonhealing wounds that can adequately mimic the cellular and molecular changes seen in human clinical situations, such as the venous ulcer ***(13,14)***. In addition, there are no rodent models of keloid or hypertrophic scars ***(15)***. This chapter describes an excellent model of acute healing and scar formation in rodents. This model is readily adaptable, for example, to mimic burns, skin grafts, and wounds at other sites. It also allows for the manipulation of wounds by administration of substances, for example growth factors, which will alter the wound healing response and may lead to important clinical findings.

2. Materials

2.1. In Vivo Wounding

1. Wella Contura hair clippers (IMS, Industrial Medical Supplies, Congleton, Cheshire, UK).

2. 70% alcohol and swabs or alcohol wipes.
3. No. 11 scalpel blades and holder.
4. Sterile biopsy punches from Stiefel (Wooburn Green, Bucks, UK). (These are available in 2- to 8-mm diameter.)
5. 15-cm ruler.
6. Nontoxic and permanent marker pens (Secureline 2 marker pens; Raymond Lamb, Eastbourne, East Sussex, UK).
7. Inhalation anesthetic (*see* **Note 1**).
8. 35-mm or digital camera with flash for macroscopic record of scar.

2.2. Histological Analysis of Wounds

2.2.1. Tissue Fixation and Processing

1. Phosphate-buffered 10% formaldehyde (Sigma).
2. Vacuum Infiltration Processor (Beckman).
3. Industrial methylated spitits (IMS).
4. Toluene.
5. Embedding wax (Cellpath) (*see* **Note 2**).

2.2.2. Histological Stains

1. Mayer's Hematoxylin (Sigma).
2. Eosin Y (Sigma).
3. Masson's Trichrome (Sigma).
4. Picro Sirius Red (Sigma).

2.2.3. Immunohistochemical Staining

1. Optimal cutting temperature (OCT) embedding medium (Cellpath).
2. Methanol/Acetone fixative.
3. Primary antibodies to inflammatory markers (Serotec and Pharmingen).
4. Fluorecsent-labeled secondary antibodies (Serotec).

3. Methods

3.1. Animals

The following protocols are designed for adult mice (10–12 wk or 20–25 g) and adult rats (180–250 g). In order to eliminate the influence of female hormones on wounding which is known to affect wound parameters, it is desirable to use male rodents. In order to prevent skin lesions from fighting males, which may interfere with wound repair, animals are housed singly (1 wk pre- and for the entire period postwounding).

The number and size of incisional and excisional wounds described in this protocol are routinely used in our wound healing studies; however, the number and size of these wounds may be varied subject to appropriate ethical and regulatory approval.

The spatial positions of the wounds on the dorsal surface have been derived over a number of years to minimize differences in the wound gape and interference from the cage environment, or from the normal behavior of the animal, e.g., scratching or grooming.

A combination of incisional and excisional wounds can be applied to the same animal, again subject to ethical and regulatory approval.

3.1.1. Incisional Wounds

The procedure is carried out under general anesthesia with recovery (*see* **Note 1**).

1. Shave the entire dorsal surface area to be wounded and swab with 70% alcohol.
2. In mice, from the base of the skull, measure and mark two points 3 and 4 cm along the midline using a nontoxic marker pen (**Fig. 1**). Mark two further points 1 cm either side of the midline, at the 3- and 4-cm marks. This will form the template for two 1-cm incisional wounds running parallel to the midline.
3. In rats, measure and mark four points 5, 6, 8, and 9 cm from the base of the skull along the midline (**Fig. 2**). Mark eight further points 1 cm either side of the midline, at the 5-, 6-, 8-, and 9-cm marks. This will form the template for four 1-cm incisional wounds running parallel to the midline.
4. To make a 1-cm incisional wound, take the skin of the animal between the finger and thumb of one hand, slightly above the cranial marked point. Insert the tip of the scalpel blade at the marked point and cut piercing the epidermis, dermis, and panniculus carnosus. Applying even pressure, pull the scalpel blade between the marked points in a cranial/caudal direction, making sure to keep the incision linear.
5. Lift the skin on either side of the wound and pull apart gently, checking that a full thickness incision has been made and that the underlying muscle is visible. Cut through any remaining connective tissue strands. There should be little or no bleeding from the wound.
6. Repeat for the remaining wounds. Allow the animal to recover form the anesthetic and house singly. The wounds are allowed to heal by primary intention.

3.1.2. Excisional Wounds

1. Anesthetise and shave animal as in **Subheading 3.1.1.**
2. In mice, from the base of the skull, measure and mark a point 3.5 cm along the midline. Mark two further points, 1 cm either side of this point. These delineate the centers of two excisional wounds.
3. In rats, measure and mark two points 5.5 and 8.5 cm from the base of the skull along the midline. Mark four further points, 1 cm either side of the midline, two at each of the marked points. These delineate the centers of four excisional wounds.
4. Align the biopsy punch vertically over the center of a mark and pierce the epidermis, dermis, and panniculus carnosus by applying pressure and twisting at the same time. Remove the skin plug (*see* **Note 4**).

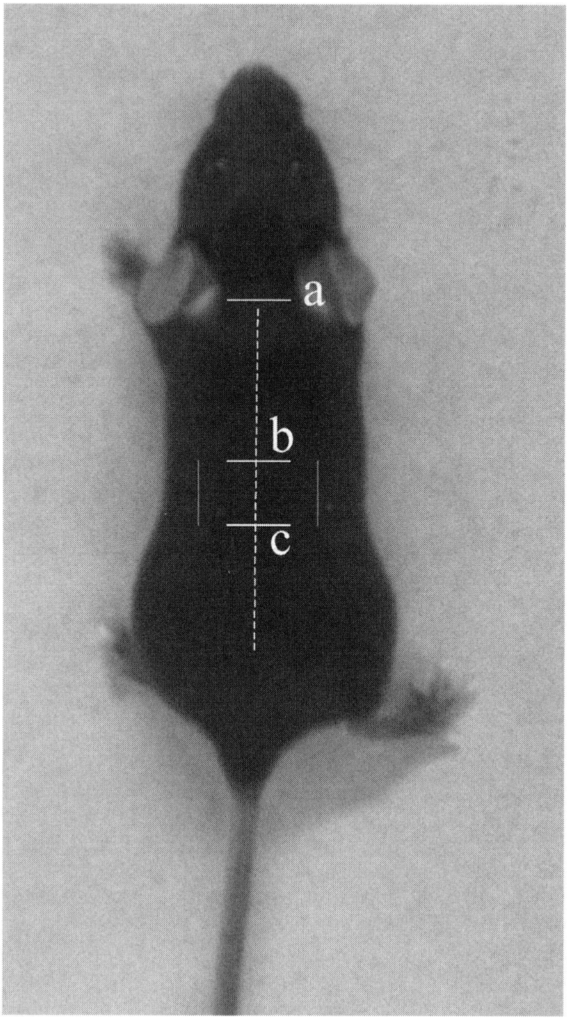

Fig. 1. Incisional wounding template on the dorsum of a mouse. Distance a to b is 3 cm from nape of neck along the midline (dotted line). Distance a to c is 4 cm. Two linear incisions are made, 1 cm in length and positioned 1 cm to either side of the midline.

5. Lift the skin to ensure a full thickness excisional wound has been made and that the underlying muscle is visible. Cut through any remaining connective tissue strands. There should be little or no bleeding from the wound.
6. Repeat for the remaining wounds. Allow the animal to regain consciousness and house singly. The wounds are allowed to heal without further procedures.

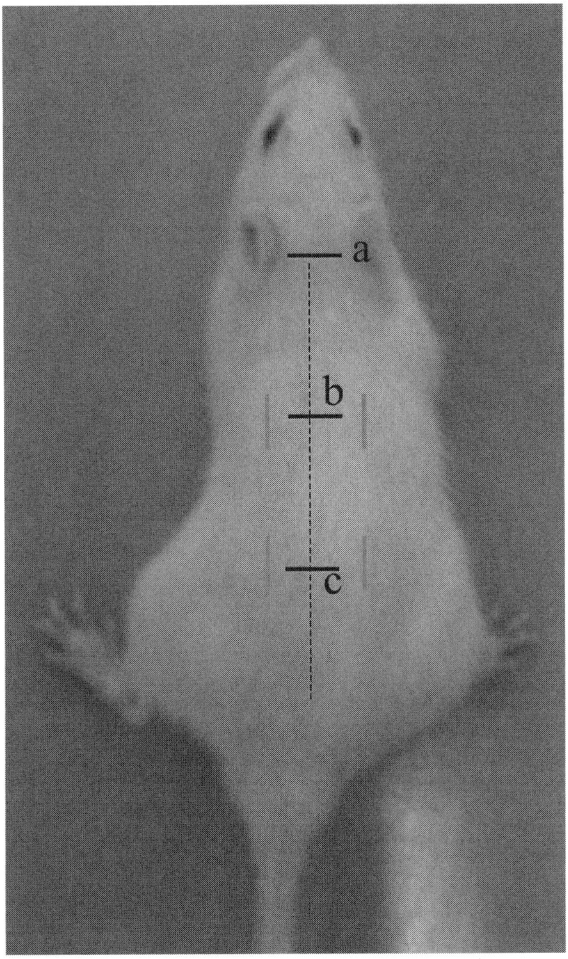

Fig. 2. Incisional wounding template on the dorsum of a rat. Distance a to b is 5 cm from nape of neck along the midline (dotted line). Distance a to c is 8 cm. Four linear incisions are made, 1 cm in length and positioned 1 cm to either side of the midline.

3.1.3. Administration of Agents to Wounds

The optimal method of delivering therapeutic agents to incisional and excisional wounds is by intradermal injection. The dosing regimen has to be experimentally derived, but there are a number of basic principles. If the animal is to be dosed prior to wounding, the agent can be injected intradermally into the skin where the incision or excision is to be made. The skin is then wounded through the "bleb."

By injecting different substances into each wound, a single animal can act as its own control and thereby minimize intra-animal variability. For example, two of the four incisional wounds in a rat can be injected with the test substance (at two doses), the third wound injected with the vehicle, and the fourth left unmanipulated. The injection treatments can be situated around the wound sites in different areas, thus controlling for any effects of wound site on the healing outcome.

3.2. Harvesting and Processing Wounds

The time of harvesting postwounding depends on the parameter to be evaluated; however, the overall method for harvesting is essentially the same for each time point.

Evaluation of the inflammatory response is carried out in wounds from 1 h to 14 d postwounding. A typical time course would be 1, 6, 12, 24, and 48 h and 3, 5, 7, 10, and 14 d. Measurement of re-epithelialization can be carried out from immediately postwounding up to d 7. Assessment of vascularization would cover 1 to 7 d. Appraisal of scar quality is carried out at least 70 d postwounding in mice and 80 d in rats. Measurement of wound breaking strength and image analysis of wounds can take place throughout the above times.

1. The animal is killed by a legally recognized method (In the United Kingdom, guidance notes can be obtained from the Animal Scientific Procedures Committee at the Home Office). The dorsum is shaved and the top and bottom of the incisional wound marked. The orientation of excisional wounds with respect to the dorsum can also be marked with a pen, which will survive subsequent processing for histology.
2. A photographic record of the wound or scar may be taken at this point using suitable apparatus such as a 35-mm or digital camera, with a 60-mm lens and flash.
3. Excise the wound including 3 to 4 mm of surrounding tissue, cutting through the body wall to give support to the excised wound.
4. At this stage, tissues can be fixed and processed for histology (*see* **Note 2**). Hematoxylin and eosin are stains used for inflammatory infiltrates, and Masson's or Mallory's trichrome and Picro Sirius Red are used to illustrate ECM deposition (**Fig. 3**). Alternatively, wounds can be frozen for immunocytochemistry. A convenient method is to bisect the wound and freeze the tissue, cut surface down, in OCT in small foil receptacles.

3.3. Evaluation of Wound Parameters

1. *Inflammation.* Markers to antigens expressed on neutrophils, T- and B-lymphocytes, and macrophages can be used to quantify the temporal and spatial expression in untreated, control and treated wounds. Cell numbers can be quantified in

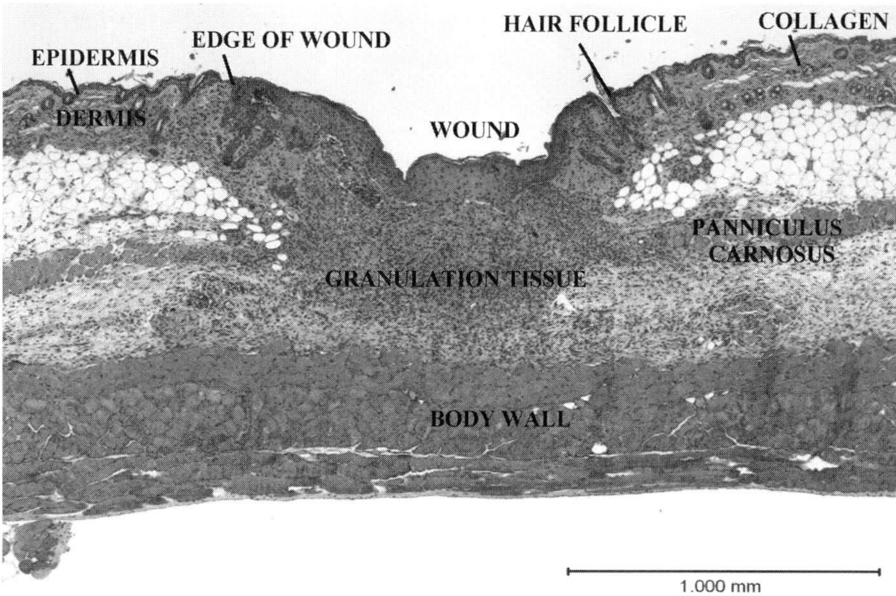

Fig. 3. Masson's trichrome-stained micrograph of full thickness incisional wound 7 d postwounding.

immunolabeled frozen or wax sections by image analysis. Antibodies are available that identify the state of maturation, activation or subset marker of macrophages, either resident within the skin or newly elicited from the blood at different times during the healing process *(15)* (*see* **Note 5**).

2. *Re-epithelialization.* Re-epithelialization can be easily identified in stained sections by the proliferating and migrating epidermis at either side of the wound.

3.4. Image Analysis

1. Using image analysis software, or manually on micrographs, measure the distance from the junction between normal and proliferating epidermis on one side of the wound, across the healing surface to the similar junction on the opposite wound margin.
2. Measure the length of proliferating epidermis on both sides and express this as a percentage of the total length. Measurement of the rate of re-epithelialization can be compared at various times during postwounding.

3.5. Vascularization

The newly formed blood vessel component of granulation tissue can be measured by image analysis in immunolabeled sections at various times postwounding. Antibodies to CD31 can be used to evaluate the development of

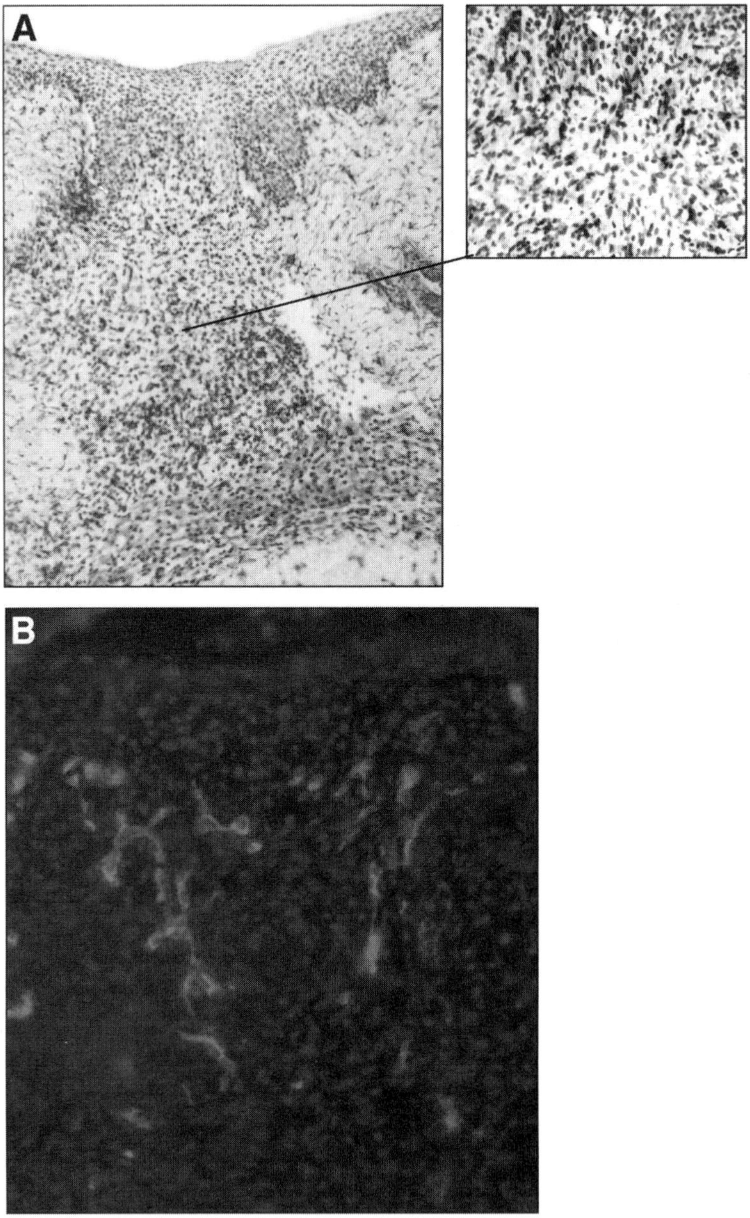

Fig. 4. Murine skin showing CD34+ string-like structures in the wound **(A)** peroxidase staining and **(B)** by immunohistochemistry (TRITC with DAPI nuclear stain), 7 d postwounding.

angiogenic response from existing blood vessels. CD34 can be used as a marker of vasculogenesis from precursor cells (**Fig. 4**).

3.6. Scarring

Dermal scarring is quantified on macroscopic and histological appearance. Evaluation of the macroscopic appearance involves allocating a score of 0 to 10 by placing a mark on a 10-cm line, 0 indicating normal skin and 10 indicating a severe scar. This is termed a visual analog scale, and the data can be subjected to statistical analysis.

Compilation of a standard set of micrographs of the macroscopic and histological appearance of scars, selected to be representative of all severities of scar quality encountered, is used for training personnel and minimizing inter and intra-observer variability. A second set of data slides generated from wounds, which are unmanipulated, is representative of the normal distribution of macroscopic and histological appearance. Each set of macroscopic and histological data should be scored by a number of observers blind to the experimental intervention.

When the histological appearance of a scar is assessed, various parameters within the wound area can be scored individually on the visual analog scale. These include wound width at the epidermis, midwound and panniculus carnosus; wound perimeter; orientation of collagen bundles; and size of collagen fibers and spacing between fibers. Alternatively, the observer can allocate an overall score, taking into account all of the aforementioned parameters. Normal surrounding dermis, i.e., ECM in a basket weave pattern, with similar fiber size and spacing, would score at the lower end of the scale. A wide scar with densely packed linear collagen would conversely score highly.

3.7. Analysis of Wound Strength

Traditional methods of measurement of wound strength involved subjecting excised tissues to disruption and tensiometry. The preferred method is now to assess the breaking strength by applying stress to wounds in vivo. Briefly, multi-axial stress is applied to wounds in an anesthetized animal. A plastic ring is secured over the wound area using cyanoacrylate adhesive, two infrared reflective markers are positioned over the plastic ring, and negative pressure applied. Displacement of the infrared targets is videotaped when the wound is deformed and ultimately ruptured and the change in pressure and skin deformation analyzed to determine wound mechanical properties and strength ***(16,17)***.

4. Notes

1. Inhalation anesthetics such as isoflurane delivered with O_2 are suitable for incisional and excisional wounding and recovery is rapid. If required, Buprenophine (15 mg/kg delivers adequate pain relief) may be given 15 to 45 min prior to surgery for analgesia postrecovery.

2. The recommended protocol for skin processing is as follows: dehydration in IMS from 50 to 100%, clearing in Toluene starting with a 50%/50% IMS/Toluene mix, and finally wax impregnation over four cycles using fresh wax each time.
3. As rodents do not have tethered skin, it is sometimes necessary to do wounding in pigs such as Yucatan. Pigs have fixed skin more closely resembling human tissue. Pigs also allow a greater number of wounds, compounds and dose ranges to be used in one animal ***(18)***.
4. In addition to using punch biopsies to create an excisional wound it is also possible to make a square excisional wound if this is preferable. Incisional and excisional wounds can also be done on the same animal, allowing for a direct comparison of the healing phenotype in different types of wounds.
5. When planning experiments and deciding on which rodent species to use, it is important to note that for immunocytochemical studies, there is a greater range of antibodies available for mouse than rat.

Acknowledgments

The authors would like to thank Miss Hayley Willis for her invaluable help in preparing the figures.

References

1. Clark, R. A. F. (ed.) (1996) Wound repair overview and general consideration, in *The Molecular and Cellular Biology of Wound Repair*, Plenum, New York, pp. 3–35.
2. Chettibi, S. and Ferguson, M. (1999) Wound repair: an overview, in *Inflammationl Basic Principles and Clinical Correlates,* 3rd ed., Lippincott Williams and Wilkins, pp. 865–877.
3. Ferguson, M. W. J and Leigh, I. M. (1998) Wound Healing, in Rook/Wilkinson/Ebling, *Textbook of Dermatology* 6th ed. (Champion, R. H., Burton, J. L., Burns, D. A., and Breathnach, S. M., eds.), Blackwell Science, Oxford, UK, pp. 337–356.
4. Cowin, A. J., Brosnan, M. P., Holmes, T. M., and Ferguson, M. W. J. (1998) Endogenous inflammatory response to dermal wound healing in the fetal and adult mouse. *Dev. Dyn.* **212,** 385–393.
5. Gilitzer, R. and Goebeler, M. (2001) Chemokines in cutaneous wound healing. *J. Leuk. Biol.* **69,** 513.
6. Alberts, B., Bray, D., Lewis, J., Raff, M., Roberts, K., and Watson, J. (1994) *Molecular Biology of the Cell.* Garland, London, p. 1157.
7. Bucala, R., Spiegel, L., Chesney, J., Hogan, M., and Cerami, A. (1994) Circulating fibrocytes define a new subpopulation that mediates tissue repair. *Mol. Med.* **1(1),** 71–81.
8. McCallion, R. L. and Ferguson, M. W. J. (1996) Fetal wound healing and the development of antiscarring therapies for adult wound healing, in *The Molecular and Cellular Biology of Wound Repair* (Clark, R. A. F.,ed), Plenum, New York, pp. 561–600.

9. Ashcroft, G. S., Horan, M. A., and Ferguson, M. W. J. (1997) The effects of ageing on wound healing: immunolocalisation of growth factors and their receptors in a murine incisional model. *J. Anat.* **190,** 351–365.
10. Ashcroft, G. S., Horan, M. A., and Ferguson, M. W. J. (1998) Aging alters the inflammatory and endothelial cell adhesion molecule profiles during human cutaneous wound healing. *Lab. Invest.* **1,** 47–58.
11. O'Kane, S. and Ferguson, M. W. J. (1997) Transforming growth factor betas and wound healing. *Int. J. Biochem. Cell. Biol.* **29,** 63–78.
12. Herrick, S. E., Sloan, P., McGurk, M., Freak, L., McCollum, C. N., and Ferguson, M. W. J. (1992) sequential changes in histologic pattern and extracellular matrix deposition during the healing of chronic venous ulcers. *Am. J. Pathol.* **141,** 1085–1095.
13. Ferguson, M. W. J., Herrick, S. E., Spencer, M. J., Shaw, J. E., Boulton, A. J., and Sloan, P. (1996) The histology of diabetic foot ulcers. *Diabetic. Med.* **13,** S30–S33.
14. Morris, D. E., Wu, L., Bolton, L., Roth, S. I., Ladin, D. A., and Mustoe, T. A. (1997) acute and chronic animal models for excessive dermal scarring: quantitative studies. *Plast. Reconstruct. Surg.* **100,** 674–681.
15. Leenen. P. J. M., de Bruijn, M. F. T. R., Voerman, J. S. A., Campbell, P. A., and van Ewijk, W. (1994) Markers of mouse macrophage development detected by monoclonal antibodies. *J. Immunol. Meth.* **174,** 5–19.
16. Charles, D., Williams, K., Perry, L. C., Fisher, J., and Rees, R. S. (1992) An improved method of in vivo wound disruption and measurement. *J. Surg. Res.* **52,** 214–218.
17. Clugston, P. A., Vistnes, M. D., Perry, L. C., Maxwell, G. P., and Fisher, J. (1995) Evaluation of silicone-gel sheeting on early wound healing of linear incisions. *Ann. Plast. Surg.* **34,** 12–15.
18. Sullivan, T. P., Eaglestein, W. H., Davis, S. C., and Mertz, P. (2001) The pig as a model for human wound healing. *Wound. Rep. Regener.* **9,** 66–76.

14

Modeling Liver Fibrosis in Rodents

Christothea Constandinou, Neil Henderson, and John P. Iredale

Summary

Animal models of hepatic fibrosis provide a means to study the cell and molecular mediators of fibrosis in a serial manner during both progression and recovery.

Several approaches to induction of fibrosis have been described. Of these, CCl_4 intoxication in rats and mice is probably the most widely studied. In addition, the CCl_4 model is the best characterized with respect to histological, biochemical, cell, and molecular changes associated with the development of fibrosis. CCl_4 can be given intraperitoneally or by oral gavage; it induces zone III necrosis and hepatocyte apoptosis with associated hepatic stellate cell activation and tissue fibrosis. With repetitive dosing CCl_4 can be used to induce bridging hepatic fibrosis (4 wk of twice-weekly dosing), cirrhosis (8 wk of twice-weekly dosing) and advanced micronodular cirrhosis (12 wk of twice-weekly dosing). In addition, for each of these models spontaneous recovery from fibrosis can be studied after cessation of dosing. Mechanistic studies using gene knockout and transgenic animals can also be established using CCl_4. Together these models have provided unparalleled insights into the mechanisms underlying hepatic fibrosis.

Key Words: Liver fibrosis; CCl_4; rodents; hepatic stellate cell; collagen.

1. Introduction

Animal models are essential to the investigation of liver fibrosis and other fibrotic diseases because they provide the only model in which the serial sampling of tissue, which facilitates the dissection of the cell and molecular processes that underlie fibrosis, can be made. The importance of studying human models of disease cannot be overemphasized. Nevertheless, at best they can only provide a snapshot of a disease process which may develop over weeks or months. In addition, the morbidity, potential mortality, and ethical issues associated with liver biopsy in humans, significantly limits the use of biopsy material for research. Finally, it is, of course, ethically impossible to manipulate the pathogenic process of liver fibrosis experimentally in vivo in human beings.

From: *Methods in Molecular Medicine, Vol. 117: Fibrosis Research: Methods and Protocols*
Edited by: J. Varga, D. A. Brenner, and S. H. Phan © Humana Press Inc., Totowa, NJ

For these reasons, animal models of liver fibrosis remain a vital experimental tool.

Many experimental models of hepatic fibrosis have been described. These include those associated with toxic damage (e.g., carbon tetrachloride, diamethylnitrozamine, thioacetamide *[1–10]*), immunological damage (e.g., that mediated by heterologous serum and experimental schistosomiasis *[11–13]*), biliary fibrosis (e.g., common bile duct ligation *[14,15]*), and alcoholic liver disease (e.g., the baboon ethanol diet or the Tsukamoto/French model in rats *[16]*).

Carbon tetrachloride-induced fibrosis and cirrhosis is one of the oldest and probably the most widely used toxin-based experimental model for the induction of fibrosis. It has the advantages that it has been clearly characterized and in many respects mirrors the pattern of disease seen in human fibrosis and cirrhosis associated with toxic damage (detailed review in **refs. *16*** and ***17***). In addition, there is extensive experience with this model with respect to the characterization of histological and biochemical changes and changes associated with injury, inflammation, and fibrosis ***(17,18)***. Most specifically, the cellular sources of key matrix components, including collagen-1 in addition to the matrix degrading metalloproteinases (matrix metalloproteinases [MMPs]) and their inhibitors (tissue inhibitors of metalloproteinases [TIMPs]), have been determined ***(18–20)***. Finally, in experienced hands, and even with outbred rats or mice, this model elicits a reproducible and predictable fibrotic response, making it a valuable basis for study. For these reasons, there is a relatively extensive experience and growing literature in which CCl_4-induced fibrosis is used as a basis for mechanistic study, either though the use of genetically modified mice ***(21)*** or the manipulation of the process via a drug or other mediator ***(1,7,13,22)***.

Of course, the CCl_4 model has disadvantages. In comparison, as a model, it has no direct human disease counterpart ***(17)***. Additionally, unlike human liver fibrosis, there is more pronounced cholangiolar cell hyperplasia in advanced CCl_4 fibrosis and, in rats, in the presence of CCl_4-induced cirrhosis, and there is failure to progress to the development of hepatocellular carcinoma (this has been reported in mice subjected to CCl_4 injury, however) ***(17)***. A final consideration is that, in comparison with studies of human tissue and murine tissue, the availability of protein-based reagents such as antibodies, which work effectively in rat models, is relatively limited. These comments notwithstanding, this article will describe the methods for using CCl_4 as an in vivo model of fibrosis in rats.

Carbon tetrachloride, like other halokanes, is activated by oxidases to yield a trichloromethyl radical ***(16,17)***. This free radical initiates lipid peroxidation and can react with the sulphydrol group of proteins ***(16,17)***. CCl_4 has been administered to rodents by inhalation, gastric gavage, and by subcutaneous and intraperitoneal injections ***(16,17)***. Because of the necessity for bioactivation, the severity of CCl_4 injury will be strongly influenced by the type of diet and the presence of other xenobiotics. Specifically, microsomal cytochrome p450 induction significantly enhances CCl_4-mediated damage ***(16,17)***. Thus, diet or drugs that activate cytochrome p450 enhance CCl_4 toxicity and the speed of development of fibrosis. This evidence has been used to increase the speed of development of fibrosis via the addition of barbiturates to drinking water in conjunction with CCl_4 intoxication ***(16)***. Conversely, of course, p450 inhibitors will reduce the toxicity and fibrosis induced by CCl_4 intoxication.

In our laboratory, we have used CCl_4 experiments in a series of experimental models of liver injury and fibrosis. These include using CCl_4: to induce acute injury characterized by self-limiting hepatic stellate cell (HSC) activation and hepatocellular regeneration ***(23)***, to develop early and established fibrosis (4–6 wk of CCl_4, administered as described later ***[19,20]***), to develop early reversible cirrhosis (8 wk of CCl_4 intoxication), and to develop cirrhosis that demonstrates only partial reversibility (12 wk CCl_4 intoxication, unpublished at present) (**Fig. 1**). Because of concerns over the confounding effects of xenobiotics, we do not anesthetize animals for CCl_4 injection.

2. Materials

The use of animals in biomedical research is subject to statutory considerations in most countries. The important legal and environmental considerations are discussed in **Subheading 2.1.** The stock materials that are required are listed under **Subheading 2.2.**

2.1. Legal, Health and Safety, and Environmental Considerations

1. *Legal and statutory considerations:* any work with animals must conform to regulations laid down by relevant local and national statutory bodies. For example, in the United Kingdom, the investigator must hold a relevant UK Home Office project license and personal license. The investigator must be properly trained in the handling and manipulation of experimental animals and the work must take place in an appropriate animal research facility.
2. *Environment:* carbon tetrachloride is toxic to humans by inhalation and ingestion. Preparation of carbon tetrachloride should take place in a fume hood. Injection of animals should take place, where possible, in a fume hood; although for experienced users, if a sealed stock solution of CCl_4 is being used and only opened for filling syringes, then use in a well-ventilated room is probably acceptable. All unused solutions containing CCl_4 should be disposed of in accordance with local regulations.
3. Handling of animals: it is self-evident that anyone undertaking such work should be experienced in handling animals and, where necessary, have attended appro-

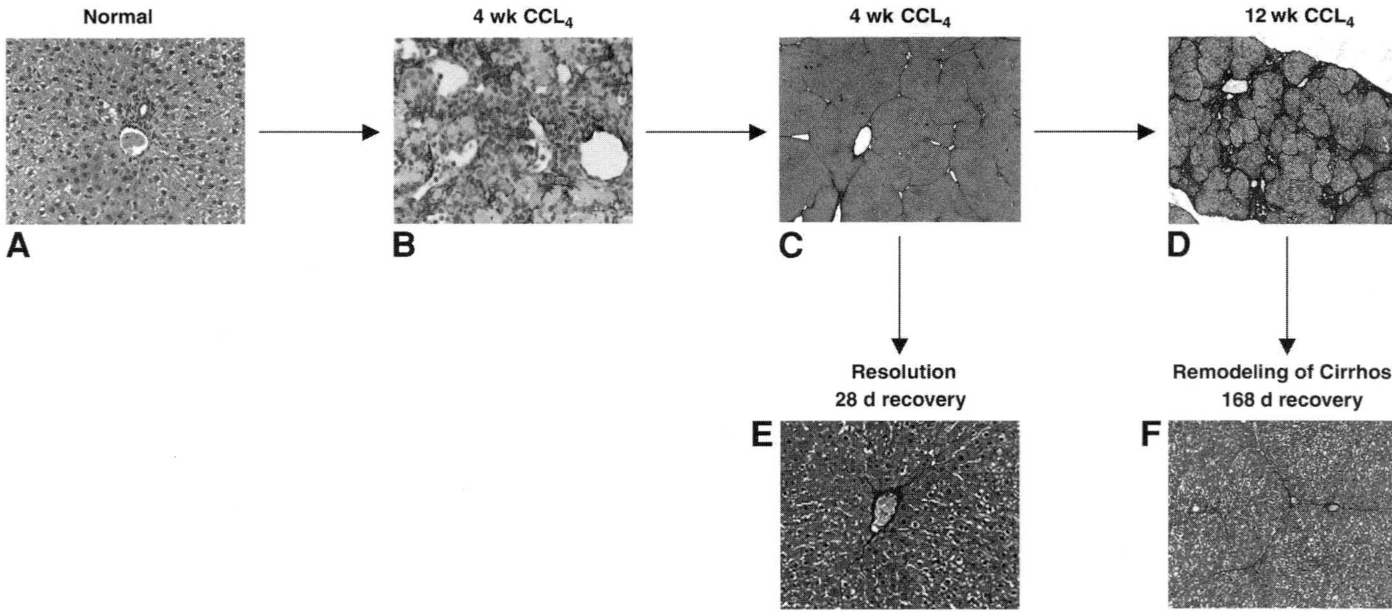

Fig. 1. Examples of CCL_4-induced liver injury of variable duration and periods of recovery in Sprague-Dawley rats, illustrating also the different immunochemical stains used for analysis. **A** shows normal liver. **B** shows activated hepatic stellate cells identified by α-smooth muscle actin staining in areas of inflammation and damage after CCL_4 intoxication. An established fibrosis can be induced after 4 wk **(C)** and an advanced cirrhosis by 12 wk of CCL_4 intoxication **(D)** as described in the text. Spontaneous recovery from each of these injuries will occur although in more advanced fibrosis the extent of recovery may be limited (**F** and **E**, respectively). Reproduced in ammended form from **ref. *25***.

priate animal handling courses. We have found that the routine administration of anesthesia results in an unnecessary stress to the animals and potentially introduces the confounding variable of a xenobiotic.

We, therefore, routinely administer CCl_4 without anesthetic, but in animals that have been regularly handled for a week prior to commencing an experiment. This results in the rats being relaxed and calm at the time of injection.

2.2. Induction of Fibrosis

1. Stock CCl_4 and olive oil vehicle (Sigma-Aldrich).
2. Stock sterile glassware.
3. Nitrile gloves, appropriate eye protection.
4. Equipment for weighing animals.
5. Fume hood with sufficient space for injecting of animals. *Consideration*: CCl_4 will solubilize plastic rubber and leach dye from other chemicals and other articles of apparatus. Therefore, CCl_4 and CCl_4-containing mixtures must be prepared and kept in sterile glass containers under aseptic conditions.
6. 1-mL disposable syringes, 5/8 × 23-gage needles, sterile disposable Hamilton glass syringe.
7. Rat and mouse stock: Sprague-Dawley rats, 250- to 350-g young male adults. For mice, C57 black, male 6 wk of age. See comments on strains below.
8. Mix CCl_4 with olive oil in a fume hood. For rats, mix equal parts of CCl_4 and olive oil (i.e., 1:1); for mice, add one part olive oil to seven parts CCl_4 (i.e., 1:7).
9. Administration of CCl_4: for rats, if use of CCl_4 mixture is immediate, disposable syringes can be used—1 mL with a 5/8 ×23-gage disposable needle. For mice, the CCl_4 mixture should be administered from a 100-µL Hamilton syringe with a 5/8 × 23-gage disposable needle. All used syringes and needles should be disposed of safely in a sharps bin. The Hamilton syringe should be sterilized by autoclaving after use.

2.3. Assessment of Tissue and Histological Techniques

1. Dulbecco's phosphate-buffered saline, pH 7.4 (D-PBS; Sigma-Aldrich, D5652).
2. 10% Formalin (Formaldehyde solution approx 38% in 1X D-PBS, BDH, 101134A).
3. Industrial methylated spirits (IMS) GPR (BDH, 30244 4E).
4. Xylene (BDH, 10293 4F).
5. Paraffin wax (Histoplast wax, Shandon, 67740060), heat to 60°C before use.
6. Acetone (BDH, 10003 3P).
7. Phenylmethylsulfonyl fluoride (Sigma-ALDRICH, P7626).
8. Iodoacetamide (Sigma-Aldrich, 57670).
9. JB4-embedding kit (Park Scientific, 0226).
10. Microtome (Shandon AS200-Innovative base sledge microtome, 0200).
11. VECTABOND™ (Vector Laboratories, SP-1800).
12. Microscope slides (2.6 × 7.6 × 1.0 cm, Surgipath Europe Ltd, 08108G).

13. Mayer's Hemalum (BDH, 35060 4T).
14. Scott's tap water (Surgipath Ltd., 02900).
15. Eosin (BDH, 35084 4K).
16. DPX (BDH, 36029 4H).
17. Cover slips (Surgipath Ltd., 00146).
18. Ehrlich's hematoxylin (Raymond Lamb, AS047-C).
19. 0.5% Aqueous phloxine (Raymond Lamb, S282-2).
20. 0.2% Phosphomolybdic acid (Sigma-Aldrich, P7390).
21. Saturated aqueous picric acid (Sigma-Aldrich, P6744).
22. 0.01% Hydrochloric acid (Sigma-Aldrich, H7020).
23. 0.1% Trypsin (Autogen Bioclear UK Ltd., TRYPE-102012).
24. 0.6% Hydrogen peroxide (H_2O_2) solution (Sigma-Aldrich, H1009), diluted in methanol (BDH, 10158 5A).
25. VECTASTAIN™ Universal Quick kit: Vector Laboratories Ltd., PK-8800).
26. Monoclonal anti-α-smooth muscle actin (α-sma) (Vector Laboratories Ltd., NCL-SMA).
27. Monoclonal anti-α-sma 1A4 fluorescein isothiocyanate (FITC) conjugate antibody (Sigma-Aldrich, F3777).
28. Humidity chamber: Shandon Sequenza™-immunostaining center (Thermo Shandon Inc., 73300001) with Coverplates™ (7211013).
29. Mouse immunoglobulin (Ig)G2a culture supernatant (DakoCytomation Ltd., X0943).
30. Diaminobenzidine substrate kit (DAB) (Vector Laboratories Ltd., SK-4100).
31. 0.1% Sodium azide solution (Sigma-Aldrich, S2002).
32. Blocking kit (Vector Laboratories Ltd., SP-2001).
33. Dulbecco's modified Eagle's medium (DMEM) (Cambrex Bio Science Wokingham Ltd., BE12-604F).
34. Fetal bovine serum (FBS), heat inactivated (Invitrogen Ltd., 10108-165).
35. Bovine serum albumin (BSA) fraction V (Sigma-ALDRICH, A-7906).
36. Penicillin/atreptomycin liquid (Invitrogen Ltd., 15140-122).
37. Rabbit anti-FITC antibody (DakoCytomation Ltd., V0403).
38. Swine anti-rabbit immunoglobilins/Biotinylated, Swine $F(ab')_2$, antibody (DakoCytomation, E0431).
39. Avidin/biotin complex (from the Elite standard VECTASTAIN ABC kit, Vector Laboratories Ltd., PK-6100).

3. Methods

3.1. Dosage and Animal Numbers

In this section, the techniques for administering CCl_4 to induce liver fibrosis are described. **Subheading 3.2.** describes the necessary duration of injection. The techniques required for harvesting of fibrotic rat or mouse liver are described in **Subheading 3.3.** together with the key initial techniques for analyzing the harvested livers.

1. Calculating animal numbers: Lehr's formula can be used as a power calculation to determine the number of animals required for specific experimental groups (*see* **Note 1**). In our experience, in comparative analyses of treated groups of rats, a number of 6 to 8 is required in each group.
2. CCl_4 dosage and frequency: for rats, inject 0.2 mL/100 g of the 1:1 ratio CCl_4:olive oil mix, previously described, twice weekly at equal intervals, i.e., Monday and Thursday for 2 wk followed by 0.1 mL of the 1:1 mix for the duration specified by project (i.e., rats received 0.1 mL/100 g of CCl_4 for 2 wk followed by 0.05 mL CCl_4/100 g for the duration specified by the project). For mice, inject 1 μL/g body weight of the 1:7 ratio CCl_4:olive oil mix previously described every 5 d (i.e., mice receive 0.125 mL/g of CCl_4 for the duration of the project). *See also* **Note 2.**
3. Pre-injection assessment: rats and mice are weighed and the dose of CCl_4 calculated (a previously drawn-up chart of weight/dosages is useful here; *see* **Note 3**). The rat/mouse is restrained as described.
4. Injection technique: rat intraperitoneal injections require two investigators. One investigator gently but firmly holds the animal while another injects. Immobilize the rat by grasping gently but firmly around the shoulder region with the thumb under the lower jaw. The other hand supports the lower body and the tail is kept out of the way with the fingers. The animal's body should be kept taut, with the head held lower than the rest of the body so that the viscera move towards the diaphragm. Make the injection in the lower middle of the abdomen with a single, firm thrust, taking care to avoid the bladder and diaphragm.

   For mice, there are several differences in technique and one person should be able to restrain and inject simultaneously. The mouse should be gently but firmly scruffed behind the neck region between the thumb and forefinger. The hand is turned over so that the mouse is supported on the palm against the base of the thumb with the third and/or fourth finger resting over the pelvic region. The abdomen should be kept taut by extending the hand. Other precautions are as for the rats.

3.2. Duration of Injection

1. For a self-limiting injury, resulting in activation of HSCs and expression of fibrotic genes: inject rats with two doses of CCl_4 as previously described; harvest 24 h after final injection.
2. For an established early fibrosis (**Fig. 1**): inject rats with CCl_4 as above for 4 wk (i.e., 8 doses in total); harvest 3 d after final injection.
3. For established but reversible fibrosis: inject rats with CCl_4 twice weekly as above for 6 wk (i.e., 12 doses in total); harvest 3 d after final injection. This model can also be used to study spontaneous recovery, which will occur over the subsequent 28 to 56 d following withdrawal of CCl_4.
4. For established but reversible cirrhosis: inject rats with CCl_4 as above for 8 wk (i.e., 16 doses in total); harvest 3 d after final injection at 8 wk. This cirrhosis will undergo spontaneous regression over the subsequent 84 d. For an established

micronodular cirrhosis: inject rats with CCl_4 for 12 wk (i.e., 24 doses in total); harvest liver 3 d after final injection. Although substantive remodeling of fibrosis will occur if this model is allowed to recover spontaneously over the subsequent 84 to 168 d, persistent macronodular features will be present even after 366 d of recovery (**Fig. 1**).

5. For control rats: cohorts should be injected with an identical volume of olive oil (i.e., 0.2/mL × mL 100 g for 2 wk followed by 0.1 mL/100 g for the duration of the project).
6. For mice (C57B), an established fibrosis can be induced by 4 wk of injection with the 1:7 CCl_4:olive oil mix. Harvest 3 d after final injection. An early cirrhosis can be induced by 8 wk treatment with the 1:7 CCl_4:olive oil mix. Harvest 3 d after final injection.

3.3. Harvest

1. Animals are intoxicated with carbon dioxide and subjected to cervical dislocation.
2. Laparotomy is performed and the liver removed for analysis as described below. In addition, the spleen can be removed and weighed as an indirect index of portal hypertension and other viscera removed and stored as necessary.
3. A single blood sample is taken by direct cardiac puncture for measure of liver enzymes and bilirubin. In addition, in more advanced models of hepatic fibrosis, ascites should be measured using a syringe and needle.

3.4. Assessment of Tissues

Clearly individual experimental techniques will be undertaken to address the questions underlying the research developed by particular individuals. Nevertheless, routine assessment of the extent and distribution of fibrosis will be necessary and common to all models (**Fig. 1**). The routine histological amount of fibrosis is described as follows:

1. The liver is divided and two lobes sectioned regularly at 2 to 4 mm intervals and fixed in 10% buffered formalin. Tissues are routinely processed through a series of alcohols followed by xylenes before embedding in paraffin wax.
2. Further tissue can be fixed overnight in cold acetone containing 2 m*M* phenylmethylsulfonyl fluoride and 20 m*M* iodoacetamide. These tissues are routinely processed using the JB4-embedding kit finally embedding in Glycol methacrylate (GMA) resin. This method fixation is useful for specific immunohistochemical and *in situ* interrogation.
3. The remaining tissue is snap-frozen in liquid nitrogen.

3.4.1. Routine Histological Analysis of Fibrosis

Obtain 2 to 4 μm tissue sections from the formalin-fixed, paraffin-embedded GMA and frozen tissues using a microtome. Tissue sections are placed onto VECTABOND-treated microscope slides, ready for immunohistochemical analysis.

3.4.2. Histological Staining Techniques

Before immunohistochemistry, tissue sections should be treated in the following way:

1. Paraffin-embedded tissue should be deparaffinized through xylene twice, followed by IMS twice, each time for 5 min before rehydrating in tap water.
2. GMA tissue sections can be used immediately for immunohistochemical techniques.
3. Frozen tissue sections must be thawed for 20 min at room temperature before fixing for 5–10 min in cold acetone, or an alternative fixative for specific immunohistochemical or *in situ* interrogation. Tissue sections are then left to air dry for a further 20 min before performing immunohistochemical techniques.

3.4.3. Hematoxylin and Eosin Staining

Hemotoxylin and eosin staining provides a specimen in which the overall architecture, degree of inflammation, necrosis, cellular apoptosis, and cellular mitosis can be assessed.

For paraffin-embedded and frozen tissue sections:

1. Dip tissue sections in filtered Mayer's Haemalum for approx 30 s to 1 min.
2. Thoroughly wash tissue sections in tap water until the water is clear.
3. Blue tissue sections in Scott's tap water for 1 min.
4. Thoroughly wash tissue sections in tap water.
5. Dip tissue sections in eosin for 30 s.
6. Thoroughly wash tissue sections in tap water until the water is clear.
7. Dehydrate tissue sections through IMS twice, followed by xylene twice, each time for 5 min.
8. Sections were mounted using cover slips with distrene, plasticizer, xylene (DPX) medium.

For GMA-processed tissue sections:

1. Place tissue sections in preheated Ehrlich's hematoxylin for 20 min at 60°C.
2. Thoroughly wash tissue sections in tap water until the water is clear.
3. Differentiate tissue sections in 1% acid alcohol for up to 5 s.
4. Thoroughly wash tissue sections in tap water
5. Blue tissue sections in Scott's tap water for 1 min.
6. Counterstain tissue sections in 0.5% aqueous phloxine for 5 min.
7. Thoroughly wash tissue sections in tap water until the water is clear.
8. Dehydrate tissue sections through IMS twice, followed by xylene twice, each time for 5 min.
9. Mount tissue sections using cover slips with DPX.

*3.4.4. Sirius Red Staining (see **Note 4**)*

Sirius Red staining identifies the collagens in a section and provides an excellent visual index of the extent and distribution of fibrosis (**Fig. 1**). The following protocol is for paraffin-embedded GMA and frozen tissue sections. GMA tissue sections have a longer incubation time and are shown parenthetically:

1. Thoroughly wash all tissue sections in distilled water.
2. Place tissue sections into 0.2% phosphomolybdic acid at room temperature for 5 min (GMA: 30 min).
3. Transfer tissue sections into picro-Sirius Red solution (0.1 g Sirius Red F3B in 100 mL saturated aqueous picric acid for 2 h [GMA: 24 h]).
4. With the exception of the GMA tissue samples, briefly wash tissue sections in 0.01% hydrochloric acid.
5. Thoroughly wash ALL tissue sections in tap water.
6. Counterstain tissue sections in filtered Mayer's Hemalum for approx 30 s to 1 min.
7. Thoroughly wash tissue sections in tap water until the water is clear.
8. Blue tissue sections in Scott's tap water for 1 min.
9. Thoroughly wash tissue sections in tap water.
10. Dehydrate tissue sections through IMS twice, followed by xylene twice, each time for 5 min.
11. Mount tissue sections using cover slips with DPX.

3.4.5. α-Sma Staining (see **Note 4**)

α-Sma staining will identify activated HSCs and other tissue myofibroblasts in liver sections. It provides a excellent visual index of the extent and distribution of activated HSCs in areas of liver injury and fibrosis (**Fig. 1**).

For paraffin-embedded and frozen tissue sections:

1. Wash all tissue section in 1X D-PBS for 5 min at room temperature.
2. Retrieval of antigens masked by crosslinkages occurring during the tissue fixation process can be accomplished by placing tissue sections in preheated 0.1% trypsin in 1X D-PBS and incubating at 37°C for 20 min.
3. Thoroughly wash all tissue sections in 1X D-PBS.
4. Endogenous peroxidase activity can be blocked by placing tissue sections into 0.6% hydrogen peroxide in methanol solution for 15 min at room temperature.
5. Thoroughly wash all tissue sections in 1X D-PBS.
6. To reduce background secondary staining, add 100 μL of normal horse blocking serum (from the VECTASTAIN Universal Quick kit) diluted 1:40 in 1X D-PBS to the tissue section and incubate at room temperature for 10 min.
7. Remove excess serum and add 100 μL of α-sma diluted 1:40 in 1X D-PBS. Incubate the tissue sections in a humidity chamber at 4°C overnight. No primary antibody and/or equivalent concentrations of mouse IgG2a can be added to tissue sections to act as negative controls. Vascular structures in the liver tissue sections or muscle tissue can act as positive controls.
8. Wash tissue sections in 1X D-PBS for 5 min.
9. Add 100 μL of biotinylated universal secondary antibody (from the VECTASTAIN Universal Quick kit) diluted 1:20 in 1X D-PBS with blocking serum diluted 1:10. Incubate the tissue sections at room temperature for 15 min.

10. Wash tissue sections in 1X D-PBS for 5 min.
11. Add 100 μL of streptavidin/peroxidase preformed complex antibody (from the VECTASTAIN Universal Quick kit) diluted 1:40 in 1X D-PBS. Incubate the tissue sections at room temperature for 10 min.
12. Wash tissue sections in 1X D-PBS for 5 min.
13. Antigen visualization can be performed adding 100 μL of DAB (from the DAB substrate kit, to 5 mL distilled water add two drops of buffer, pH 7.5; four drops of DAB; and two drops of H_2O_2). α-sma antigen bound substrate is converted to an insoluble brown product.
14. Wash tissue sections thoroughly in tap water.
15. Dip tissue sections in filtered Mayer's Hemalum for approx 30 s to 1 min.
16. Thoroughly wash tissue sections in tap water until the water is clear.
17. Blue tissue sections in Scott's tap water for 1 min.Thoroughly wash tissue sections in tap water.
18. Dehydrate tissue sections through IMS twice, followed by xylene twice, each time for 5 min.
19. Mount tissue sections using cover slips with DPX.

For GMA-processed tissue sections:

The following protocol is applicable to GMA tissue sections from all species. This same protocol can also be applied to mouse formalin-fixed paraffin embedded tissue.

1. Wash all tissue section in 1X D-PBS for 5 min at room temperature.
2. Endogenous peroxidase activity can be blocked by placing tissue sections into 1% hydrogen peroxide in 0.1% sodium azide solution for 30 min at room temperature.
3. Wash tissue sections in 1X D-PBS for 5 min.
4. Add 100 μL of Avidin D solution (from the Blocking kit) and incubate at room temperature for 15 min.
5. Wash tissue sections in 1X D-PBS for 5 min.
6. Add 100 μL of biotin solution (from the Blocking kit) and incubate at room temperature for 15 min.
7. Add 100 μL of blocking medium (80 mL DMEM, 20 mL FBS, 1 g BSA) to the tissue sections. Incubate at room temperature for 30 min (mouse tissue: incubate at 37°C for 20 min).
8. Add 100 μL of monoclonal anti α-sma 1A4 FITC conjugate antibody diluted 1:7000 in 1X D-PBS (mouse tissue: dilute 1:16000 in 1X D-PBS). Incubate the tissue sections in a humidity chamber, place in the dark at 4°C overnight.
9. Wash tissue sections in 1X D-PBS for 5 min.
10. Add 100 μL of rabbit anti-FITC antibody diluted 1:1500 in 1X D-PBS. Incubate the tissue sections in the dark for 90 min. For mouse tissue, dilute antibody 1:4000 in 1X D-PBS and incubate for 30 min in the dark.
11. Add 100 μL of Swine anti-rabbit immunoglobilins/biotinylated, Swine $F(ab')_2$, antibody diluted 1:10,000 in 1X D-PBS. Incubate the tissue sections in the dark

for 90 min. For mouse tissue, dilute antibody 1:200 in 1X D-PBS and incubate for 30 min in the dark.

12. Wash tissue sections in 1X D-PBS for 5 min.
13. Add 100 μL of avidin/biotin complex (from the Elite standard VECTASTAIN ABC kit, to 5 mL of 1X D-PBS add 100 μL reagent A and 100 μL reagent B, prepare 30 min in advance) and incubate the tissue sections for 90 min (mouse tissue: incubate for 30 min).
14. Wash tissue sections in 1X D-PBS for 5 min.
15. Antigen visualization can be performed using the DAB substrate kit according to manufacturers instruction, whereby α-sma antigen-bound substrate is converted to an insoluble brown product.
16. Wash tissue sections thoroughly in tap water.
17. Dip tissue sections in filtered Mayer's Hemalum for approx 30 s to 1 min.
18. Thoroughly wash tissue sections in tap water until the water is clear.
19. Blue tissue sections in Scott's tap water for 1 min.
20. Thoroughly wash tissue sections in tap water.
21. Dehydrate tissue sections through IMS twice, followed by xylene twice, each time for 5 min.
22. Mount tissue sections using cover slips with DPX.

4. Notes

1. Although the power calculations and recommendations of absolute numbers of experimental animals described here are a guide (*see* **Subheading 3.1.**), the use of a pilot study to determine the response and likely outcome of any specific experimental manipulations is strongly recommended.
2. For mice, strain-specific differences in CCl_4 sensitivity represent a significant and unpredictable variable. The potential mechanisms for strain variation are reviewed in **ref. *24***. For example, both 129SV and BALB/C strains appear to be relatively unresponsive to CCl_4 compared with C57B blacks. For this reason, we strongly recommend a pilot study for any experiment involving inbred mice (e.g., gene knockout or transgenic mice) whatever the originating background strain.
3. When injecting mice or rats, it is useful to have a table listing the injection volumes for a range of rat/mouse weights. This enables the injection to be undertaken with little or no delay after the animal is weighed, thus minimizing stress and unnecessary handling.
4. Use the presence of collagen and smooth muscle cells in the vascular structures as a positive control for Sirius red and α-sma staining, respectively, when characterizing tissues histologically.

Acknowledgments

The authors gratefully acknowledge the support of the MRC UK (Snr Clinical Fellowship to JPI), The Childrens Liver Disease Foundation (project grant to JPI), and the Welcome Trust (Clinical Fellowship to NH).

References

1. Ala-Kokko, L., Stenback, F., and Ryhanen, L. (1989) Preventative effect of malotilate on dimethylnitrosamina-induced liver fibrosis in rats. *J. Lab. Clin. Med.* **113,** 177–183.
2. Cameron, G. R. and Karunaratne, W. A. E. (1936) Carbon tetrachloride cirrhosis in relation to liver regeneration. *J. Pathol. Bacteriol.* **42,** 1–21.
3. Igarashi, S., Hatahara, T., and Nagai, Y. (1986) Anti-fibrotic effects of Malotilate on liver fibrosis induced by carbon tetrachloride in rats. *Jpn J. Exp. Med.* **56,** 235–245.
4. Madden, J. W., Gertman, P. M., and Peacock, E. E. (1970) Dimethylnitrosamine induced hepatic cirrhosis – a new canine model of an ancient human disease. *Surgery* **68,** 260–268.
5. Marrione, T. G. (1949) Factors influencing the collagen content in experimental cirrhosis. *Am. J. Pathol.* **25,** 273–285.
6. Martinez-Hernandez, A. (1985) The hepatic extracellular matrix 11 Electron immunohistochemical studies in rats with CCl4 induced cirrhosis. *Lab. Invest.* **53,** 166–186.
7. Nakamura, N., Fusamoto, H., and Koizumi, T. (1975) The effects of aminoacetonitrile and its derivative on components of hepatic connective tissue in rats with chronic hepatic injury. *Acta Hepatogastroenterol.* **22,** 78–84.
8. Rojkind, M. and Dunn, M. A. (1979) Hepatic fibrosis. *Gastroenterology* **76,** 849–863.
9. Rubin, E., Hutterer, F., and Popper, H. (1963) Cell proliferation and fibrous formation in chronic carbon tetrachloride intoxication. *Am. J. Pathol.* **42,** 715–728.
10. Zimmerman, H. (1976) Experimental hepatotoxicity, in *Experimental Production of Disease, Part 5: Liver.* (Eiciler, O., ed.), Springer-Verlag, Berlin: pp. 1–120.
11. Ballardini, G., Degli, E. S., and Bianchi, F. B. (1983) Correlation between Ito cells and fibrogenesis is in an experimental model of hepatic fibrosis. A sequential stereological study. *Liver* **3,** 58–63.
12. Dunn, M. A., Rojkind, M., and Warren, K. S. (1977) Distribution of Ito cells in experimental hepatic fibrosis. *J. Clin. Invest.* **59,** 666–674.
13. Yokoi, Y., Namihisa, T., Matsuzaki, K., Miyazaki, A., and Yamaguchi, Y. (1988) Distribution of Ito cells in experimental hepatic fibrosis. *Liver* **8,** 48–52.
14. Issa, R., Williams, E., Trim, N., et al. (2001) Apoptosis of hepatic stellate cells: involvement in resolution of biliary fibrosis and regulation by soluble growth factors. *Gut* **48,** 548–557.
15. Tams, E. G. (1957) Morphological and functional changes in the livers of rats after ligation and excision of the common bile duct. *Am. J. Pathol.* **33,** 13–27.
16. Tsukamoto, H., Matsuoka, M., and French, S. W. (1990) Experimental models of hepatic fibrosis: A review. *Semin. Liver Dis.* **10,** 56–65.
17. Tamayo, R. P. (1983) Is cirrhosis of the liver experimentally produced by CCl4 an adequate model of human cirrhosis? *Hepatology* **3,** 112–120.
18. Maher, J. J. and McGuire, R. F. (1990) Extracellular matrix gene expression increases preferentially in rat lipocytes and sinusoidal endothelial cells during hepatic fibrosis in vivo. *J. Clin. Invest.* **86,** 1641–1648.

19. Iredale, J. P., Benyon, R. C., Arthur, M. J. P., et al. (1996) Tissue inhibitor of metalloproteinase-1 messenger RNA expression is enhanced relative to interstitial collagenase messenger RNA in experimental liver injury and fibrosis. *Hepatology* **24,** 176–184.
20. Iredale, J. P., Benyon, R. C., Pickering, J., et al. (1998) HSC apoptosis and reduced hepatic expression of metalloproteinase inhibitors. *J. Clin. Invest.* **102,** 538–549.
21. Issa, R., Zhou, X., Trim, N., et al. (2003) Mutation in collagen-1 that confers resistance to the action of collagenase results in failure of recovery from CCl4 induced liver fibrosis, persistence of activated hepatic stellate cells, and diminished hepatocytes regeneration. *FASEB J.* **17(1),** 47–49.
22. Wright, M. C., Issa, R., Smart, D. E., et al. (2001) Gliotoxin stimulates the apoptosis of human and rat hepatic stellate cells and enhances the resolution of liver fibrosis in rats. *Gastroenterology* **121,** 685–698.
23. Oakley, F., Trim, N., Constandinou, C. M., et al. (2003) Hepatocytes express nerve growth factor during liver injury: evidence for paracrine regulation of hepatic stellate cell apoptosis. *Am. J. Pathol.* **163(5),** 1849–1858.
24. Zengdun, S., Wakil, A. E., and Rockey, D. C. (1994) Strain specific differences in mouse hepatic wound healing are mediated by divergent T. helper cytokine responses. *Proc. Natl. Acad. Sci. USA* **94(20),** 10663–10668.
25. Iredale, J. P. (2003) Cirrhosis: new research provides a basis for rational and targeted treatments. *BMJ* **327(7407),** 143–147.

15

Animal Models of Pulmonary Fibrosis

Mehrnaz Gharaee-Kermani, Matthew Ullenbruch, and Sem H. Phan

Summary

In general, there are two types of animal models: natural and experimental. Because there are no natural models for pulmonary fibrosis, an experimental model that reproduces key aspects of the human disease would be useful for the study of this form of lung disease, the natural history of which is not always known. To date, a variety of animal models have been used to investigate mechanisms of pulmonary and other types of fibrosis, including the intratracheal instillation of bleomycin, fluorescein isothiocyanate, or particulate matter, such as silica and asbestos. This chapter will describe two commonly used techniques, namely bleomycin and silica-induced, which have been developed for the study of pulmonary fibrosis in animal models.

Key Words: Pulmonary fibrosis; animal model; bleomycin; silica; intratracheal instillation.

1. Introduction

Idiopathic pulmonary fibrosis is associated with an extremely poor prognosis, the median survival rate being approx 5 yr *(1–2)*. It is characterized by some degree of lung inflammation and abnormal tissue repair, resulting in the replacement of normal tissue with abnormal accumulation of fibroblasts and deposition of extracellular matrix in the interstitium and alveolar spaces *(3–14)*. This process is now known to involve the activation of an intricate cytokine network, resulting in the elevation of collagen gene expression and abnormal deposition of collagen in the lung *(3–14)*.

Although in the past two decades we have increased our understanding of the pathogenesis of idiopathic pulmonary fibrosis, the importance of inflammation remains controversial. This is partly a result of the fact that the inflammatory component is variably present at the time of diagnosis, and even the most potent antiinflammatory drugs do not seem to control or arrest the progression

From: *Methods in Molecular Medicine, Vol. 117: Fibrosis Research: Methods and Protocols*
Edited by: J. Varga, D. A. Brenner, and S. H. Phan © Humana Press Inc., Totowa, NJ

of fibrosis. This highly lethal disorder continues to pose major clinical challenges because an effective therapeutic regimen has yet to be determined.

Much of our knowledge about the pathogenesis of pulmonary fibrosis has benefited from studies using animal models of lung fibrosis in multiple species ***(6–31)***. These models have exploited a number of agents, which are known to cause some degree of lung injury, inflammation, and fibrosis, such as bleomycin, silica, asbestos, fluorescein isothiocyanate, and radiation ***(6–31)***. As is evident, much valuable information has been generated from these animal models of pulmonary fibrosis. The accumulated data cover a broad base of information, from biochemistry and cellular and molecular biology to pulmonary function testing and therapeutic interventions. In this chapter, two commonly used and well-characterized methods of induction of lung fibrosis in animal models will be described. The first relies on bleomycin, an anti-tumor antibiotic that causes DNA strand scission and cellular/tissue injury. This is usually restricted to the lungs and skin as a result of lower levels of bleomycin hydrolase in these organs. The ensuing inflammation is followed by fibrosis that develops commonly over a 2- to 3-wk period. The other common model induced by particulate matter to mimic the pneumoconioses is induced by silica. Injury resulting from the silica particles and the inability to clear the particles by phagocytes lead to sustained chronic inflammation and subsequent fibrosis. These two models, one based on soluble and the other on insoluble inducing agents will be described in this chapter.

2. Materials

2.1. Animals

A number of animal species, including mice, rats, hamsters, rabbits, dogs, and nonhuman primates have been used for models of pulmonary fibrosis. In this chapter, we focus on the use mice and rats, which are readily available, including transgenic strains, and relatively inexpensive compared with other species. Moreover, an exhaustive list of reagents for studies in these species, especially mice, is also readily available to assist in in vitro as well as in vivo studies. Use of these relatively small animals also affords savings in the use of reagents that are often expensive.

2.1.1. Mice

Pathogen-free mice of multiple different strains (e.g., CBA/J, C57BL/6, BALB/C) can be directly purchased from Jackson Laboratory (Bar Harbor, ME). They should be housed in positive-pressure, air-conditioned units (25°C, 50% relative humidity) on a 12-h light–dark cycle. They usually weigh between 20 and 22 g at approx 8 wk of age when used in the described animal model studies (*see* **Note 1**).

2.1.2. Rats

Specific pathogen-free Fisher 344 rats of 2 to 3 mo of age and weighing 150 to 200 g are obtained from Charles River Breeding Laboratories, Inc. (Wilmington MA) (*see* **Note 2**). The animals should arrive in filtered cages, and be maintained in clean animal quarters, separate from other laboratory animals. They should be maintained using microisolator techniques with daily veterinarian monitoring.

2.2. Anesthetic Drugs

For the induction of pulmonary fibrosis via endotracheal instillation of agents, the animals are anesthetized using a combination of ketamine and rompun via intraperitoneal injection. In order to make 10 mL of the stock solution of the anesthetic drugs for rats, mix 8 mL of ketamine (50 mg/mL) and 2 mL of rompun (xylazine, 20 mg/mL Bayer). The dosage for the rat is 0.1 mL of this mixture per 100 g body weight (*see* **Note 3**). To make 10 mL of the stock solution of the drugs for mice, mix 0.87 mL of the ketamine and 0.65 mL of rompun mixed with 8.48 mL of phosphate-buffered saline (PBS). The dosage for mice is 0.1 mL of this mixture per 10 g body weight. The ketamine and the rompun maybe stored at room temperature in a locked box.

2.3. Agents for Induction of Pulmonary Fibrosis

2.3.1. Bleomycin

Much information has been generated from animal model studies of bleomycin-induced pulmonary fibrosis ***(6–14,17,18,22–25)***. For induction of pulmonary fibrosis in this animal model, bleomycin sulfate (Blenoxane, Mead Jackson, NJ) is suspended in sterile saline at either 5 or 1 U/mL. The bleomycin stock solution can be stored frozen at –20°C until administration (*see* **Note 4**).

2.3.2. Silica

A suspension of crystalline silica particles in sterile 0.9% saline at a dose of 2.5 mg per 20 g body weight should be used in the mouse. Because the silica particles may contain traces of endotoxin, particles are heated at 200°C for 2 h immediately before suspension and administration ***(15,26)***.

2.4. Materials Needed for Surgery

The materials needed for surgery are as follows: sterile scissors, forceps, auto-suture clips (AUTOCLIP 9 mm, Becton Dickinson, Sparks, MD), surgery board (at an approx 70° angle), blade, 1-mL syringes with 26-gage needles (*see* **Note 5**), warmer pads, sheets for warmer pads, bedding and surgical vinyl bags, adhesive tape, and paper towels; gloves, marker and masks, ethanol swabs, and providone swabs; shaver, balance, sterile 0.9% saline, and ice.

3. Methods

3.1. Bleomycin-Induced Pulmonary Fibrosis in Rodent Models

3.1.1. Routes of Administration

Clinically, the major route of bleomycin administration is parenterally except in cases where intrapleural injection is used. Although early animal models used parenteral routes such as intravenous, intraperitoneal, and intramuscular ***(28–30)*** to mimic the clinical application, many subsequent animal models used a single intratracheal injection of bleomycin ***(6–14,17,18,22–25)***. The cumulative doses used in the parenteral models were in the 100 to 200 mg (units)/kg range, whereas the intratracheal single-injection models used a single dose in the 1.5 to 7.5 mg/kg range ***(6–14,17,18,22–25)***.

The intratracheal bleomycin animal models were not only shown to induce lung fibrosis similar to the parenteral models, but also to have several advantages such as use of less bleomycin, a quicker kinetic development, and a clear start time for lung injury. In addition to intratracheal injection, recently bleomycin was administered by transoral instillation in mice ***(27)***. This method of administration is not only easy and quick, but also does not involve surgery ***(27)***. In the following section, we describe the intratracheal and transoral bleomycin administration methods in detail.

3.1.2. Intratracheal Bleomycin Instillation

Mice or rats should be matched by age, weight, and sex and randomly allocated into bleomycin-treated and control groups. The animals are anesthetized with a combination of ketamine and rompun via intraperitoneal injection as described in **Subheading 2.2.** Within 10 min, the animals will be anesthetized; then the neck area is shaved and sterilized using a betadine scrub. The animals are then placed on the surgery board, and their tails immobilized with adhesive tape. Following this, a 1-cm midline incision is made in the neck area with sterile scissors, while the skin is held with sterile forceps. Care is taken to prevent cutting the neck muscles. The trachea is exposed through the incision, using a sterile surgical probe. A sterile 1-mL syringe fitted with a 26-gage needle is filled with the appropriate amount of bleomycin sulfate (1–10 U/kg body weight for mice or 7.5 U/kg for rats). The needle is introduced into the visualized trachea at an oblique angle and directed caudally (*see* **Fig. 1**) and the bleomycin solution is then quickly injected during inspiration. After withdrawing the needle, the incision is sutured with an auto suture clip. The animals are then placed on warmer pads to stabilize temperature and allowed to

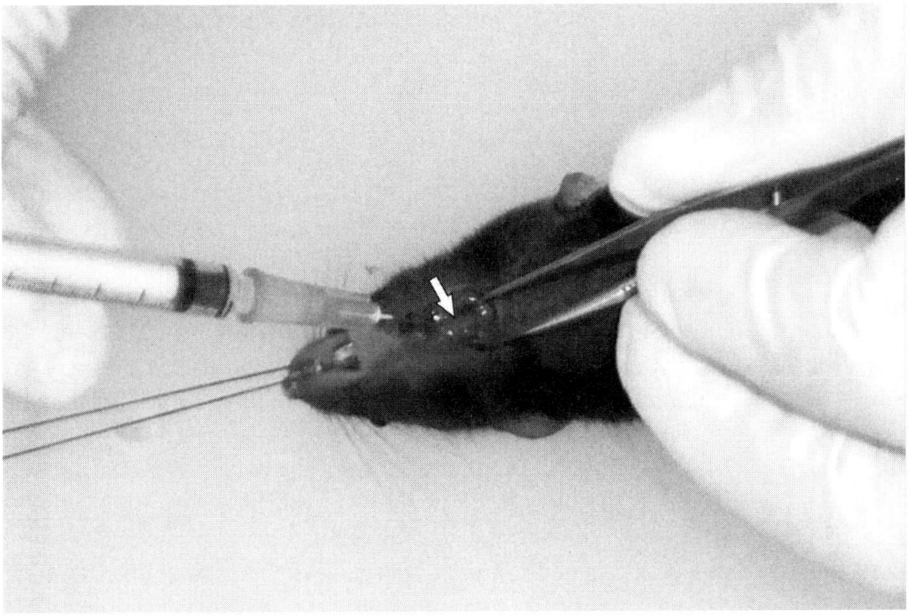

Fig. 1. Intratracheal bleomycin instillation in mouse. View of exposed trachea (arrow) through a midline incision is shown. The overlying muscles have been pushed aside by the forceps, and a 1-mL syringe with 26-gage needle is shown just penetrating the trachea.

recover. The animals are monitored until fully awake from the anesthesia. Usually, the entire procedure takes about 15 min, and the animals become fully awake within an hour after induction of anesthesia. Control animals receive an equal volume of sterile saline instead of the bleomycin solution.

Animals are examined daily, and body weights and survival rates may be recorded at the same time if needed. The specified control and experimental groups are sacrificed at the time points of interest under ketamine overdose anesthesia, commonly on d 1, 3, 7, 14, 21, and 28 post-bleomycin or saline injection when key pathogenetic events are known to occur ***(5–14)***. After the abdominal cavity is opened using scissors, the abdominal aorta is transected to achieve exsanguination. Then the chest cavity is quickly exposed by removal of the rib cage using scissors and sterile saline is injected gently into the right ventricle of the heart using a 5- or 10-mL syringe and 21-gage needle, until the lungs are blanched. Then the lung tissue can be harvested for cell, RNA, and/or protein isolation as well as miscellaneous biochemical analysis. Bronchoalveolar lavage can also be performed with sterile saline at this stage. For morphological examination, the lungs are rapidly inflated with fixative and then embedded in paraffin *(6–14)*.

3.1.3. Transoral Bleomycin Instillation

Recently, an alternative nonsurgical technique has been reported for intratracheal instillation of bleomycin via a trans-oral route. (**27**). After anesthesia as under **Subheading 3.1.2.**, the animal is laid on the surgery board and suspended on the angled surgery board with surgical thread via its incisors, and the tail is immobilized with adhesive tape. Then with sterile forceps the mouth is nudged open and, with the same forceps, the tongue is gently pulled out and toward the mandible and lower incisors. This maneuver allows visualization of the vocal cords with the assistance of adequate lighting, and the bleomycin can then be delivered through the vocal cords using a sterile 100-μL pipet during inspiration. The animals are then allowed to recover from the anesthesia as described under **Subheading 3.1.2.** Not only does the transoral bleomycin administration induce lung injury similar to the intratracheal model, it also has several advantages, such as being an easier and faster technique, plus the fact that the animals recover more quickly from the procedure without the side effects/disadvantages of surgery.

3.1.4. Usefulness and Disadvantage of the Models

Rapid limited development of lung fibrosis occurs in mice or rats following a single injection of bleomycin using either approach. Regardless of the route of administration, lung injury in each model progressed uniformly in a similar manner with the development of pulmonary fibrosis. Although these models represent very quick ways to study the mechanisms of fibrosis, they do not produce a chronic progressive type of lesion as seen in patients with idiopathic pulmonary fibrosis. However, it may be possible to have a more progressive type of model by using a continuous infusion method of bleomycin delivery via a subcutaneously implanted osmotic pump *(31)*. With this approach, mice receiving bleomycin continuously over 1 wk exhibit significantly more lung collagen that is more evenly distributed at 6 wk compared with animals receiving a similar dose through daily subcutaneous injection. The study also suggests that animals receiving continuous infusion may have evidence of progressive disease, but that longer time periods are needed before a true progressive lesion can be established.

3.2. Silica-Induced Pulmonary Fibrosis

Animals are anesthetized as described under **Subheading 3.1.2.** The silica particle suspension (2.5 mg in 60 μL sterile saline) is administered intratracheally into each mouse as described under **Subheading 3.1.2.** *(16,26)*.

The use of silica in animals caused the development of a slowly progressive form of pulmonary fibrosis accompanied by granulomatous inflammation. Longer time periods (months) are needed for significant fibrosis to develop relative to the bleomycin (weeks) model, but the silica model has the advantage of a clearer dependence on macrophages and other mononuclear phagocytes.

4. Notes

1. It is important to use strain-, age-, sex-, and weight-matched control mice for induction of pulmonary fibrosis. Nonmatched animals have variable responses to pulmonary fibrosis-inducing agents. Among mice, the CBA/J strain is the highest responder to bleomycin, with the C57Bl/6 being a moderate responder, and the Balb/c a non- or low-responder. Hence the recommended doses for bleomycin are 1, 5, and 10 U/kg body weight, respectively for these three strains. Too high a dose will kill the mice at earlier time points, commonly before fibrosis has a chance to fully develop, and may involve different pathogenetic mechanisms than at doses which do not cause significant fatality but allow fibrosis to fully develop.
2. Previous studies have generally used male rats and female (less cannibalism toward sick litter mates than males) mice for the study of pulmonary fibrosis, but it is recognized that gender could play a significant role in determining responsiveness to fibrosis inducing agents.
3. Mice and rats with differing ages, sexes, or backgrounds have different responses to anesthetic drugs and therefore the anesthetic dosages may need to be fine-tuned by the investigator.
4. Make an aliquot of bleomycin and store it at –20°C. Avoid freeze–thaw, which tends to diminish its effectiveness in inducing the model. Keep the bleomcin vial on ice until the time of administration.
5. All instruments for surgery need to be autoclaved. Avoid using nonsterile equipment so as to minimize the risk of infection.

Acknowledgments

This work was supported in part by the American Lung Association of Michigan (grant to MG-K) and by National Institutes of Health grants HL28737, HL31963, HL52285, and HL 77297 (to SHP).

References

1. Hiwatari, N., Shimura, S., Sasaki, T., et al. (1991) Prognosis of idiopathic pulmonary fibrosis in-patients with mucous hypersecretion. *Am. Rev. Respir. Dis.* **143**, 182–185.
2. Mannino, D. M., Etzel, R. A., and Parrish, R. G. (1996) Pulmonary fibrosis deaths in the United States, 1979-1991; an analysis of multiple-cause mortality data. *Am. J. Respir. Crit. Care Med.* **153**, 1548–1552.
3. Gross, T. J. and Hunninghake, G. W. (2001) Idiopathic pulmonary fibrosis. N. Engl. J. Med. **345**, 517–525.

4. Piguet, P.F., Collart, M. A., Grau, G. E., Sappino, A. P., and Vassalli, P. (1990) Requirement of tumor necrosis factor for development of silica-induced pulmonary fibrosis. *Nature* **344**, 245–247.
5. Gharaee-Kermani, M. and Phan, S. H. (2001) Role of cytokines and cytokine therapy in wound healing and fibrotic diseases. *Curr. Pharm. Des* **7**, 1083–1103.
6. Gharaee-Kermani, M., Nozaki, Y., Hatano, K., and Phan, S. H. (2001) Lung interlukin-4 gene expression in a murine model of bleomycin-induced pulmonary fibrosis. *Cytokine*. **5**, 138–147.
7. Huaux, F., Liu, T., McGarry, B., Ullenbruch, M., and Phan, S. H. (2003) Dual roles of interleukin-4 (IL-4) in lung injury and fibrosis. *J. Immunol.* **170**, 2083–2092.
8. Gharaee-Kermani, M. and Phan, S. H. (1997) Lung Interleukin-5 expression in murine bleomycin-induced pulmonary fibrosis. *Am. J. Respir. Cell Mol. Biol.* **16**, 438–447.
9. Zhang, K., Gharaee-Kermani, M., McGarry, B., and Phan, S. H. (1994) In situ hybridization analysis of rat lung al (I), and a2 (I) collagen gene expression in pulmonary fibrosis induced by endotracheal bleomycin injection. *Lab. Invest.* **70**, 192–202.
10. Zhang, K., Gharaee-Kermani, M., Jones, M. L., Warren, J. S., and Phan, S. H. (1994) Lung monocyte chemoattractant protein-1 gene expression in bleomycin-induced pulmonary fibrosis. *J. Immunol.* **153**, 4733–4741.
11. Zhang, K., Gharaee-Kermani, M., McGarry, B., Remick, D., and Phan, S. H. (1997) TNF-a mediated lung cytokine networking and eosinophil recruitment in pulmonary fibrosis. *J. Immunol.* **158,** 954–959.
12. Zhang, K., Flanders, K. C., and Phan, S. H. (1995) Cellular localization of transforming growth factor-b expression in bleomycin-induced pulmonary fibrosis. *Am. J. Pathol.* **147**, 352–361
13. Gharaee-Kermani, M., McCullumsmith R. E., Charo, I. F., Kunkel, S. L., and Phan, S. H. (2003) CC-Chemokine receptor 2 required for bleomycin-induced pulmonary fibrosis. *Cytokine* **24**, 266–276.
14. Gharaee-Kermani, M., McGarry, B., Lukacs, N., Huffnagle, G., Egan, R. W., and Phan, S. H. (1998) The role of IL-5 in bleomycin-induced pulmonary fibrosis. *J. Leukocyte Biol.* **64**, 657-666.
15. Barbarin, V., Arras, M., Misson, P., et al. (2204) Characterization of the effect of interleukin-10 on silica-induced lung fibrosis in mice. *Am. J. Respir. Cell Mol. Biol.* **31**, 78–85.
16. Kolodsick, J. E., Toews, G. T., Jakubzick, C., et al. (2004) Protection from fluorescein isothiocyanate-induced fibrosis in IL-13 deficient, mice results from impaired collagen synthesis by fibroblasts. *J. Immunol.* **172,** 4068–4076.
17. Kelley, J., Newman, R. A., and Evans, J. N. (1980) Bleomycin-induced pulmonary fibrosis in the rat. Prevention with an inhibitor of collagen synthesis. *J. Lab. Clin. Med.* **96**, 954–964.
18. Reid, L. M. (1980) needs for animal models of human diseases of the respiratory system. *Am. J. Pathol.* **101(3)**, *S* 89–101.

19. Coin, P. G., Osornio-Vargas, A. R., Roggli, V. L., and Brody, A. R. (1996) Pulmonary fibrogenesis after three consecutive inhalation exposures to chrysotile asbestos. *Am. J. Respir. Crit Care Med.* **154**, 1511–1519.
20. Karvonen, R. L., Fernandez-Madrid, F., Maughan, R. L., Palmer, K. C., and Fernandez-Madrid, I. (1987) An animal model of pulmonary radiation fibrosis with biochemical, physiologic, immunologic, and morphologic observations. *Radiat. Res.* **111**, 68–80.
21. Last, J. A., Gelzleicher, T. R., Pinkerton, K, E., Walker, R. M., and Witschi, H. (1993) A new model of progressive pulmonary fibrosis in rars. *Am. Rev. Respir. Dis.* **111**, 68–80.
22. Hashimoto, N., Jin, H., Liu, T., Chensue, S. W., and Phan, S. H. (2004) Bone marrow-derived progenitor cells in pulmonary fibrosis. *J. Clin. Invest.* **113**, 243–252.
23. Park, S-H., Saleh, D., Giaid, A., Michel, R. P. (1997) Increased endothelin-1 in bleomycin-induced pulmonary fibrosis and the effect of an endothelin receptor antagonist. *Am. J. Respir. Crit Care Med.* **156**, 600–608.
24. Umeda, Y., Marui, T., Matsuno, Y., et al. (2004) Skeletal muscle targeting *in vivo* electroporation-mediated HGF gene therapy of bleomycin-induced pulmonary fibrosis in Mice. *Lab. Invest.* **84**, 836-844.
25. Gharaee-Kermani, M. and Phan, S. H. (2004) Role of fibroblasts and myofibroblasts in idiopathic pulmonary fibrosis, in *Pulmonary Fibrosis* (Lynch, J. P., ed.) Dekker, New York: pp. 509–563.
26. Huaux, F., Louahed, J., Hudspith, B., Meredith, C., Delos, M., Renauld, J.-C., and Lison, D. (1998) Role of interleukin-10 in the lung response to silica in mice. *Am. J. Respir. Cell. Mol Biol.* **18**, 51–59.
27. Huaux, F., Liu, T., McGarry, B., Ullenbruch, M., Xing, Z., Phan, S. H. (2003) Eosinophils and T lymphocytes possess distinct roles in bleomycin-induced lung injury and fibrosis. *J. Immunol.* 1**71**, 5470–5481.
28. Feischmann, R. W., Barber, J. R., Thompson, G. R., et al. (1971) Bleomycin induced interstitial pneumonia in dogs. *Thorax.* **26**, 675–682.
29. Adamson, I. Y. R. and Bowden, D. H. (1974) The pathogenesis of bleomycin-induced pulmonary fibrosis in mice. *Am. J. Pathol.* **77**, 185–190.
30. McCullough, B., Collins, J. F., Johanson, W, G., and Grover, F. L. (1978) Bleomycin induced diffuse interstitial pulmonary fibrosis in baboons. *J. Clin. Invest.* **61**, 79–88.
31. Harrison, J. H. and Lazo, J. S. (1987) High dose continuous infusion of bleomycin in mice: a new model for drug-induced pulmonary fibrosis. J. *Pharmacol. Exp. Ther.* **243**, 1185–1194.

16

Animal Models of Renal Fibrosis

Michael Zeisberg, Mary A. Soubasakos, and Raghu Kalluri

Summary

Most of the present knowledge on pathomechanism of renal fibrosis is based on experimental studies with laboratory animals. Today, a variety of genetic and inducible animal models that mimic primary causes of human disease such as diabetes mellitus, glomerulonephritis, or lupus erythematodes are available. However, only few of these models progress consistently to interstitial fibrosis in the kidney involving interestitial fiberosis, tubular atrophy, and glomerulosclerosis, which are common features of renal fibrogenesis. In this chapter, the mouse models of nephrotoxic serm nephritis, COL4A3-deficiency, and unilateral urethral obstruction, which all result reliably into renal fibrosis, are described.

Key Words: Renal fibrosis; Tubulointerstitial fibrosis; tubular atrophy; fibroblasts; epithelial-mesenchymal transition (EMT); nephrotoxic serum, unilateral ureteral obstruction (UUO); collagen; basement membrane; Alport syndrome.

1. Introduction

The most common diseases that cause end-stage renal failure (ESRF) differ significantly in their underlying primary pathomechanisms *(1,2)*. Glomerulonephritis resulting from primary glomerular inflammation, metabolic diseases such as diabetes mellitus, cystic nephropathies such as polycystic kidney disease, interstitial nephritis resulting from primary interstitial inflammation, and vasculopathies are among the leading causes of ESRF *(1)*. Despite the diversity of primary pathomechanisms associated with these different kidney diseases, they all lead to an indistinguishable scarred/fibrotic kidney *(1)*. The observation that chronic renal failure seems to possess common patterns independent of the underlying disease has resulted in the speculation for the existence of a common pathogenic pathway leading to ESRF associated with fibrosis *(1,3)*.

Most of the present knowledge on pathomechanisms of renal fibrosis is based on experimental studies with laboratory animals. Today, a variety of genetic and inducible animal models that mimic primary causes of human dis-

From: *Methods in Molecular Medicine, Vol. 117: Fibrosis Research: Methods and Protocols*
Edited by: J. Varga, D. A. Brenner, and S. H. Phan © Humana Press Inc., Totowa, NJ

ease, such as diabetes mellitus, glomerulonephritis, or lupus erythematodes, are available. However, only few of these models progress consistently to interstitial fibrosis in the kidney involving interestitial fibrosis, tubular atrophy, and glomerulosclerosis, which are common features of renal fibrogenesis. In this chapter, three different mouse models of human kidney disease, COL4A3-deficiency, nephrotoxic serum nephritis (NSN), and unilateral ureteral obstruction are described, highlighting their utility for studying pathways leading to renal fibrosis (*see* **Note 1**).

2. Materials

1. CD-1 mice (i.e., Charles River Laboratories, Cambridge) at a weight of approx 30 g.
2. Nephrotoxic serum.
3. Normal sheep immunoglobulin (Ig)G (i.e., Sigma, St. Louis, MO).
4. Complete Freund's adjuvant.
5. COL4A3-deficient mice (Jackson Laboratories, Bar Harbor, ME).
6. DNA-isolation kit (i.e., DNeasy purification kit, Qiagen, Hilden, Germany).
7. Oligonucleotide primers.
8. Polymerase chain reaction (PCR) equipment.
9. Agarose and gel documentation equipment.
10. Anesthetics (ketamine, xylazine, lidocain).
11. Suture material (i.e., 7-0 silk, 6-0 absorbable, 6-0 nylon).
12. Surgical area (temperature controller with rectal probe, heating pad).
13. Surgical equipment (tissue forceps, fine point forceps, straight operating scissors, delicate scissors).
14. Analgesics (buprenophin).
15. Histology equipment and microscope.
16. Antibodies (i.e., type I collagen, type IV collagen, fibroblast-specific protein 1 [FSP1], α-smooth muscle actin [α-sma], E-cadherin).

3. Methods

3.1. Nephrotoxic Serum Nephritis

Currently, glomerulonephritis is the underlying cause of about 10% of end-stage renal disease (ESRD) cases in the United States. NTN is a commonly used model for anti-glomerular basement membrane (anti-GBM) disease or *in situ* immune-complex glomerulonephritis, which features a primary glomerular insult that can then lead to tubulointerstitial injury and subsequent fibrosis *(4)*. NTN is characterized by two distinct disease phases: an early heterologous phase resulting from linear anti-GBM antibody deposition in the glomerulus that resembles anti-GBM disease and a subsequent autologous immune response against the planted antibodies resulting in an *in situ* immune complex formation that resembles, e.g., postinfectious glomerulonephritis *(4)*.

Preimmunization with rabbit/sheep IgG in CFA prior to administration of a subnephritic dose of nephrotoxic serum (NTS) results in an augmentation of the autologous phase, leading to nephrotic range proteinuria and interstitial fibrosis within 3 to 6 wk *(4,5)*.

NTN has been successfully utilized as a model for fibrosis using CD-1 mice, C57BL/6 mice, and various gene knockout mice. NTS is classically raised in sheep or rabbits against crude preparations of rat glomeruli and hence contains polyclonal antibodies against multiple GBM, endothelial, mesangial, and podocyte cell wall antigens. In order to induce fibrosis in CD1 mice, these mice are pre-immunized by subcutaneous injection of normal sheep IgG followed by intravenous NTS injection. Fibrotic lesions (interstitial collagen deposition, increased fibroblasts, epithelial-mesenchymal transition [EMT]) appear after 1 to 2 wk of NTN. Severe tubulointerstitial fibrosis is observed between 3 and 6 wk, and reaches ESRF after 4 to 6 wk (**Fig. 1**).

3.1.1. Pre-Immunization

Pre-immunize mice a single subcutaneous injection of sheep IgG (200 μg) emulsified in CFA. Prepare a stock solution of sheep IgG of 4 mg/mL sterile in isotonic NaCl. To prepare the emulsion, load equal amounts of sheep IgG and CFA in a Hamilton syringe. Lock a second syringe with a double-hub microemulsifying needle to the filled syringe and pump the liquid between the two syringes to produce a uniform mixture. The emulsion is ready when it appears homogenous and viscous. Mice should be anesthetized for the injection and monitored for signs of distress and necrosis at the site of injection (*see* **Note 3**).

3.1.2. Immunization

Immunize mice 5 d after pre-immunization by three intravenous injections of NTS. Anesthetize mice and inject them intravenously with 100 μL on three consecutive days (*see* **Note 3**).

3.1.3. Monitoring of NTN

Monitor mice for signs of renal failure and inflammation of the injection site. Progression of NTN is reflected by proteinuria and decreased excretory renal function. Mice injected with NTS are significantly proteinuric by d 3 and become progressively more so during the course of disease *(5)*. Blood urea nitrogen levels rise rapidly during the acute phase of immunologic injury, but then return to baseline values by d 10. However, concomitant with the development of progressive interstitial and glomerular fibrosis, blood urea nitrogen levels rise progressively from d 14 until the death of these mice *(5)*. In our experience, mice will appear normal for a long time and will only appear sick

Nephrotoxic Serum Nephritis (NTN)

Day 1:	**Pre-immunization of CD-1 mice (30 gr.) with 200 μg sheep IgG in 200 μL in complete Freund's adjuvant (s.c.)**
Day 5:	**Injection of 50 μL NTN i.v.**
Day 6:	**Injection of 50 μL NTN i.v.**
Day 7:	**Injection of 50 μL NTN i.v.**
Day 14:	**Start of fibrosis**
Day 28:	**Severe interstitial fibrosis**

Fig. 1. Time-course of nephrotoxic serum nephritis. s.c., subcutaneously; i.v., intravenously.

after the disease has led to ESRF. At this stage, mice lose weight rapidly and appear lethargic. Some mice develop edema as a result of the loss of proteins in their urine.

3.1.4. Progression of NTN

Twelve hours after the first injection of NTS, protein casts are present in renal tubules, coinciding with the onset of proteinuria. After 24 h, leukocytes are evident within the interstitium and by d 3, prominent perivascular infiltrates are observed. At this point the glomeruli are clearly hypercellular with focal areas of necrosis. On d 5, some glomeruli contain crescents, and interstitial and perivascular infiltrates are also pronounced *(5)*. On d 7, about two-thirds of glomeruli exhibit prominent cellular crescents and marked abnormalities are present within the tubules and interstitium *(5)*. These include severely dilated tubules with flattened or denuded epithelia and expansion of the interstitium resulting from edema, interstitial infiltrates, and the onset of fibrosis. On d 14, the fibrotic process is more diffuse throughout the interstitium *(5)*. Severe tubulointerstitial fibrosis then progresses to ESRD between wk 2 and 6.

3.2. COL4A3-Deficient Mice

Mice with a targeted disruption of the *COL4A3* gene, which encodes for the α3 chain of type IV collagen (COL4A3), were originally generated as a model for Alport syndrome *(6,7)*. These mice lack normal composition of α3(IV), α4(IV), and α5(IV) type IV collagen chains in the GBM and display hearing defects and progressive renal disease *(6,8)*. The renal disease is initially characterized by splitting of the GBM (similar to the human disease), but then leads to crescentic glomerulonephritis and severe renal fibrosis *(6,9)*. Depending on their genetic background, these mice develop ESRD between 14 wk (129 background) and 32 wk (C57BL/6 background) ***(6,7)***. The progression of renal fibrosis in these mice stems from a defined genetic lesion, which makes interpretation of newly generated data transparent. Additionally, the progression of fibrosis within a particular genetic background is remarkably consistent without any further manipulations. Therefore, these mice represent a reproducible genetic mouse model, which is an excellent tool with which to study the progression of fibrosis in the kidney ***(10)***.

The COL4A3-deficient mice on a 129Sv background have a normal phenotype until 4 wk of age ***(7,9,11)***. At this age, the foot processes of podocytes are unaltered, the urine contains normal levels of protein, which indicates an intact glomerular filtration barrier; and no pathological alterations in the tubulointerstitium can be detected ***(9)***. After 8 wk of age, significant splitting of the GBM is observed, associated with podocyte effacement and increased urine protein levels, indicating a malfunction within the glomerular filtration barrier. At this stage, tubulointerstitial fibrosis, the common pathway associated with several chronic nephropathies, is observed ***(6,7,12)***. Interstitial fibrosis at this stage is indicated by a widening of the interstitial space, associated with an increase in the number of interstitial fibroblasts ***(1,3,12,13)***. Fibrosis is furthermore characterized by an increased remodeling of the interstitial extracellular matric (ECM), resulting in excessive deposition of fibrillar ECM ***(1,13,14)***.

3.2.1. Mouse Line and Maintenance

COL4A3-deficient mice on a 129Sv background are available from the Jackson Laboratories (Bar Harbor, ME). Because the lifespan of the homozygous COL4A3-deficient mice is short, we generate knockout mice by breeding heterozygous-deficient mice. Breeding of heterozygous-deficient COL4A3 mice yields offspring that are wild-type, heterozygous, or homozygous for the COL4A3-deletion in Mendelian ratio. The mice are housed under standard conditions. At the age of 10 to 12 wk, mice can exhibit edema as a result of nephrotic range proteinuria and they can become lethargic as a result of renal insufficiency. The mice can be easily genotyped by PCR of genomic DNA, which is obtained from tail biopsies.

3.2.2. Isolation of Genomic DNA From Mouse Tail Tissue

1. Cut a 5 to 10 mg piece of mouse tail tissue into a 1.5-mL microcentrifuge tube (*see* **Note 4**). Add 180 μL of buffer ATL and 20 μL proteinase K. Mix by vortexing and incubate the tissue is completely lysed. Disperse the tissue by vortexing and place on a rocking platform.
2. Add 400 μL of buffer AL-ethanol mixture to the sample and mix vigorously by vortexing. Pipet the mixtue into the spin column placed into a new 2-mL collec-

tion tube and centrifuge at 6000*g* for 1 min. The flow-through and the collection tube can be discarded. Repeat the washing step with 500 µL of buffer AW1.

3. Place the spin column in a new 2-mL collection tube, add 500 µL of Buffer AW2, centrifuge at 20,000*g* and discard the tube with the flow-thrugh.
4. Place the DNeasy spin column in a clean 1.5-mL or 2-mL microcentrifuge tube and pipet 200 µL of Buffer AE onto the memebrane. Incubate for 1 min a room temperature and elute the DANN by centrifuging for 1 min at 6000*g*.

3.2.3. Genotyping by PCR

1. Primers. Genotyping is then performed by two separate PCR reactions using the common reverse primer (3'- CCT GCT AAT ATA GGG TTC GAG A -5') and primers for the knockout allele (5'-CCA GGC TTA AAG GGA AAT CC -3') or the wildtype allele (5'- TTC CCC TGT CAC CAG GAT TTC CC -3').
2. PCR mixture. The PCR mixture contains 250 m*M* of each primer, 200 µ*M* of each deoxynucleotide triphosphate, 0 m*M* Kcl, 10 m*M* Tris-HCl, pH 8.3, 1.5 *M* magnesium acetate, 1.25 U of Taq DNA polymerase, and 3 µL of genomic tail DNA in a total volume of 50 µ*M*.
3. PCR conditions include an initial incubation at 95°C for 3 min followed by 30 cycles of 95°C (30 s), 58°C (40 s), 72°C (3 min), with a final incubation for 7 min at 72°C.
4. Analyze PCR products by electrophoresis in agarose gel. The wild-type allele (900 bp) can be distinguished from the knockout allele (1050 bp).

3.2.4. Monitoring of Disease in COL4A3-Deficient Mice

Progression of renal disease in COL4A3-deficient mice is reflected by proteinuria and decreased excretory renal function. Analysis of urinary protein excretion reveals the onset and progression of disease in these mice, whereas occurrence of hematuria is inconsistent in these mice. Blood urea nitrogen levels and serum creatinine levels increase significantly, starting between 6 and 8 wk of age.

3.3. Unilateral Ureteral Obstruction

Unilateral ureteral obstruction (UUO) is a model resembling human obstructive nephropathy, which represents an inducible model of interstitial fibrosis secondary to a nonimmune insult. UUO is induced by ligation of a ureter of one kidney, while the contra-lateral kidney serves as a control. In order to obtain reliable obstruction usually two ligatures about 5 mm apart are placed in the upper two-thirds of the ureter. An additional feature of this model is that regeneration of established lesions occurs if the obstruction is relieved within the first 3 d of disease. In order to allow relief of the obstruction in a second surgery, the ureter can be protected during obstruction with a small piece of polyethylene tubing. Interstitial fibrosis, indicated by the widening of the interstitial space, associated with interstitial deposition of type IV collagen and tubular cell apoptosis can be observed as early as 3 d after obstruction ***(15)***. If the ureteral ligation is maintained, within 2 wk severe fibrosis is noticed.

3.3.1. Preparation of the Surgical Site

Shave the surgical exceeding the planned incision by approx 150%. Prep the surgical site with 70% ethanol and wipe it with betadine. Cover the surgical site with a sterile drape and cover the entire mouse sparing the head with sterilized surgical crepe paper. Sterile instruments should be used for the entire procedure.

3.3.2. Surgical Procedure

Anesthetize the mice with a mixture of ketamine (100 mg/kg) and xylazine (10 mg/kg) given at 0.1 mL intraperitoneally. Keep the mice at 36 to 37°C using a heating pad and monitor the body temperature using a temperature controller connected to a rectal probe. Introduce 0.1 mL of 1% lidocaine under the skin and open the flank by an incision. Use a retractor to facilitate the view of the ureter if necessary. Prepare the ureter from the surrounding tissue and place two ligatures about 5 mm apart in the upper two-thirds of the ureter of the left kidney in order to obtain reliable obstruction (i.e., with 7-0 silk suture). After the ligation, close the incision. Muscles and skin are closed layer by layer with 6-0 nylon and 6-0 absorbable (for muscles) sutures. The duration of the whole procedure takes about 5 to 10 min. The sutures should be removed 10 d after the surgical procedure.

3.3.3. Postsurgical Care

After the surgery, watch the mice constantly until they recover from anesthesia. Mice should be kept warm until they recover using heating pads. For the first 6 h during recumbency, observe the mice hourly (*see* **Note 5**). The mice should be examined twice daily for evidence of wound dehiscence, separation of layers, infection, or lethargy. Allow the mice to drink water immediately after recovery and maintain them on their normal diet from 12 h after surgery. For the first 48 h after surgery, administer analgesics (i.e., Buprenorphin 1.0 mg/kg subcutaneously every 48 h). Weigh the mice daily for the first 6 d after surgery.

3.3.4. Monitoring of UUO

As the contralateral unligated kidney compensates for the functional loss of the obstructed kidney, functional parameters are insufficient to monitor disease progression in these mice. However, the progression of disease in these mice is extremely stable if the ureter is ligated sufficiently and can be followed by histological assessment.

3.4. Histopathology and Morphometric Analysis

In order to compare the disease progression among different mouse models and different treatment protocols, a standardized procedure that evaluates interstitial fibrosis, tubular atrophy, and glomerulosclerosis by morphometric analysis is required. In our laboratory, we have established a standardized algorithm, which is applied to all our renal fibrosis studies (**Fig. 2**).

3.4.1. Sacrifice of Mice and Harvest of the Kidneys

The mice should be killed by CO_2 asphyxiation using a glas cylinder (optionally mice can be injected with a lethal dose of sodiumbarbital). Open the abdominal cavity with a longitudinal incision and collect the kidneys (*see* **Note 6**). Make a coronary cut with a razor blade to cut both kidneys in halves. Place one half into a cryo mold with Tissue-Tek® (Sakura Finetek) and snap-freeze it immediately in isopentane (or liquid nitrogen). Snap-freeze the second half in an RNase-free microcentrifuge tube in liquid nitrogen. Place the third half in fresh 4% paraformaldehyde at 4°C. Fix the fourth half in glutaraldehyde if electron microscopy is required.

3.4.2. Histology and Morphometric Analysis

Stain paraffin-embedded kidney sections with periodic acid-Schiff (PAS), hematoxylin eosin (H&E), and Masson's Trichrome staining. In order to quantify pathologic lesions, determine the interstitial volume (as an indicator of interstitial fibrosis), the tubular atrophy index, glomerulosclerosis, and glomerular cellularity (as parameters for glomerular injury) ***(10)***.

3.4.2.1. Interstitial Volume

Determine the interstitial volume by a point-counting technique on tissue sections stained by the Masson's Trichrome method and express it as the mean percentage of grid points lying within the interstitial area within five fields of renal cortex. View a 1-mm^2 graded ocular grid at approx ×200 magnification to delineate each of these fields. Evaluate five randomly selected cortical areas that include glomeruli for each animal. In order to distinguish between acute inflammation and chronic fibrosis, evaluate the interstitial area containing blue-stained fibrous material.

3.4.2.2. Tubular Atrophy

To determine the "tubular atrophy index" ***(10)***, stain kidney sections with PAS. Identify atrophic tubules by their thickened and sometimes duplicated

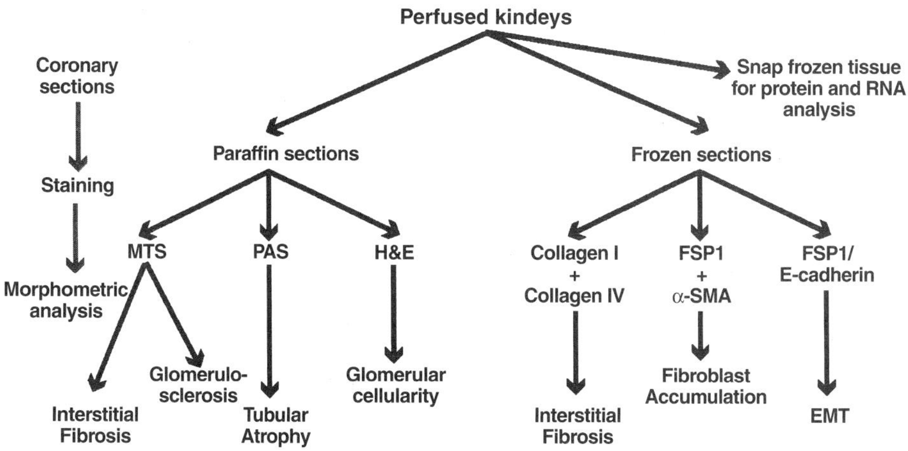

Fig. 2. Standardized analysis of renal fibrosis.

basement membranes, flattening of the epithelial cells, and widening of the tubular lumen. Count the number of atrophic tubules per field at approx ×400 magnification and analyze about 10 to 20 fields per kidney cortex section. The number of atrophic tubules is then expressed as percentage of all tubules.

3.4.2.3. Glomerulosclerosis

In order to quantify glomerulosclerosis, use a semiquantitative grading system, in which glomerulosclerotic lesions are scored for severity (0–4, 0 = normal, 4 = maximum severity) as described by Raij ***(16)***. Additionally, count all nuclei in 50 glomeruli of similar size in each kidney to estimate glomerular cellularity.

3.4.3. Immunohistochemistry

In order to further characterize the fibrotic lesions in a kidney, perform immunohistochemistry on frozen sections. Stain sections with antibodies to type I collagen (to assess interstitial collagen deposition), type IV collagen (to assess disruption of tubular basement membrane and ectopic expression in the interstitium), FSP1 (to determine to accumulation of fibroblasts), α-SMA (to assess fibroblast activation), and FSP1/E-cadherin double staining (to evaluate the occurrence of EMT [*see* **Note 7**]).

4. Notes

1. Which is the best model to use? We have used each of these mouse models to study the progression of fibrosis in the kidney. Each of these models consis-

tently results in severe tubulointerstitial fibrosis. In our experience. the genetic model of COL4A3-deficient mice is a reliable, consistent model of fibrosis. This model is associated with slow progression rate, and thus might also reflect the fibrotic process in humans with kidney diseases. However, this model is currently limited to only few mouse strains, which differ substantially in their rate of progression for reasons unknown at the moment. The model of UUO is also quite consistent; it has been induced in various genetic backgrounds and it yields results in a relatively short period of time. Furthermore, this model is widely used and thus well-characterized, which allows a comparison of the newly obtained results with numerous previously published studies. However, the relevance of this model to human disease is unknown, as obstruction of the ureter is less likely to lead to fibrosis in humans. Furthermore, the underlying pathomechanisms in this model differ substantially from the underlying pathomechanisms in most renal diseases associated with fibrosis. NSN, results in renal fibrosis as a result of a primary insult in the glomerulus, which is representative of a majority of underlying diseases leading to renal fibrosis. Progression of disease towards fibrosis occurs within 4 to 6 wk, which represents an intermediate time-course as compared with UUO and COL4A3-deficient mice. Even though this model is easily inducible, its utility can be limited because of substantial variation in disease progression. However, this model has been successfully used in several treatment studies that attempted to test the therapeutic potential of novel drugs.

2. CFA emulsion should be of viscous consistency. Injections containing CFA should be given subcutaneously because intravenous injections can damage the lung by rapid embolism. The inoculum containing the adjuvant should be divided into fractions of 50 µL per injection site. The injection sites should be clean to decrease any risk of injection-site infection.
3. NTS is usually prepared by immunizing male sheep with a lysate of rat glomeruli, isolated by differential sieving. The sheep serum is heat inactivated at 56°C, absorbed with rat red blood cells and serum proteins, and then filter-sterilized. NTS has moderate reactivity to type IV collagen and laminin and substantial reactivity to glomerular cell membrane proteins, particularly integrins. Alternatively, NTS can be also raised in rabbits.
4. Optimally, tail biopsies are obtained from mice at the age of 2 wk and no later than 4 wk of age. Do not forget to mark the mice, i.e., by ear clipping.
5. In order to reduce the risk of aspiration, we cover the bedding of the mice with a paper towel for the first 6 h postsurgery.
6. Perfusion. Better results are obtained when the animal is perfused with 4% paraformaldehyde before the kidneys are collected. In order to perfuse the mouse, open the thoracic cavity immediately after the mouse is dead and puncture the left ventricle with a 26-gage needle. Make a small incision (in the liver) to allow removal of blood. Allow approx 30 mL of phosphate-buffered saline (PBS) to drip into the ventricle until most blood is flushed out of the mouse (notice that the fluid rinsing from the incision turns clear). Perfuse the mouse slowly with 15 mL

of 4% paraformaldehyde. Notice a more rigid consistency when the organs are properly fixed.

7. Double staining with epithelial markers and mesenchymal markers (i.e., E-cadherin and FSP1) allows for detection of early stages of EMT. The origin of interstitial fibroblasts can only be delineated if resident fibroblasts and tubular cells are genetically marked.

References

1. Remuzzi, G. and Bertani, T. (1998) Pathophysiology of progressive nephropathies. *N. Engl. J. Med.* **339,** 1448–1456.
2. Pastan, S. and Bailey, J. (1998) Dialysis therapy. *N. Engl. J. Med.* **338,** 1428–1437.
3. Zeisberg, M., Strutz, F., and Muller, G. A. (2001) Renal fibrosis: an update. *Curr. Opin. Nephrol. Hypertens.* **10,** 315–320.
4. Lloyd, C. M., Minto, A. W., Dorf, M. E., et al. (1997) RANTES and monocyte chemoattractant protein-1 (MCP-1) play an important role in the inflammatory phase of crescentic nephritis, but only MCP-1 is involved in crescent formation and interstitial fibrosis. *J. Exp. Med.* ***185,*** 1371–1380.
5. Zeisberg, M., Hanai, J., Sugimoto, H., Mammoto, T., Charytan, D., Strutz, F., and Kalluri, R. (2003) BMP-7 counteracts TGF-beta1-induced epithelial-to-mesenchymal transition and reverses chronic renal injury. *Nat. Med.* ***9,*** 964–968.
6. Cosgrove, D., Meehan, D. T., Grunkemeyer, J. A., Kornak, J. M., Sayers, R., Hunter, W. J., and Samuelson, G. C. (1996) Collagen COL4A3 knockout: a mouse model for autosomal Alport syndrome. *Genes Dev.* ***10,*** 2981–2992.
7. Miner, J. H. and Sanes, J. R. (1996) Molecular and functional defects in kidneys of mice lacking collagen alpha 3(IV): implications for Alport syndrome. *J. Cell Biol.* **135,** 1403–1413.
8. Kalluri, R. and Cosgrove, D. (2000) Assembly of type IV collagen. Insights from alpha3(IV) collagen-deficient mice. *J. Biol. Chem.* **275,** 12,719–12,724.
9. Hamano, Y., Grunkemeyer, J. A., Sudhakar, A., et al. (2002) Determinants of vascular permeability in the kidney glomerulus. *J. Biol. Chem.* **30,** 30.
10. Zeisberg, M., Bottiglio, C., Kumar, N., Maeshima, Y., Strutz, F., Muller, G. A., and Kalluri, R. (2003) Bone morphogenic protein-7 inhibits progression of chronic renal fibrosis associated with two genetic mouse models. *Am. J. Physiol. Renal Physiol.* **285,** F1060–1067.
11. Andrews, K. L., Betsuyaku, T., Rogers, S., Shipley, J. M., Senior, R. M., and Miner, J. H. (2000) Gelatinase B (MMP-9) is not essential in the normal kidney and does not influence progression of renal disease in a mouse model of Alport syndrome. *Am. J. Pathol.* **157,** 303–311.
12. Cosgrove, D., Rodgers, K., Meehan, D., et al. (2000) Integrin alpha1beta1 and transforming growth factor-beta1 play distinct roles in alport glomerular pathogenesis and serve as dual targets for metabolic therapy. *Am. J. Pathol.* **157,** 1649–1659.
13. Eddy, A. A. (1996) Molecular insights into renal interstitial fibrosis [editorial]. *J. Am. Soc. Nephrol.* **7,** 2495–2508.

14. Border, W. A. and Noble, N. A. (1995) Targeting TGF-beta for treatment of disease. *Nat. Med.* **1,** 1000–1001.
15. Iwano, M., Plieth, D., Danoff, T. M., Xue, C., Okada, H., and Neilson, E. G. (2002) Evidence that fibroblasts derive from epithelium during tissue fibrosis. *J. Clin. Invest.* **110,** 341–350.
16. Raij, L., Azar, S., and Keane, W. (1984) Mesangial immune injury, hypertension, and progressive glomerular damage in Dahl rats. *Kidney Int.* **26,** 137–143.

17

Animal Models of Cardiac Fibrosis

Yao Sun and Karl T. Weber

Summary

A collagen network, composed largely of type I and III fibrillar collagens, is found in the heart's interstitial space. This network has multiple functions, including the preservation of tissue architecture and chamber geometry. Given its tensile strength, type I collagen is a major determinant of tissue stiffness. Its disproportionate accumulation, expressed in morphological terms as tissue fibrosis, increases myocardial passive and active stiffness and contributes to ventricular diastolic and systolic dysfunction. Various animal models of cardiac fibrosis have been used to study its functional consequences and to elucidate factors regulating the cellular and molecular biology of fibrogenesis. Herein, we present our experience and findings with several models of cardiac fibrosis.

Key Words: Cardiac fibrosis; myocardial infarction; aldosterone; angiotensin II; myofibroblasts.

1. Introduction

The myocardium is composed of cardiomyocytes and nonmyocyte cells, such as fibroblasts and vascular endothelial and vascular smooth muscle cells. A fibrillar collagen scaffolding preserves tissue architecture and chamber geometry. Low-level collagen turnover is normally provided by fibroblasts located in interstitial and perivascular spaces. Collagen synthesis and degradation coexist in the heart, and their balanced equilibrium determines its collagen concentration. Collagen is continuously synthesized and degraded; its half-life is 80 to 120 d *(1)*. Collagen degradation involves proteolytic enzymes, particularly matrix metalloproteinases (MMPs), and tissue inhibitors of metalloproteinases (TIMPs), each of which reside in latent form within the matrix *(2,3)*.

An adverse accumulation of collagen, secondary to either increased synthesis or inadequate degradation, leads to cardiac fibrosis. Fibrosis can be defined from various perspectives. In morphological terms, it includes: a reactive peri-

From: *Methods in Molecular Medicine, Vol. 117: Fibrosis Research: Methods and Protocols*
Edited by: J. Varga, D. A. Brenner, and S. H. Phan © Humana Press Inc., Totowa, NJ

vascular and/or interstitial fibrosis that appears in the absence of cardiomyocyte necrosis; and a replacement fibrosis, or scarring, that may occur at macroscopic or microscopic levels in response to the loss of necrotic cardiomyocytes *(4)*. Apoptotic cell death does not lead to fibrosis. From a biochemical perspective, an increased concentration of tissue hydroxyproline, an amino acid specific to collagen, can be used to define fibrosis *(5,6)*. Fibrous tissue is primarily composed of type I and III fibrillar collagens and where type I collagen represents three-quarters of all fibrillar collagens *(7–11)*.

Cardiac fibrosis creates heterogeneity in tissue structure that impairs ventricular function and predisposes to arrhythmias. Various animal models have been used to study functional consequences of fibrosis and factors regulating fibrous tissue formation, including the cellular and molecular biology of fibrogenesis. Those models we have used include: tissue repair in response to coronary artery ligation with myocardial infarction; insertion of a foreign body (i.e., silk ligature) into the myocardium; manual handling of the heart's surface, or visceral pericardium; and the heart's response to infusions of various hormones, such as aldosterone (ALDO), angiotensin (Ang)II, and a catecholamine (i.e., isoproterenol). Herein, we present our experience with each of these models: method of induction; means used to study fibrous tissue responses; cells responsible for cardiac fibrosis; and factors regulating fibrogenesis.

2. Fibrosis Following Myocardial Infarction

2.1. Animal Model

A transmural infarction of the anterior left ventricle of 8-wk-old male Sprague-Dawley rats (Harlan, Indianapolis, IN) is created by ligation of the left coronary artery using silk ligature *(12,13)*. Rats are anesthetized with isoflurane, intubated and ventilated with a rodent respirator (Harvard apparatus, Waukesha, WI). After left thoracotomy and pericardiotomy, the heart is rapidly exteriorized and 6-0 silk suture placed around the left coronary artery (*see* **Note 1**). The vessel is ligated and the heart returned to the chest. The chest is closed and the lungs reinflated using positive end-expiratory pressure. Coronary artery occlusion with myocardial infarction (MI) is confirmed by microscopic evidence of lost cardiomyocytes with replacement of fibrosis and grossly visible scarring of the left-ventricular free wall. Mortality from ventricular arrhythmias and pulmonary edema within 24 h of coronary artery ligation is about 30 to 40%; thereafter it is less than 5%. Sham operation includes each of the previously described procedures except ligation of the coronary artery. We have used this model to study the foreign-body fibrosis, which surrounds the silk ligature.

2.2. Morphology

Connective tissue can be selectively stained with Masson's Trichrome or Picrosirius Red stain and viewed by light microscopy. We prefer Picrosirius Red staining because it is specific for fibrillar collagen and its volume fraction can be quantified with an image analysis system. Moreover, details of the fibrillar collagen network can be viewed under both direct and polarized light. As detected by Picrosirius Red staining, we find a small amount of collagen in the interstitial and perivascular spaces of the normal rat heart, whose collagen volume is 2 to 3% of total cardiac volume (**Fig. 1A**).

Transmural MI leads to macroscopic scarring of the anterior left ventricle. By Picrosirius Red staining, fibrillar collagen begins to appear at the infarct site by d 7 post-MI and it continues to accumulate for weeks thereafter. At wk 4, a dense fibrillar collagen network has formed at the infarct site (**Fig. 1B**) *(14)*. Collagen volume can account for as much as 70 to 80% of total volume of the infarcted myocardium. Infarct scar thinning appears after wk 6.

Fibrous tissue also appears over time in noninfarcted myocardium. This includes a perivascular/interstitial fibrosis of the right ventricle and interventricular septum; a pericardial fibrosis after manual handling of the heart (**Fig. 1C**); as an endocardial fibrosis of the left ventricle (**Fig. 1D**); and foreign-body fibrosis around the silk ligature placed under the left coronary artery *(15)*. Perivascular/interstitial fibrosis is first seen in noninfarcted myocardium at wk 2 and becomes more evident at wk 4. Quantitative analysis reveals that interstitial collagen volume fraction in noninfarcted myocardium can increase to 6% over the course of 4 wk post-MI. Endocardial fibrosis, pericardial fibrosis, and foreign-body fibrosis also first appear at wk 1 and become more evident over ensuing weeks.

2.3. Cellular and Molecular Biology

After coronary artery ligation, a process of tissue repair follows the necrotic loss of cardiomyocytes at the infarct site. It begins with an activation of latent MMPs that degrade the existing extracellular matrix and coronary vasculature. Circulating inflammatory cells arrive at the infarct site within hours after MI where they too contribute to the proteolytic digestion and phagocytosis of infarcted tissue. MMP-1, or collagenase, is a major enzyme for fibrillar collagen degradation. MMP-1 mRNA and activity are significantly increased in the infarcted myocardium during the end of wk 1 and decline thereafter *(14,16,17)*. The expression of TIMPs is significantly increased in the infarcted myocardium at wk 1 post-MI and remained elevated over the course of 4 wk *(14,16,17)*. The early elevation of MMP synthesis is responsible for existing collagen degradation in the necrotic myocardium, whereas the following suppression of

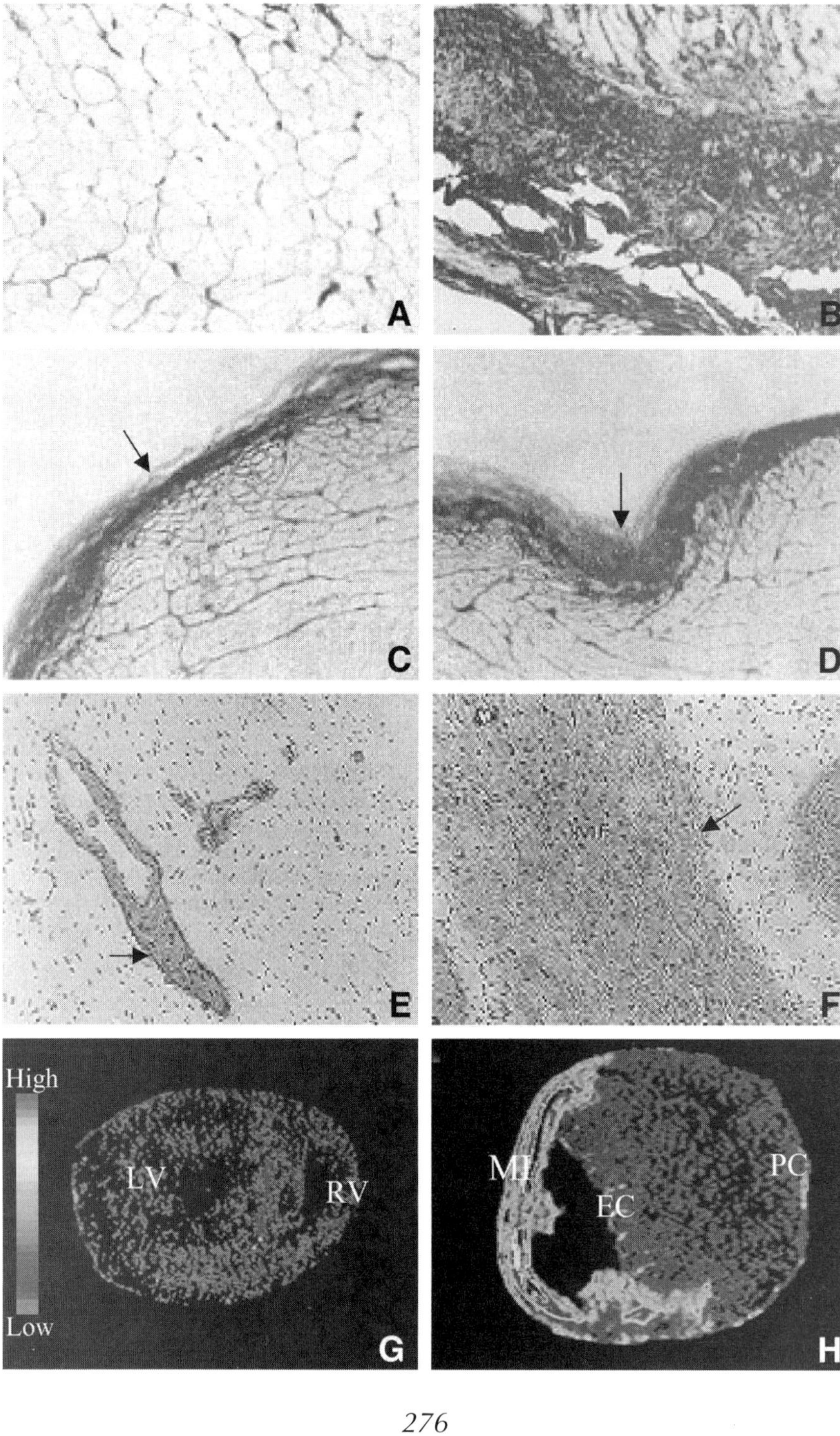
A
B
C
D
E
F
High
Low
LV
RV
G
MI
EC
PC
H

MMP activity and upregulation of TIMPs contribute to collagen accumulation at the infarct site.

Following the initial phase of collagen degradation, the accumulation of fibrillar collagen replaces lost parenchymal cells. Expression of type I and III collagen genes is upregulated as early as d 3 post-MI (**Fig. 1H**), whereas collagen fibers appear by light microscopy by d 7. An organized assembly of these fibers in the form of scar tissue becomes evident by d 14 ***(18–20)***. Collagen continues to accumulate at the site of MI over 8 wk. Hydroxyproline concentration at the infarct site increases over 6 to 8 wk as does collagen crosslinking.

In situ hybridization localizes and identifies increased type I and III collagen mRNAs at remote sites in noninfarcted myocardium, endocardium of interventricular septum, pericardium, and myocardium containing the silk ligature. Endocardial fibrosis, pericardial fibrosis, and foreign-body fibrosis are secondary to tissue inflammation. The perivascular/interstitial fibrosis which appears at remote site involving noninfarcted myocardium likewise does not appear in response to cardiac damage. The cause of this perivascular/interstitial fibrosis remains uncertain. Our recent studies have identified clustered CD4-positive lymphocytes in noninfarcted myocardium, which peaks at wk 3 and is sustained, albeit at lower levels, until wk 8 post-MI ***(21)***. This observation suggests the possibility of an autoimmune response that arises from exposure to self-antigen at the time of MI. Such ongoing inflammation may contribute to myocardial remodeling following MI.

Cells responsible for fibrous tissue formation at the infarct site consist principally of phenotypically transformed fibroblast-like cells having distinctive morphological features and phenotypic characteristics. They are termed myofibroblasts (myoFb) (**Fig. 1F**) ***(22–24)***. These cells are larger than normal fibroblasts, and have a prominent endoplasmic reticulum and a large nucleus, often wrinkled in keeping with cell contraction, and α-smooth muscle actin (α-sma) microfilaments acquired during phenotypic transformation ***(25)***. Pre-

---

Fig. 1. Cardiac fibrosis following coronary artery ligation. Detected by Picrosirius Red staining, a small amount of collagen is observed in the interstitial space of the normal myocardium (**A**). At 4 wk post-MI, collagen is accumulated at the site of MI (**B**), pericardium (**C**, arrow) and endocardium (**D**, arrow). **E** shows immunohistochemical α-smooth muscle actin (sma) labeling in the normal myocardium, where only vascular smooth muscle cells are positively labeled (arrow) and myofibroblasts (myoFb) are not found. In the infarcted myocardium (**F**) and other sites of repair (not shown), myoFb (arrow) become abundant. By quantitative *in situ* hybridization, type I collagen mRNA is largely increased at the site of MI, endocardium (EC) and pericardium (PC) at d 3 post-MI (**H**) compared with controls (**G**). **A–F**: ×120.

cursor cells that account for the appearance of myoFb are uncertain. They may include: interstitial fibroblasts; adventitial fibroblasts; pericytes; a population of circulating fibroblasts known as fibrocytes; circulating monocytes; or circulating bone marrow-derived progenitor cells, which are mobilized at the time of injury and home to the infarct site where they that transdifferentiate. It is presumed that transforming growth factor (TGF)-β_1, elaborated by macrophages, governs the appearance of the myoFb phenotype ***(26–28)***. MyoFb are responsible for formation of scar tissue via their expression (at mRNA and protein levels) of type I and III fibrillar collagens. **Figure 1F** identifies the presence of α-sma-positive myoFb residing within the 4-wk-old scar of the infarcted rat heart. After their appearance, myoFb persist in the infarcted myocardium for years in man and months in rodents ***(29,30)***; however, their number is less than that found at wk 4. The decline in myoFb number may be secondary to programmed cell death (apoptosis).

MyoFb, identified by α-sma labeling, are also found in the fibrosed visceral pericardium, endocardial fibrosis, microscopic scars, and the site of foreign-body fibrosis surrounding silk suture. They too are responsible for collagen deposition at these sites. MyoFb are not observed in noninfarcted septum and right ventricle, where perivascular/interstitial fibrosis is contributed by fibroblasts.

2.4. De Novo *Angiotensin II and Fibrosis*

MyoFb have a diverse portfolio of metabolic activities that provide autocrine and paracrine regulation of cell behavior at and remote to MI. *In situ* hybridization, in vitro autoradiography, and immunohistochemistry have shown these cells express renin ***(30)***, angiotensin-converting enzyme (ACE) ***(22)***, and Ang receptors ***(13)*** at the infarct site. In the infarcted rat heart, AngII receptors are found to be predominantly of the AT_1 subtype ***(13)***. Ou et al. ***(31)*** have shown high-density ACE binding and ACE activity of fibrosed pericardium in the infarcted heart is responsible for AngII production from AngI precursor and which is abrogated by an ACE inhibitor. Yamagishi et al. ***(32)*** have reported an increased content of AngII in the infarcted myocardium. These observations suggest the potential autocrine role of AngII on myoFb growth and collagen turnover. Pharmacological agents that interfere with AngII generation (i.e., ACE inhibitors) or which bind to AT_1 receptors support a role for locally generated AngII in regulating myoFb collagen synthesis at the infarct site by induction of TGF-β_1. Chronic treatment with an AT_1 receptor antagonist, losartan, significantly attenuated the expression of TGF-β_1 and type I collagen at and remote to the infarct ***(19)***. Administration of an ACE inhibitor, either captopril or enalapril, for 6 wk attenuates infarct size and prevents fibrosis remote to the MI in rats ***(33,34)***.

Similar findings have been reported for losartan, indicating that locally produced AngII contributes to fibrogenesis ***(35)***. ACE inhibitors, captopril or perindopril, initiated at the time of MI, prevent interstitial fibrosis in noninfarcted myocardium ***(35)***. A similar response was observed for losartan ***(36,37)***. Pericardial fibrosis, which appears both in the infarcted rat heart and in sham-operated hearts following manual handling, is attenuated by chronic treatment with lisinopril. Persistent elevations in circulating AngII and ALDO have not been observed following MI in rats ***(38,39)***, suggesting that the beneficial role of ACE inhibition or AT_1 receptor blockade on cardiac fibrosis post-MI is related to AngII produced at sites of repair.

3. Fibrosis in Response to Aldosterone Treatment

3.1. Animal Model

A model of chronic aldosteronism, such as that seen in congestive heart failure (CHF), is created in uninephrectomized rats with ALDO infusion by implanted minipump and 1% NaCl/0.4%KCl in drinking water ***(40,41)***. Eight-wk-old male Sprague-Dawley rats are anesthetized with isoflurane and the left abdomen shaved. After opening the abdomen, the left kidney is exposed, its renal artery and vein ligated, and the kidney removed and abdominal incision closed. Dorsal skin is then shaved, a 1-cm incision is made, and an osmotic minipump (Durect, Cupertino, CA) loaded with ALDO (Fisher Scientific, Pittsburgh, PA) is implanted subcutaneously and the skin incision is closed (*see* **Note 2**). The minipump releases ALDO at the rate of 0.75 μg/h, raising plasma ALDO levels to those seen in CHF. The amount of solvent used to make the ALDO solution is 7% of 95% ethanol, 5.5% of double-distilled water, and 87.5% polyethylene glycol. Following surgery, rats receive regular laboratory chow together with 1% NaCl and 0.4% KCl in drinking water. Animals are treated with this regimen, termed ALDO/salt treatment (ALDOST), for four or more weeks. During wk 1 and 2 ALDOST, animals are active, eating, drinking, and gaining weight comparable to age-/gender-matched, untreated controls. Lethargy and anorexia appear at wk 3 and beyond. Mortality is zero within 4 wk and about 20 to 30% from wk 4 to 6. Arterial pressure rises gradually after 2 wk of ALDOST and left-ventricular hypertrophy is evident at wk 4.

3.2. Morphology

This model represents a time-dependent induction of fibrosis involving the normotensive, nonhypertrophied right and left atria, right ventricle, and pulmonary artery, as well as the hypertensive, hypertrophied left ventricle and aorta ***(40,42)***. Cardiac fibrosis is first seen at 4 wk of ALDOST. Two morphological forms of fibrous tissue formation are seen: a proinflammatory vascular phenotype that involves intramural coronary arteries and leads to a perivascular fibrosis;

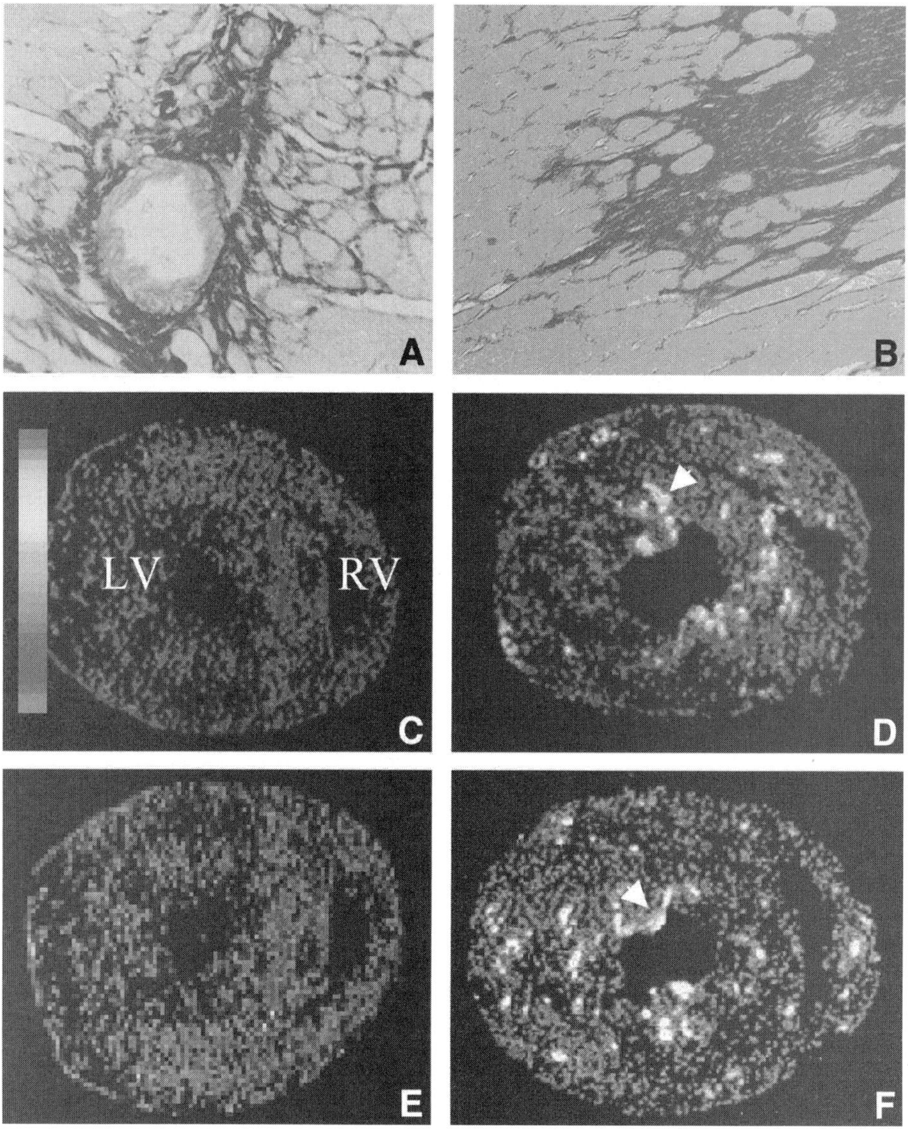

Fig. 2. Cardiac fibrosis induced by aldosterone/salt treatment (ALDOST). At 4 wk treatment, perivascular fibrosis (**A**) and microscopic scars (**B**) are seen in both atria and ventricles by Picrosirius Red staining. As detected by *in situ* hybridization, low-level expression of type I collagen mRNA (**C**) and transforming growth factor (TGF)-α_1 mRNA (**E**) are seen in both ventricles of the normal heart. At 4 wk of ALDOST, high-level expression of type I collagen (**D**, arrow) and TGF-β_1 mRNAs (**F**, arrow) are observed at sites of fibrosis.

and microscopic scarring, or reparative fibrosis, that follows cardiomyocyte necrosis (**Fig. 2A** and **B**) *(40,42,43)*. These changes are not observed in the first 3 wk of ALDO treatment. At wk 5 and 6, cardiac fibrosis becomes more extensive involving progressively more sites in both the left and right heart.

The etiological basis of cardiomyocyte necrosis in this model is likely multifactorial and not fully understood. Depleted intracellular potassium has been excluded throught the supplementation of the diet with KCl.

3.3. Cellular and Molecular Biology

Immunohistochemistry identifies the presence of oxidative and nitrosative stress within inflammatory cells that have invaded the intramural coronary vasculature and microscopic sites of injury, together with activation of a redox-sensitive nuclear factor (NF)-κB and upregulated mRNA expression of a proinflammatory mediator cascade that it regulates, and which includes intercellular adhesion molecule (ICAM)-1 and monocyte chemoattractant protein (MCP)-1 *(44)*. This is accompanied by increased expression of TGF-β_1 and type I collagen (**Fig. 2D** and **F**), each of which contribute to the appearance and composition of fibrous tissue by myoFb *(44)*. The upregulated expression of these adhesion molecules and chemokines leads to the appearance of ED-1^+ monocytes/macrophages, $CD4^+$ lymphocytes, and α-sma^+ myoFb at these sites *(44,45)*. This inflammatory cell response is followed by a perivascular fibrosis and microscopic scars in both right and left ventricles. This is accompanied by increased expression of tumor necrosis factor (TNF)-family ligands and oxidative stress in peripheral blood mononuclear cells (PBMCs) *(45,46)*. These monocytes and lymphocytes are activated prior to tissue invasion by induction of an altered redox state as evidenced by H_2O_2 production in these cells and upregulated expression of antioxidant defenses *(45,46)*. Aldosteronism, therefore, is accompanied by an immunostimulatory state based on an activation of circulating immune cells induced by iterations in PBMC divalent cations ($Mg^{2+}$and Ca^{2+}) and transduced by oxidative/nitrosative stress. ALDO receptor antagonism and antioxidant modulate this neuroendocrine–immune interface *(45,46)*.

3.4. De Novo *AngII and Fibrosis*

ALDO-induced proinflammatory/fibrogenic cardiac phenotype is spatially concordant with the expression of ACE and AT_1 receptors by activated macrophages and myoFb at sites of repair. Tissue ACE regulates the biochemical milieu found at these sites through its conversion of substrates that contribute to healing. This would include not only AngII generation from AngI, but in its dual capacity as a kininase the degradation of bradykinin, substance P, enkephalins, and a recently described inhibitor of cell growth, AcSDKP *(47)*.

We were not able to measure AngII levels at sites of cardiac injury in the ALDO/salt model given the microscopic size of these lesions. However, our previous study implicated tissue AngII, produced *de novo* at sites of repair in the injured rat heart, in contributing to inflammatory and fibrogenic responses *(48)*. Robert et al. *(49)* have demonstrated that AT_1 receptor antagonist prevents perivascular fibrosis of the coronary vasculature in the ALDO/salt model in which circulating AngII is suppressed. Our recent study has demonstrated that AT_1 receptor antagonism with valsartan attenuates the expression of proinflammatory/fibrotic meadiators of repair and the extent of fibrosis *(45)*. These observations implicate AT_1-mediated actions of tissue AngII in regulating cardiac fibrosis. We did not address and therefore cannot exclude a role for the AT_2 receptor. However, the great majority of receptors found at sites of repair in the adult Sprague-Dawley rat heart are of the AT_1 subtype *(13)*.

4. Fibrosis in Response to AngII Treatment

4.1. Animal Model

Eight-week-old male Sprague-Dawley rats are anesthetized with isoflurane and the dorsal skin shaved in preparation for a 1-cm skin incision. An osmotic minipump (Durect, Cupertino, CA) loaded with AngII (Sigma, St. Louis, MO) is implanted subcutaneously and skin is closed (*see* **Note 3**). The minipump releases AngII at the rate of 9 μg/h. AngII is loaded into the minipump dissolved in normal saline *(50,51)*. Following surgery, rats receive regular chow with 0.4% KCl in drinking water. During the first week of AngII treatment, lethargy and anorexia appear. Arterial pressure rises on the secondary day after AngII treatment and left-ventricular hypertrophy is evident at wk 2. Mortality is 10 to 20% within the first 4 wk and more than 50% from wk 4 to 6.

4.2. Morphology

Cardiac fibrosis is well developed at 2 wk of AngII treatment and presents in two morphological forms involving the right and left heart: a perivascular fibrosis of intramural coronary arteries; and reparative fibrosis, or microscopic scarring (**Fig. 3B** and **C**) *(40)*. In rats receiving AngII for 2 wk, fibrosis is observed in both left and right atria and ventricles and becomes more widely distributed within these structures at 4 and 6 wk of continued treatment.

Fig. 3. Cardiac fibrosis induced by either angiotensin (Ang)II infusion or isoproterenol administration. In the normal rat heart, a certain amount of collagen is found within the perivascular space (**A**, arrow) by Picrosirius Red staining. In rats receiving AngII infusion for 2 wk, perivascular fibrosis (**B**) and microscopic scars (**C**) are observed in both atria and ventricles. At 2 wk following isoproterenol administration, endomyocardial fibrosis is evident in both ventricles (**D**, arrow) by Picrosirius Red staining. Abundant α-smooth muscle actin$^+$ myoFb are located at these sites (**E**, arrow).

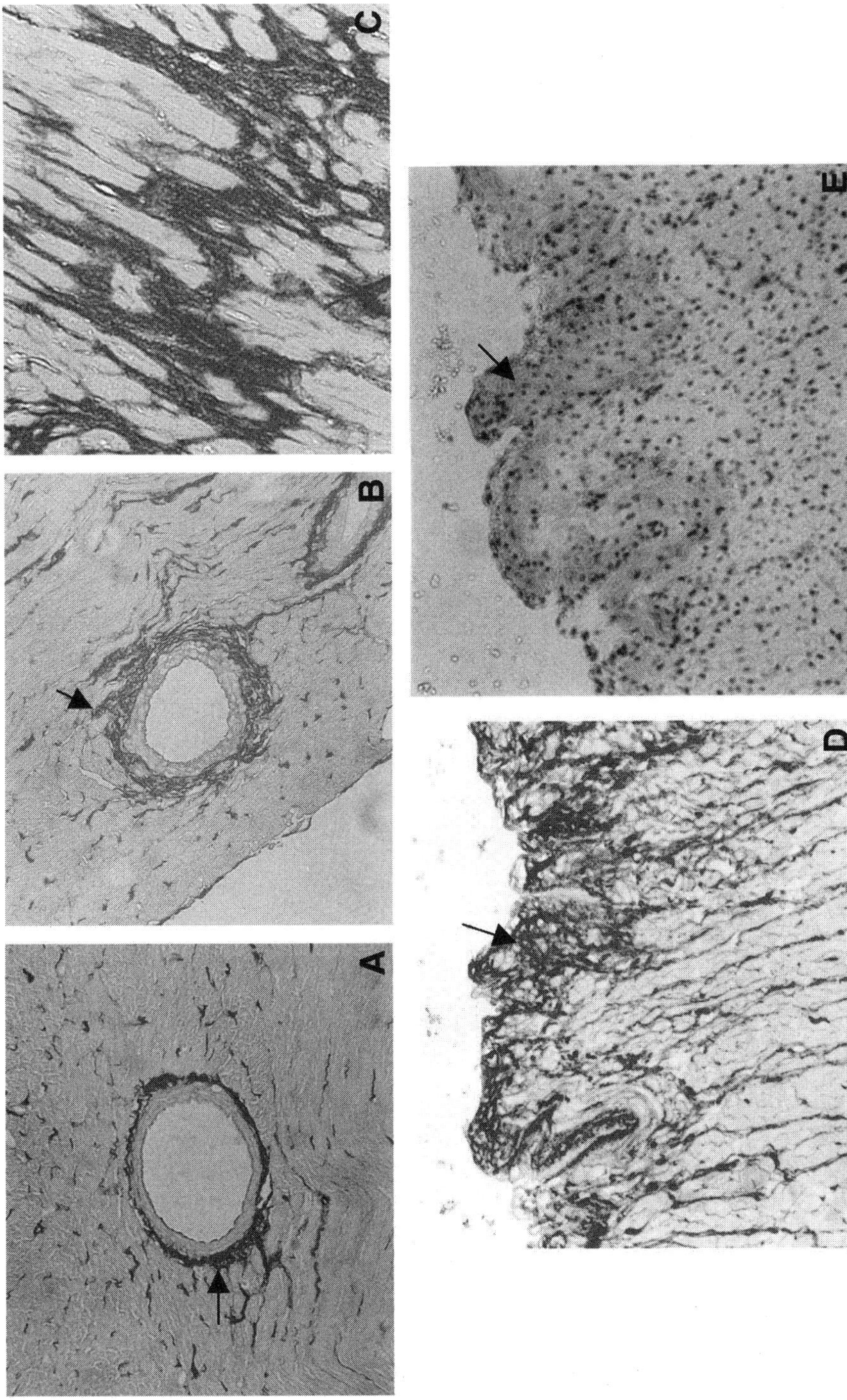
A
B
C
D
E

4.3. Cellular and Molecular Biology

Chronic elevations in circulating AngII are associated with an activation of circulating PBMC and endothelial cells, thereby promoting a proinflammatory/fibrogenic vascular phenotype involving the heart, kidneys, and other systemic organs ***(52–54)***. Type I collagen mRNA expression is increased in the rat right and left ventricles between d 4 and 7 of a 2-wk AngII infusion and localized by *in situ* hybridization to affected intramural arteries and sites of cardiomyocyte loss. By Picrosirius Red staining, a perivascular fibrosis, and microscopic scars are evident by light microscopy on d 14. The pathophysiological basis of cardiac fibrosis in this model appears to be similar to ALDOST. AngII is associated with nicotinamide adenine dinucleotide phosphate (NADPH) oxidase, activation and the generation of reactive oxygen species (ROS) ***(55,56)***. ROS act as signal transduction messengers for several important transcription factors, including NF-κB ***(57,58)***. Activation of NF-κB enhances the expression of numerous proinflammatory and profibrogenic genes and triggers tissue repair/remodeling, as noted earlier.

AngII is implicated in the development of pathological lesions in multiple tissue and organs, including blood vessels, heart, and kidneys. AngII exerts its actions through two receptors: AT_1 and AT_2. Characterization of these receptors and their functions has led to an understanding of the role that AngII plays in vascular remodeling and has opened new avenues for pharmacological intervention. The AT_1 receptor mediates most of the deleterious effects of AngII, such as vasoconstriction, endothelial damage, and cell growth. Selective inhibition of the AT_1 receptor not only inhibits these effects, but also leaves the AT_2 receptor unopposed for stimulation by AngII. Among the many potential effects mediated by stimulation of the AT_2 is the cellular regeneration after injury and inhibition of pathological cell growth. Thus, AT_1 receptor blockade appears to offer both active and passive therapeutic benefits.

4.4. De Novo *AngII and Fibrosis*

AngII-induced cardiac perivascular fibrosis and microscopic scars are colocolized with expression of ACE and AT_1 receptors, suggesting the potential autocrine and paracrine role of AngII on cardiac repair in this model. MyoFb and macrophages are primarily responsible for ACE and AT_1 receptor expression at these sites. Lijnen et al. have reported that AT_1 receptor antagonist treatment abolished AngII infusion-induced cardiac fibroblast proliferation and perivascular fibrosis in rats ***(59,60)***. Our previous study has demonstrated that an ACE inhibitor, lisinopril, attenuated cardiac fibrosis induced by AngII infusion ***(51)***.

5. Fibrosis in Response to Isoproterenol Treatment

5.1. *Animal Model*

Eight-week-old male Sprague-Dawley rats are given a single injection (1 mg/kg) of isoproterenol hydrochloride subcutaneously for 2 d *(61)*. Isoproterenol is a β-adrenergic receptor agonist, which induces cardiomyocyte necrosis primarily within the endomyocardium followed by fibrosis. There is no sign of lethargy and anorexia during the 2 wk of treatment. Mortality is 20% in rats receiving isoproterenol at the above dosage (*see* **Note 3**).

5.2. *Morphology*

Two weeks after isoproterenol administration, evidence of lost cardiomyocytes to necrosis has been followed by a reparative fibrosis, or scarring. It is found in the endomyocardium of both ventricles. **Figure 3D** illustrates fibrillar collagen accumulation at this site. α-sma$^+$ myoFb are abundant and co-localized with fibrillar collagen that presents as an endomyocardial fibrosis (**Fig. 3E**). Such cardiac fibrosis is not progressive and intramural vessels are not involved.

5.3. *Cellular and Molecular Biology*

After isoproterenol administration, a process of tissue repair follows the necrotic endomyocardial loss of cardiomyocytes. Inflammatory cells and myoFb contribute to the repair process. As detected by *in situ* hybridization, the expression of type I and III collagen genes is upregulated at d 3 and collagen fibers are morpholocally evident by d 14. MyoFb contribute to enhanced type I and III mRNAs in the endomyocardium.

5.4. De Novo *AngII and Fibrosis*

By quantitative in vitro autoradiography, we studied ACE binding density in the model and found it to be markedly increased at the site of endomyocardial fibrosis, where the cells expressing ACE are primarily macrophages and myoFb *(61)*. These findings further support supposition AngII production is enhanced at sites of cardiac repair, irrespective of its location or etiological basis of injury.

6. Conclusions

Cardiac fibrosis creates heterogeneity in cardiac tissue structure which impairs ventricular function. It is represented as a reactive perivascular and/or interstitial fibrosis and as reparative fibrosis. Various models have been used to study cardiac fibrosis. That includes coronary artery ligation-induced extensive fibrosis in both infarcted and noninfarcted myocardium, ALDO or AngII infusion-induced perivascular and interstitial fibrosis, and isoproterenol-induced endomyocardial fibrosis. Cells responsible for collagen synthesis at these various sites of fibrosis are primarily myoFb irrespective of the nature of injury. ACE and AngII receptors are increased at sites of fibrosis in each of these models and pharmacological intervention with ACE inhibitors or AT_1 receptor antagonists attenuates cardiac fibrosis, indicating the role of local AngII in cardiac fibrogenesis.

7. Notes

1. The left-ventricular infarct size is dependent on the location of the coronary artery ligation. Ligation of the main left coronary artery will lead to 40 to 50% left ventricle infarction, whereas ligation of the left coronary artery branch will cause 10 to 30% left ventricle infarction.
2. Different minipumps release ALDO or AngII for 1, 2, or 4 wk based on the needs of the experiment. The mean fill volume of a minipump is 210 µL and the mean pumping rate is 0.25 µL/h (4 wk pump), 0.5 µL/h (2 wk pump), and 1 µL/h (1 wk pump). Therefore, ALDO and AngII concentrations must be adjusted by using different pumps.
3. Higher doses of isoproterenol hydrochloride will cause up to 100% mortality. The dosage of isoproterenol (1 mg/kg) must be strictly followed.

Acknowledgments

This work was supported in part by National Institutes of Health National Heart, Lung, and Blood Institute grants R01-HL67888 (to Y.S.), and R01-HL62229 (to K.T.W.), and grants from the University of Tennessee Health Science Center Center of Excellence in Connective Tissue Diseases (to Y.S. and K.T.W.).

References

1. Laurent, G. J. (1987) Dynamic state of collagen: pathways of collagen degradation *in vivo* and their possible role in regulation of collagen mass. *Am. J. Physiol.* **252,** C1–C9.
2. Docherty, A. J. and Murphy, G. (1990) The tissue metalloproteinase family and the inhibitor TIMP: a study using cDNAs and recombinant proteins. *Ann. Rheum. Dis.* **49,** 469–479.
3. Tyagi, S. C., Ratajska, A. and Weber, K. T. (1993) Myocardial matrix metalloproteinase(s): localization and activation. *Mol. Cell. Biochem.* **126,** 49–59.
4. Weber, K. T., Sun, Y. and Katwa, L. C. (1997) Myofibroblasts and local angiotensin II in rat cardiac tissue repair. *Int. J. Biochem. Cell Biol.* **29,** 31–42.
5. Jugdutt, B. I. and Amy, R. W. M. (1986) Healing after myocardial infarction in the dog: changes in infarct hydroxyproline and topography. *J. Am. Coll. Cardiol.* **7,** 91–102.

6. Brilla, C. G., Matsubara, L. S., and Weber, K. T. (1993) Anti-aldosterone treatment and the prevention of myocardial fibrosis in primary and secondary hyperaldosteronism. *J. Mol. Cell. Cardiol.* **25,** 563–575.
7. Medugorac, I. (1980) Collagen content in different areas of normal and hypertrophied rat myocardium. *Cardiovasc. Res.* **14,** 551–554.
8. Weber, K. T., Pick, R., Janicki, J. S., Gadodia, G., and Lakier, J. B. (1988) Inadequate collagen tethers in dilated cardiopathy. *Am. Heart J.* **116,** 1641–1646.
9. Bishop, J., Greenbaum, J., Gibson, D., Yacoub, M., and Laurent, G. J. (1990) Enhanced deposition of predominantly type I collagen in myocardial disease. *J. Mol. Cell. Cardiol.* **22,** 1157–1165.
10. Chapman, D., Weber, K. T., and Eghbali, M. (1990) Regulation of fibrillar collagen types I and III and basement membrane type IV collagen gene expression in pressure overloaded rat myocardium. *Circ. Res.* **67,** 787–794.
11. Mukherjee, D. and Sen, S. (1990) Collagen phenotypes during development and regression of myocardial hypertrophy in spontaneously hypertensive rats. *Circ. Res.* **67,** 1474-1480.
12. Pfeffer, M. A., Pfeffer, J. M., Fishbein, M. C., Fletcher, P. J., Spadaro, J., Kloner, R. A., and Braunwald, E. (1979) Myocardial infarct size and ventricular function in rats. *Circ. Res.* **44,** 503–512.
13. Sun, Y. and Weber, K. T. (1994) Angiotensin II receptor binding following myocardial infarction in the rat. *Cardiovasc. Res.* **28,** 1623–1628.
14. Sun, Y., Zhang, J. Q., Zhang, J., and Lamparter, S. (2000) Cardiac remodeling by fibrous tissue after infarction in rats. *J. Lab. Clin. Med.* **135,** 316-–323.
15. Sun, Y., Cleutjens, J. P. M., Diaz-Arias, A. A., and Weber, K. T. (1994) Cardiac angiotensin converting enzyme and myocardial fibrosis in the rat. *Cardiovasc. Res.* **28,** 1423–1432.
16. Cleutjens, J. P. M., Kandala, J. C., Guarda, E., Guntaka, R. V., and Weber, K. T. (1995) Regulation of collagen degradation in the rat myocardium after infarction. *J. Mol. Cell. Cardiol.* **27,** 1281–1292.
17. Peterson, J. T., Li, H., Dillon, L., and Bryant, J. W. (2000) Evolution of matrix metalloprotease and tissue inhibitor expression during heart failure progression in the infarcted rat. *Cardiovasc. Res.* **46,** 307–315.
18. Cleutjens, J. P. M., Verluyten, M. J. A., Smits, J. F. M., and Daemen, M. J. A. P. (1995) Collagen remodeling after myocardial infarction in the rat heart. *Am. J. Pathol.* **147,** 325–338.
19. Sun, Y., Zhang, J. Q., Zhang, J., and Ramires, F. J. A. (1998) Angiotensin II, transforming growth factor-β_1 and repair in the infarcted heart. *J. Mol. Cell. Cardiol.* **30,** 1559–1569.
20. Wei, S., Chow, L. T., Shum, I. O., Qin, L., and Sanderson, J. E. (1999) Left and right ventricular collagen type I/III ratios and remodeling post-myocardial infarction. *J. Cardiac Failure* **5,** 117–126.
21. Gideon, P. A., Warrington, K. J., Lu, L., Sun, Y., and Weber, K. T. (2003) Autoimmune lymphocyte response at sites remote to myocardial infarction [abstract]. *Circulation* **108,** IV–69.

22. Sun, Y. and Weber, K. T. (1996) Angiotensin converting enzyme and myofibroblasts during tissue repair in the rat heart. *J. Mol. Cell. Cardiol.* **28,** 851–858.
23. Blankesteijn, W. M., Essers-Janssen, Y. P. G., Verluyten, M. J. A., Daemen, M. J. A. P., and Smits, J. F. M. (1997) A homologue of *Drosophila* tissue polarity gene *frizzled* is expressed in migrating myofibroblasts in the infarcted rat heart. *Nat. Med.* **3,** 541–544.
24. Peterson, D. J., Ju, H., Hao, J., Panagia, M., Chapman, D. C., and Dixon, I. M. (1999) Expression of $G_{i\text{-}2\alpha}$ and $G_{s\alpha}$ in myofibroblasts localized to the infarct scar in heart failure due to myocardial infarction. *Cardiovasc. Res.* **41,** 575–585.
25. Gabbiani, G., Hirschel, B. J., Ryan, G. B., Statkov, P. R., and Majno, G. (1972) Granulation tissue as a contractile organ. A study of structure and function. *J. Exp. Med.* **135,** 719–734.
26. Yokozeki, M., Moriyama, K., Shimokawa, H., and Kuroda, T. (1997) Transforming growth factor-β_1 modulates myofibroblastic phenotype of rat palatal fibroblasts *in vitro*. *Exp. Cell Res.* **231,** 328–336.
27. Khouw, I. M., van Wachem, P. B., Plantinga, J. A., Vujaskovic, Z., Wissink, M. J., de Leij, L. F., and van Luyn, M. J. (1999) TGF-β and βFGF affect the differentiation of proliferating porcine fibroblasts into myofibroblasts in vitro. *Biomaterials* **20,** 1815–1822.
28. Evans, R. A., Tian, Y. C., Steadman, R., and Phillips, A. O. (2003) TGF-β_1-mediated fibroblast-myofibroblast terminal differentiation—the role of Smad proteins. *Exp. Cell Res.* **282,** 90–100.
29. Willems, I. E. M. G., Havenith, M. G., De Mey, J. G. R., and Daemen, M. J. A. P. (1994) The α-smooth muscle actin-positive cells in healing human myocardial scars. *Am. J. Pathol.* **145,** 868–875.
30. Sun, Y., Zhang, J., Zhang, J. Q., and Ramires, F. J. A. (2000) Local angiotensin II and transforming growth factor-β1 in renal fibrosis of rats. *Hypertension* **35,** 1078–1084.
31. Ou, R., Sun, Y., Ganjam, V. K., and Weber, K. T. (1996) *In situ* production of angiotensin II by fibrosed rat pericardium. *J. Mol. Cell. Cardiol.* **28,** 1319–1327.
32. Yamagishi, H., Kim, S., Nishikimi, T., Takeuchi, K., and Takeda, T. (1993) Contribution of cardiac renin-angiotensin system to ventricular remodelling in myocardial-infarcted rats. *J. Mol. Cell. Cardiol.* **25,** 1369–1380.
33. Jugdutt, B. I., Humen, D. P., Khan, M. I., and Schwarz-Michorowski, B. L. (1992) Effect of left ventricular unloading with captopril on remodeling and function during healing of anterior transmural myocardial infarction in the dog. *Can. J. Cardiol.* **8,** 151–163.
34. Jugdutt, B. I., Khan, M. I., Jugdutt, S. J., and Blinston, G. E. (1995) Effect of enalapril on ventricular remodeling and function during healing after anterior myocardial infarction in the dog. *Circulation* **91,** 802–812.
35. Michel, J.-B., Lattion, A.-L., Salzmann, J.-L., Cerol, M. L., Philippe, M., Camilleri, J.-P., and Corvol, P. (1988) Hormonal and cardiac effects of converting enzyme inhibition in rat myocardial infarction. *Circ. Res.* **62,** 641–650.
36. van Krimpen, C., Schoemaker, R. G., Cleutjens, J. P. M., Smits, J. F. M., Struyker-Boudier, H. A. J., Bosman, F. T., and Daemen, M. J. A. P. (1991) Angiotensin I

converting enzyme inhibitors and cardiac remodeling. *Basic Res. Cardiol.* **86,** 149–155.
37. Smits, J. F. M., van Krimpen, C., Schoemaker, R. G., Cleutjens, J. P. M., and Daemen, M. J. A. P. (1992) Angiotensin II receptor blockade after myocardial infarction in rats: effects on hemodynamics, myocardial DNA synthesis, and interstitial collagen content. *J. Cardiovasc. Pharmacol.* **20,** 772–778.
38. Hodsman, G. P., Kohzuki, M., Howes, L. G., Sumithran, E., Tsunoda, K., and Johnston, C. I. (1988) Neurohumoral responses to chronic myocardial infarction in rats. *Circulation* **78,** 376–381.
39. Hirsch, A. T., Talsness, C. E., Schunkert, H., Paul, M., and Dzau, V. J. (1991) Tissue-specific activation of cardiac angiotensin converting enzyme in experimental heart failure. *Circ. Res.* **69,** 475–482.
40. Sun, Y., Ratajska, A., Zhou, G., and Weber, K. T. (1993) Angiotensin converting enzyme and myocardial fibrosis in the rat receiving angiotensin II or aldosterone. *J. Lab. Clin. Med.* **122,** 395–403.
41. Young, M., Fullerton, M., Dilley, R., and Funder, J. (1994) Mineralocorticoids, hypertension, and cardiac fibrosis. *J. Clin. Invest.* **93,** 2578–2583.
42. Sun, Y., Ramires, F. J. A., and Weber, K. T. (1997) Fibrosis of atria and great vessels in response to angiotensin II or aldosterone infusion. *Cardiovasc. Res.* **35,** 138–147.
43. Campbell, S. E., Janicki, J. S., and Weber, K. T. (1995) Temporal differences in fibroblast proliferation and phenotype expression in response to chronic administration of angiotensin II or aldosterone. *J. Mol. Cell. Cardiol.* **27,** 1545–1560.
44. Sun, Y., Zhang, J., Lu, L., Chen, S. S., Quinn, M. T., and Weber, K. T. (2002) Aldosterone-induced inflammation in the rat heart. Role of oxidative stress. *Am. J. Pathol.* **161,** 1773–1781.
45. Ahokas, R. A., Warrington, K. J., Gerling, I. C., et al. (2003) Aldosteronism and peripheral blood mononuclear cell activation. A neuroendocrine-immune interface. *Circ. Res.* **93,** e124–e135.
46. Gerling, I. C., Sun, Y., Ahokas, R. A., Wodi, L. A., et al. (2003) Aldosteronism: an immunostimulatory state precedes the proinflammatory/fibrogenic cardiac phenotype. *Am. J. Physiol. Heart Circ. Physiol.* **285,** H813–H821.
47. Rousseau-Plasse, A., Lenfant, M., and Potier, P. (1996) Catabolism of the hemoregulatory peptide *N*-Acetyl-Ser-Asp-Lys-Pro: a new insight into the physiological role of the angiotensin-I-converting enzyme *N*-active site. *Bioorg. Med. Chem.* **4,** 1113–1119.
48. Sun, Y., Zhang, J., Lu, L., Bedigian, M. P., Robinson, A. D., and Weber, K. T. (2004) Tissue angiotensin II in the regulation of inflammatory and fibrogenic components of repair in the rat heart. *J. Lab. Clin. Med.,* in press.
49. Robert, V., Heymes, C., Silvestre, J.-S., Sabri, A., Swynghedauw, B., and Delcayre, C. (1999) Angiotensin AT_1 receptor subtype as a cardiac target of aldosterone. Role in aldosterone-salt-induced fibrosis. *Hypertension* **33,** 981–986.
50. Tan, L. B., Jalil, J. E., Pick, R., Janicki, J. S., and Weber, K. T. (1991) Cardiac myocyte necrosis induced by angiotensin II. *Circ. Res.* **69,** 1185–1195.

51. Sun, Y., Ratajska, A., and Weber, K. T. (1995) Inhibition of angiotensin-converting enzyme and attenuation of myocardial fibrosis by lisinopril in rats receiving angiotensin II. *J. Lab. Clin. Med.* **126,** 95–101.
52. Brilla, C. G., Pick, R., Tan, L. B., Janicki, J. S., and Weber, K. T. (1990) Remodeling of the rat right and left ventricle in experimental hypertension. *Circ. Res.* **67,** 1355–1364.
53. Everett, A. D., Tufro-McReddie, A., Fisher, A., and Gomez, R. A. (1994) Angiotensin receptor regulates cardiac hypertrophy and transforming growth factor-β1 expression. *Hypertension* **23,** 587–592.
54. Rupérez, M., Ruiz-Ortega, M., Esteban, V., Lorenzo, O., Mezzano, S., Plaza, J. J., and Egido, J. (2003) Angiotensin II increases connective tissue growth factor in the kidney. *Am. J. Pathol.* **163,** 1937–1947.
55. Wang, H. D., Xu, S., Johns, D. G., Du, Y., Quinn, M. T., Cayatte, A. J., and Cohen, R. A. (2001) Role of NADPH oxidase in the vascular hypertrophic and oxidative stress response to angiotensin II in mice. *Circ. Res.* **88,** 947–953.
56. Harrison, D. G., Cai, H., Landmesser, U., and Griendling, K. K. (2003) Interactions of angiotensin II with NAD(P)H oxidase, oxidant stress and cardiovascular disease. *J. Renin Angiotensin Aldosterone Syst.* **4,** 51–61.
57. Barnes, P. J. and Karin, M. (1997) Nuclear factor-κB: a pivotal transcription factor in chronic inflammatory diseases. *N. Engl. J. Med.* **336,** 1066–1071.
58. Muller, D. N., Dechend, R., Mervaala, E. M., et al. (2000) NF-κB inhibition ameliorates angiotensin II-induced inflammatory damage in rats. *Hypertension* **35,** 193–201.
59. Lijnen, P. J., Petrov, V. V., and Fagard, R. H. (2001) Angiotensin II-induced stimulation of collagen secretion and production in cardiac fibroblasts is mediated via angiotensin II subtype 1 receptors. *J. Renin Angiotensin Aldosterone Syst.* **2,** 117–122.
60. Lijnen, P. J. and Petrov, V. V. (2003) Role of intracardiac renin-angiotensin-aldosterone system in extracellular matrix remodeling. *Methods Find. Exp. Clin. Pharmacol.* **25,** 541–564.
61. Sun, Y. and Weber, K. T. (1996) Angiotensin-converting enzyme and wound healing in diverse tissues of the rat. *J. Lab. Clin. Med.* **127,** 94–101.

IV

Genetic Approaches to Studying Fibrosis

18

Finding Fibrosis Genes

The Lung

Lauranell H. Burch and David A. Schwartz

Summary

Many people are exposed to environmental risk factors for fibrosis, yet only a subset go on to develop disease. It is likely that a number of tissue-specific disease genes determine the path an individual will follow upon exposure to an environmental agent, and that individuals who carry certain combinations of these genes are most susceptible. Diseases which have multiple genetic and environmental determinants, known as "complex traits," present a formidable challenge for gene discovery as the combined influence of more than one gene and one or more environmental factors decrease power to isolate the effect of any single gene. Nevertheless, the identification of the genetic differences that underlie susceptibility to fibrotic disease is crucial to understanding the disease process and to the development of effective screening tests and treatments. No single strategy or method will likely be sufficient to link a candidate disease gene to a fibrosis phenotype. Therefore, we present techniques and resources that can be used in combination to dissect the genetics of complex traits and yield viable candidate genes. Testing of candidate genes and standards for formal proof of gene discovery are discussed.

Key Words: Fibrosis; linkage; polymorphism; QTL.

1. Introduction

Approaches to identify the genetic component of disease susceptibility fall into two broad categories: positional approaches, which use genetic markers to perform an unbiased scan of all or part of the genome, and candidate gene methods, which test variants of a candidate susceptibility gene directly for association with disease. Each approach has strengths and weaknesses. Candidate gene association studies can be family-based, or use unrelated cases and controls, and offer the advantages of speed, relatively low cost, and the possibility of identifying genes with relatively small individual effects. However, prior knowledge of the biology of the disease process is a requirement for the

From: *Methods in Molecular Medicine, Vol. 117: Fibrosis Research: Methods and Protocols*
Edited by: J. Varga, D. A. Brenner, and S. H. Phan © Humana Press Inc., Totowa, NJ

candidate gene approach, and therefore limits its utility where underlying pathophysiology is not understood. Traditional linkage approaches in humans are often hindered by low power owing to difficulty in ascertaining sufficient numbers of families with multiple affected individuals. For this reason, positional cloning methods applied to mouse models of human fibrotic disease may offer the investigator a more accessible and lower-cost opportunity for gene discovery. Mouse models also offer the possibility of controlling environmental exposure and isolating genetic effects through selective breeding. In most other aspects, basic methodologies for human and mouse gene discovery projects are very similar. The major steps to finding fibrosis genes are outlined here (*see* **Fig. 1**).

1.1. Select a Model Organism and Phenotype

A single clinical diagnosis may encompass several different disorders, each with a distinct pathogenesis. To increase the likelihood of resolving this genetic complexity, a fibrosis phenotype of interest should be very narrowly defined. An even better approach may be to choose a single measurable "quantitative trait" that is a subset of the overall disease phenotype, and to pursue the genetics underlying this quantitative trait in a mouse model of fibrosis.

1.2. Obtain Expert Statistical Support

The mathematics underlying linkage analysis, particularly in human studies, is fairly complex and best handled by an experienced statistical geneticist who is involved as a co-investigator from the inception and design of the study through the data analysis component.

1.3. Mine the Literature for Candidate Genes and Loci

The rapid pace of discovery of the genes conferring susceptibility to many inherited diseases presents an opportunity to mine the literature for genes and associated polymorphisms that may be associated with fibrosis. Disease genes and markers previously associated with a fibrosis phenotype in another study can be retested as candidates in your study. In addition, genes within the same gene family or within the same or similar biological pathways as previously reported "pathogenic" sequences may serve as candidates in your study. An investigator's previous knowledge and insight into a disease process will be helpful in selecting the best candidate genes to pursue. It is also important to determine if a potential locus related to your fibrosis phenotype of interest has been mapped in any organism. Because the order of genes is conserved in blocks between species, cross-species conservation, or synteny, can be used to compare linked regions across human and animal models. Ensembl (www.ensembl.org), has excellent, easy-to-use synteny tools which will allow you to

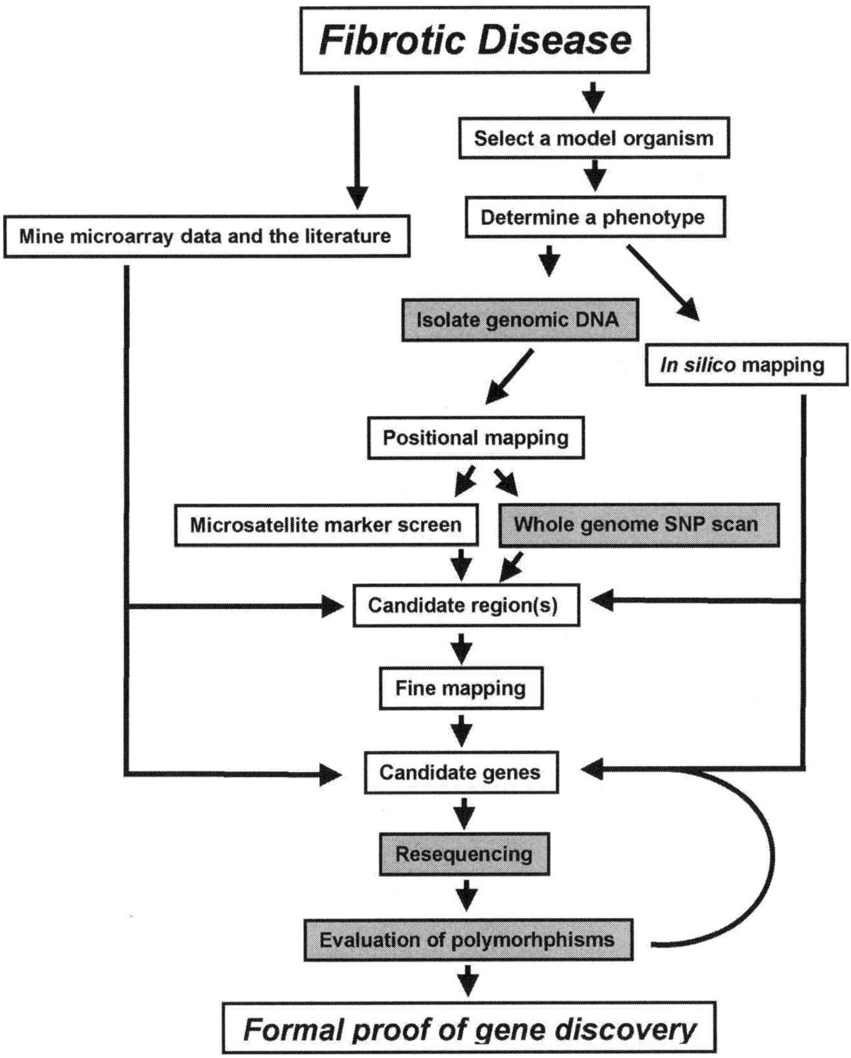

Fig. 1. Flow diagram of the fibrosis gene discovery process. Protocols provided in this manuscript are indicated in light gray.

determine whether candidate loci across a number of model organisms are likely to harbor orthologous genes.

1.4. Mine Public Microarray Data Sets

You may reap benefits from advances in microarray technology without performing your own microarray experiment. *See* the National Center for Biotechnology Information (NCBI)'s GEO (www.ncbi.nlm.nih.gov/geo/), and also Array Express (www.ebi.ac.uk/arrayexpress/), for access to several complete microarray data sets related to human and animal models of fibrosis. Data sets are fully downloadable, and may be useful in the identification of candidate genes and biological pathways that may be important in fibrosis. Most of these microarray experiments are posted on the Web as raw data (un-normalized intensities) and will require further analysis. The Institute for Genomic Research (TIGR) Web site (http://www.tigr.org/) has microarray analysis software that is free to download and is provided with detailed user manuals and tutorials to maximize ease of use. Alternatively, the Biometric Research Branch (BRB) home page (http://linus.nci.nih.gov/BRB-ArrayTools.html) offers free microarray software available as a download. BRB *ArrayTools* are compatible with an Excel format, which is convenient for most users.

1.5. Perform Your Own Microarray Study

If public microarray datasets that model your phenotype of interest are unavailable, or you have an interest in the role that specific environmental exposures may play, you may choose to conduct your own microarray experiment Another advantage of mouse models for genetic studies is the ability to challenge genetically identical individuals in separate environmental exposures. Whenever possible, it is desirable to perform an *isogenic* microarray comparison (a single individual before and after a treatment in a human study, or choose inbred animals) to eliminate noise from inter-individual variability. Microarray comparisons made against commercial reference RNAs (Stratagene) offer the opportunity to compare your data with the data of others who used this standard, and with your own future experiments. Unless you work within a group that has established microarray hybridization expertise, it is probably best to outsource your hybridizations. Many campuses have established a microarray core facility that will perform hybridizations on a fee for service basis. Agilent Technologies (www.agilent.com), Affymetrix (www.affymetrix.com), and a number of other companies offer commercially available microarray resources and support services.

1.6. Make Sense of Microarray Data

For most microarray studies, the challenge resides in deriving biological meaning from an overwhelming amount of data. Although the ability to measure large numbers of genes affords new insight by identifying genes that would not have been imagined to participate in a process, it is difficult to derive meaning from even a small experiment without the aid of sophisticated analysis tools. Some recently developed tools that can be applied to global microarray data sets are the freely available Web programs GenMAPP *(1)* (www.genmapp.org),

MAPPFinder *(2)* (www.genmapp.org/MAPPFinder.html), and EASE *(3)* (http://david.niaid.nih.gov/david/ease.html), which are used to identify biological themes present in expression data. GenMAPP is an application designed to visualize gene expression data on maps representing biological pathways and groupings of genes. An interactive tutorial for GenMAPP is available at www.genmapp.org/tutorial.html.

MAPPFinder is then used to create a global gene-expression profile across all areas of biology by integrating the annotations of the Gene Ontology (GO) project with GenMAPP–MAPPFinder finds the GO terms with the greatest change in a microarray dataset and organizes these expression changes into functional groups. EASE is a tool that identifies overrepresented functional gene categories with respect to all assayed genes using a number of categorization systems, including GO, biological pathways, chromosome location, and protein domains. The user has a choice of two statistical measures of overrepresentation: the one-tailed Fisher exact probability or "EASE score" (a variant of the Fisher exact probability). These tools, when applied to your own or previously published microarray data, may help you uncover some of the complex biology that underlies genetic susceptibility to fibrotic disease. It should be noted that microarray studies are not suitable for the study of genes for which no changes in steady state message levels occur. For this reason, expression data will likely provide much insight into the biology of a process but will not necessarily reveal underlying disease genes, as the "cause" gene residing in a linked region may not be differentially expressed in the disease state.

1.7. Conduct an Inbred Strain Survey

An inbred strain phenotype survey is an essential first step toward developing a mouse model of fibrosis. In brief, the strain/phenotype relationship for multiple inbred strains is determined in response to a challenge known to produce fibrosis, and a quantitative measurement of the phenotypic response is recorded. Strains are then ordered along the response spectrum to identify high- and low-responder strains. Once this response spectrum is determined, the genetic variability that gives rise to it can begin to be explored by *in silico* and positional mapping methods. The inbred strains representing the extremes of your phenotype of interest may have been used as progenitor strains to develop recombinant inbred (RI) lines. Recombinant inbred mouse strains are derived by successive crosses between siblings from an initial cross between two progenitor strains. These RI strains are homozygous for one or other of the progenitor DNAs at essentially every locus, but differ from one another in the representation of these strains at the various loci. RI strains can be purchased from Jackson Laboratories (http://jaxmice.jax.org), and can be used to accelerate a mapping project by circumventing costly and time-consuming experimental crosses—the genome of the progenitor strains has already been assorted across RI lines!

The next step toward gene identification in a mouse model is to perform a strain phenotype survey across an RI panel whose progenitor strains represent phenotypic extremes of your inbred strain survey, if such a panel is available. Then, a quantitative phenotype across the panel of RI strains may be entered directly in computational program that derives quantitative trait loci (QTL) from RI strain phenotype data (discussed later). You may also investigate the use of consomic panels. Consomic panels are inbred strains of mice engineered to differ by one chromosome. If you can determine which chromosome(s) confers a phenotype of interest, you have eliminated most of the genome from consideration.

1.8. In Silico *Mapping*

There are several newly developed computational methods that input phenotype values across inbred strains of mice to rapidly predict genetic susceptibility loci without the need to develop experimental intercross populations. Each of these methods uses a database of strain-specific marker genotypes for subsequent analyses. One such computational method is available on the Web at (http://mousesnp.roche.com/) *(4)*. The software provided at this Web site allows the user to view strain comparisons across the entire mouse genome, or to focus on specific regions by restricting the analysis to an individual chromosome or region of a chromosome. The search output is presented as a graphical display of each chromosome with useful links to corresponding sequences in the mouse genomic DNA, GenBank, and strain-specific genotyping assays including primer sequences and polymerase chain reaction (PCR) conditions. It is possible to return to this computational linkage Web site at any point in the project to compare strain variation in any specific chromosomal region of interest or to obtain single nucleotide polymorphism (SNP) assays for linkage or association studies. An alternative to the Roche site is the SNPview resource (http://www.gnf.org/SNP/) *(5)*, which uses strain data on physically linked SNPs inherited as blocks known as haplotypes to reveal regions of genetic diversity across eight inbred strains of mice. Inbred mice have substantially reduced genetic variation compared to the wild populations from which they were derived. Strain pairs share haplotypes across 30 to 60% of the mouse genome *(5)*. A graphical display of shared haplotype blocks across multiple strains can highlight areas of potential diversity and also reduce the number of regions of the genome that must be queried for genetic variation. Another computational shortcut for mapping complex traits without genotyping is available for RI strain data at the

WebQTL Web site (http://webqtl.org/). This software, developed at the Roswell Park Cancer Institute and University of Tennessee Health Science Center *(6)*, generates QTL by several mapping methods from trait values across an RI set. This software can also be used to generate QTL from marker data generated in your laboratory. WebQTL programs are presented with a graphical user interface that is extremely easy to use, but the underlying computational framework is hidden. For an overview of quantitative genetics with an emphasis on mathematical models for QTL determination, see *Genetics and Analysis of Quantitative Traits* by Lynch and Walsh *(7)* and **ref.** *8*.

1.9. Assemble a DNA Collection

Genomic DNA samples must be prepared for your study population before any PCR-based genotyping can take place. For human studies, whole blood samples are collected, and genomic DNA is isolated from the lysed nuclei of white blood cells present in the sample (*see* **Note 1**). For mouse studies, it is convenient to take a small tail clipping (3–6 mm) for isolation of genomic DNA.

The isolation, storage format, and database management of the DNA collection are all important to the success of the project. It is particularly desirable to automate the dispensing of DNA and reagent cocktail into assay plates. Liquid handling robots that can pick up samples from 96-well DNA sample storage boxes and dispense into 96- or 384-well assay plates represent the best investment. Robots are available with various levels of automation and a wide range of prices. Protocols for genomic DNA isolation from human blood and from mouse tail sections are provided (*see* **Subheadings 3.1.** and **3.2.**).

1.10. Microsatellite Marker Screening

Microsatellites are short repeated sequences found throughout the genome. Because these repeated regions are abundant and vary in size among individuals (and across inbred mouse strains), they are convenient for use as markers in genetic linkage studies using nonradioactive PCR-based screens. To develop microsatellite marker sets, microsatellite sequences are selected to at 5 to 10 cM intervals across the genome, and then sorted according to size, with sizes in the range of 50 to 450 bp considered most useful as markers. The heterozygosity of each marker is also important, as highly heterozygous markers are the most informative. Highly heterozygous markers with a desirable repeat size are then grouped such that the markers can be run together as a multiplex. The ability to multiplex markers is key for an efficient screening project. Ideally, all markers within a group should amplify with the same PCR profile—the primer design and concentration of commercially available screening sets have been optimized for you to make this possible. Once a group of markers are determined to be size compatible and amplify well together in a single PCR reaction, they are called a marker panel. Marker panels have been constructed throughout the genome at intervals of 3 to 10 cM to produce whole genome marker sets. Many of these marker sets can be purchased prelabeled with fluorescent tags to offer automated fluorescent DNA fragment analysis on a microcapillary sequencer (*see* **Note 2**). Fragment analysis on a microcapillary platform offers the advantages of gel-free, high-throughput capability, accurate sizing of markers, and automated allele calling. Markers are multiplexed during electrophoresis, and fragments are distinguished by the three different fluorescent dyes, FAM, VIC, and NED, used to label the PCR primers. Fluorescently labeled fragments are sized with the internal standard GenScan-500 LIZ (Applied Biosystems). Detailed protocols, reagents, and full technical support for high-throughput microsatellite marker screening on a microcapillary platform are available from Applied Biosystems (http://www.appliedbiosystems.com/). This application is available on ABI 3100 and ABI 3730 capillary sequencers. Marker data are exported to genetic mapping software such as GeneMapper 3.0 (Applied Biosystems) or MapManager QTX *(9)* to determine regions of linkage.

1.11. QTL Identification by Whole Genome SNP Scan

The rationale behind QTL identification by whole genome SNP scan is based on the knowledge that parental alleles are distributed randomly to offspring. Therefore, for any loci not contributing to a fibrosis phenotype, parental alleles will be equally represented between sufficiently large pools of fibrosis-resistant and fibrosis-susceptible mice. However, strain-specific alleles for loci that do affect susceptibility will be overrepresented in the susceptible pool. Genome-wide strain-specific SNP analyses of F2 populations can be performed by a kinetic (real-time) PCR method in a 96- or 384-well format. The use of DNA pools reduces genotyping expense and effort ***(10)***. A protocol for this procedure is provided in the methods section (*see* **Subheading 3.3.**).

1.12. Narrow the Candidate Region

Because the resolution of linkage-based mapping is poor, any linked region(s) you have identified likely spans many megabases. The identification of a recombinant individual or individuals within the critical region would narrow the candidate region, and if no such informative recombinant event has been detected, SNP association studies can be performed across the region. If your linkage project was conducted in a mouse model of fibrosis, you can return to *in silico* methods to re-examine strain-specific SNP variation and haplotype structure within a candidate region. If strain sequence data is available, proceed to direct sequence comparison to identify polymorphisms. Revisit the literature once linkage has been established to query the locus as a region for any known risk factors, and also to determine whether candidate genes from any relevant microarray studies reside within the region. Any of these approaches may yield a successful candidate gene. Finally, it is important to generate a gene list for the linked region, and to examine this list for known genes that could have a biological function related to a fibrosis phenotype. NCBI, University of California at Santa Cruz (UCSC) Genome Bioinformatics (http://genome.ucsc.edu/), and the Ensembl Genome Browser are the most popular genome browsers. These resources can be used to generate gene lists between markers, to locate high-density microsatellite markers for fine mapping, and to find SNPs for association testing. A helpful introductory guide for the use of these Web sites including worked sample exercises was recently published in *Nature* ***(11)***. Once you have exhausted the literature and computational methods for selecting candidate genes within your QTL, selective breeding strategies can be pursued in mice to harness in vivo genetic assortment and recombination to narrow your candidate region and therefore reduce the number of candidate genes you must consider. A description of common breeding strategies follows, but is by no means comprehensive. For a more complete overview of experimental crosses and other topics in mouse genetics, obtain a copy of the textbook *Mouse Genetics* by Lee M. Silver ***(12)***.

Breeding strategies:

F2 Cross: an F2 cross tests marker/trait associations in a cross of F1 siblings. Parental strains representing the phenotypic extremes in an inbred strain survey are crossed to produce F1 offspring, which are heterozygous at every locus and genetically identical to each other. F1 siblings are then crossed to produce an F2 generation where the phenotype is not uniform because genes that underlie the trait of interest are assorted. Examine the distribution of the F2 phenotype for adherence to Mendelian ratios. A continuously distributed quantitative trait in an F2 design, or across recombinant inbred strains, suggests that multiple genes contribute to the phenotype.

Backcross strategies isolate a locus of interest: congenic strains of mice are considered identical for all genetic loci except for one, which may be a transgene or a specific region of interest. Congenic strains are produced by a breeding strategy known as backcross.

Backcross projects can be accelerated by marker genotyping (*see* **Note 3**).

Conventional backcross tests marker/trait associations in progeny obtained by backcross of F_1 to one of the parental lines.

- Trait donor and background strains are crossed.
- Progeny of each generation are tested for the phenotype of interest from the donor parent and crossed back onto the background parent.
- After a number of backcross generations, the majority of the background strain genome is recovered, and the locus of interest is isolated on the background strain.

Marker-assisted backcross:

- Trait donor and background strains are crossed.
- Progeny are screened using a marker linked to the trait of interest.
- Progeny that have this trait are then screened with many markers to breed animals sharing the most markers with the background parent.
- A congenic strain is recovered in fewer generations.

1.13. Resequencing of Candidate Genes

Candidate genes are resequenced to find genetic changes that could be responsible for a phenotype. These include alterations in the coding sequence that change an amino acid sequence or the stop codon, sequence alterations in splice junctions that may affect processing of the mRNA transcript, and sequence alterations in other noncoding regulatory regions. The most efficient strategy for gene resequencing is to amplify exons individually and surrounded by enough flanking intron sequence to ensure a clear read through both donor and acceptor consensus splice sequences. Primer selection software, such as Primer3 ***(13)*** is used to ensure that primers are well-matched by melting temperature (Tm) and will likely amplify well in a standard PCR profile. Primer3 source code is available at: (http://www-genome.wi.mit.edu/genome_software/other/primer3.html) (*see* **Note 4**). Typically, a standard amplicon length of approx 500 bp is selected to reduce the need for PCR optimization. Small exons should be centered within the amplicon. For large exons, several overlapping amplicons must be designed. The read distance from the sequencing primer may vary across sequencing equipment platforms and dye terminator versions, which should be considered in the design process. Sequencing of the resulting PCR product is performed by automated capillary fluorescent sequencing. Capillary sequencers use dye-terminator chemistry, so the same unmodified oligonucleotide primers used for fragment amplification can be used individually for sequencing. Automated capillary fluorescent sequencing is now a mature technology, and the challenge resides mainly in the choice of software for downstream data handling. The program Chromas (http://www.technelysium.com.au/) is inexpensive, is downloadable from the Web, and, once installed on a PC, allows viewing and manipulation of automated sequencing file chromatograms in Windows. Several sequences from each run should be inspected visually with Chromas to assess the quality of the run before proceeding with further analysis. To enable accurate and automated sequence data analysis, we suggest installation and implementation of the Phred, Phrap, Consed, and Polyphred suite of programs (*see* the Phred/Phrap/Consed System Home Page at http://www.phrap.org/) on a Unix or Linux (desktop Unix) platform. Phred ***(14)*** reads DNA sequencer raw trace data, calls bases, assigns quality scores to the bases, and then writes base calls and quality values to output files. Phred provides superior base calling and quality filtering capability over the default base calling software provided with most sequencing instruments. Phrap ***(15)***, a sequence assembly program, is used in conjunction with the base calls and base quality scores produced by the base caller software program, Phred. Phrap does not provide editing or viewing capabilities; these are provided with a companion sequence editor/assembly viewer program, Consed ***(16)***. PolyPhred ***(17)*** is a program that analyzes sequence traces to identify heterozygous sites for single nucleotide substitutions. PolyPhred's functions are integrated with those of Phred, Phrap, and Consed. PolyPhred identifies potential heterozygotes using the base calls and peak information provided by Phred and the sequence alignments provided by Phrap. Potential heterozygotes identified by PolyPhred are marked for rapid inspection using the Consed tool. PolyPhred software is one of the few packages currently available that are designed to find heterozygous bases in sequence data, and is free to download (http://droog.mbt.washington.edu/poly_get.html). The ability to reliably detect heterozygous loci is especially useful for human studies, as the sequence changes we expect to find in candidate genes in humans are likely to be carried in the heterozygous state, although the software will find and flag any sequence differences that occur across multiple sequence alignments. We have included a resequencing protocol complete with thermal cycling parameters in the Methods section. This exon-by-exon resequencing protocol will not detect mutations in noncoding regulatory regions that lie outside the amplicon. Strategies to locate noncoding regions likely to have functional importance are discussed in the following section.

1.14. Exploit Comparative Genomics

With the availability of whole genome draft sequences for multiple species, strain-specific sequence data for several strains of inbred mice, and a host of Web-based bioinformatics tools, investigators may choose comparative genomics to evaluate sequence differences relevant to fibrosis. Strain-specific polymorphisms giving rise to QTLs in mice may be revealed on the nucleotide level by direct sequence comparison of high- and low-responder strain genomes. The genomic sequence of the C57BL/6 strain is publicly available through NCBI, Ensembl, and the UCSC. Celera (http://www.celera.com/) provides commercial and academic access by subscription to sequence data for strains 129/SvJ, DBA/2J, and A/J ***(18)***. Where available, genomic sequences corresponding to the QTL can be uploaded into the program Diffseq, which is a part of the EMBOSS (http://www.hgmp.mrc.ac.uk/Software/EMBOSS/) suite of programs. Diffseq will quickly locate even single nucleotide differences across multiple sequences with lengths of several megabases, and will run locally on a standard PC. If genomic sequence data for strains of interest are not available, individual candidate genes within the QTL may be resequenced in those strains. DNA regions can also be compared across species to highlight regions of conservation. Traditionally, sensitive local alignments and global alignments of large regions were performed by separate algorithms. LAGAN *(19)* (http://lagan.stanford.edu/), and AVID **(20)** (http://baboon.math.berkeley.edu/mavid/) alignment tools are Web-available software tools that combine the speed and sensitivity of local alignment programs with the capability of aligning several megabases of sequence at a time. The LAGAN programs include a pairwise alignment tool (LAGAN) and a multiple aligner (M-LAGAN). LAGAN multiple sequence alignments can be visualized with the Phylo-Vista tool *(21)*. VISTA *(21,22)* provides a graphical display of the degree of conservation across species. Some genes are not predicted by gene-finding algorithms and have not been identified by traditional methods. By highlighting the coding regions conserved across multiple species, the mVISTA, or "main VISTA" tools can find such genes missed in the annotation process! Sequencing of transcripts will not identify mutations in noncoding regulatory regions that may have profound effects on levels of gene transcription. The VISTA programs can also be useful in detecting which noncoding regions are conserved and therefore likely to be functionally important. rVISTA, or "regulatory" VISTA *(23)* was designed for this purpose. Regulatory regions identified by rVISTA can then be prioritized for direct sequence comparison or resequencing. The VISTA bioinformatics tools for comparative sequence analysis were developed by the Berkeley Program fro Genomic Applications (PGA) and are available online at http://www-gsd.lbl.gov/VISTA/index.html.

1.15. Evaluate Candidate Genes

Genotyping of SNPs for candidate gene association studies can be performed by TaqMan allelic discrimination assay on an ABI 7000, 7700, or 7900 Sequence Detection System (Applied Biosystems, Foster City CA). The TaqMan SNP assay is PCR-based, and utilizes the native 5' nuclease activity of Taq polymerase, which clears the way in front of the growing DNA strand, coupled with fluorescence resonance energy transfer (FRET) technology to detect allele-specific PCR amplification. A total of four oligonucleotides are designed for each assay, including unmodified forward and reverse PCR primers and a 5' labeled fluorescent probe specific for each allele. The 3' end of each probe is modified with a quencher. When the reporter and quencher are in close proximity, as they are in the intact probe, the fluorescent reporter dye is quenched by FRET. Probes with no SNP mismatch are not displaced during the amplification cycle and are degraded by the 5' nuclease activity of Taq polymerase, releasing their fluorescent reporter label. Probes with a mismatch will be displaced intact during extension and the fluorescent label will remain quenched. A different fluorescence label is attached to each allele, and the fluorescence signal of each dye is measured at the end of 40 cycles of amplification. Primer Express software (Applied Biosystems) is used to design TaqMan assays. Primer Express software has automatic assay design and batch assay design features, which save time and are easy to use. Sequences surrounding each SNP are copied and pasted into a non-rich-text format then imported into Primer Express. Sequences that fail automatic and batch design can still be used following guidelines for manual assay design, typically with a time commitment of less than 30 min per design. Assay optimization and validation must be performed on each new TaqMan primer/probe set. Optimal primer concentrations are determined first, followed by optimization of probe concentration. Data are visualized by scatter plot, and can be exported in Excel format for subsequent association testing. An association between a polymorphism and fibrosis phenotype is strong evidence for the involvement of a locus with disease. However, an associated marker may simply be "allelic" with a causative lesion in a nearby gene. The tracking of a particular polymorphism with disease in affected families (or susceptible strains of mice), and the nature of the sequence alteration with attention toward the predicted impact on protein function, will be important considerations in making a case for the involvement of a particular gene. In order to prove that a particular allele is pathogenic, functional testing must be performed.

1.16. Functional Testing of Candidate Genes

Formal proof of gene discovery requires demonstration that replacement with a gene variant produces the phenotypic variant of interest. Knock-in technology ***(24)*** or gene targeting followed by transgenic complementation in mice are two in vivo approaches that are appropriate for functional validation. The effect of some genetic variants may be species-specific, and for these variants, in vitro functional assays may be more suitable. Short interfering RNA (siRNA) technology for posttranscriptional gene silencing is an emerging technology for in vitro functional testing that may also be applied to functional validation of candidate genes ***(25,26)***.

Genetically engineered mice for your candidate gene may be available for use from several sources, which should be queried before you begin to create a mouse model *de novo*. Two databases available from Jackson Laboratories are the Transgenic/Targeted Mutation Database (TBASE) (http://tbase.jax.org/), which is a resource with emphasis placed on gene knockouts, and the Induced Mutant Resource (IMR) (www.jax.org/imr). The Bay Genomics PGA has produced a library of embryonic stem cell lines available to the scientific community for the purpose of generating knockout mice. Gene-trapping vectors carrying the β-galactosidase gene for localization expression are used in mouse embryonic stem (ES) cells to randomly inactivate genes. The list of trapped genes and endogenous expression patterns for each line are available on the Bay Genomics Web site at http://baygenomics.ucsf.edu. Thousands of genes have been trapped, many corresponding to novel genes or expressed sequence tags (ESTs). This targeted ES cell line database can be searched by accession number or on the nucleotide level by Basic Local Alignment Search Tool (BLAST) search with your sequence.

2. Materials

Minimum requirements for Web-based bioinformatics are a PC Pentium III (or better) processor and 128 Mb of random access memory (RAM) with internet access.

2.1. Genomic DNA Isolation From Human Blood

1. Purple cap blood collection tubes with ethylenediamine tetraacetic acid (EDTA), or PAXgene™ tubes (Qiagen, Valencia, CA).
2. Blood cards (Schleicher & Schuell, Keene, NH).
3. Genomic DNA isolation reagents (Gentra Systems, www.gentra.com).
4. Ultraviolet (UV) spectrophotometer.
5. 1.5-mL Polypropylene screw-cap tubes with o-rings.
6. Polypropylene tubes in 96-well format rack, with mat caps (Marsh Bio Products, Rochester NY, cat. no. T1000R).

2.2. Genomic DNA Isolation From Mouse Tail Clippings

1. Dissecting scissors and forceps.
2. DNeasy 96 Tissue Kit (Qiagen, Valencia CA; www.qiagen.com).
3. UV spectrophotometer.
4. 1.5-mL Polypropylene screw-cap tubes with o-rings.
5. Polypropylene tubes in 96-well format rack, with mat caps (Marsh Bio Products, Rochester NY, cat. no. T1000R).

2.3. Whole Genome SNP Scan

1. Unmodified oligo sets (Integrated DNA Technologies, www.idtdna.com).
2. ABI 7000 or 7900 Sequence Detection System (Applied Biosystems).
3. SYBR Green PCR Master Mix (Applied Biosystems).
4. 96- or 384-well Reaction plates.

2.4. Resequencing of Candidate Genes

1. Unmodified oligos.
2. Thermal cycler.
3. Access to an ABI 3100 or ABI3730 capillary sequencer and dye terminator reagents.
4. "Hot Start" Taq Polymerase and PCR buffer and reagents.
5. 96-Well PCR plates.

6. Agarose gel equipment.
7. PCR purification kit (QIAquick 96 PCR Purification Kit).
8. UV spectrophotometer.
9. Sequence Viewer software (Chromas).
10. Sequence Analysis software (Polyphred).

2.5. Allelic Discrimination by the TaqMan Method (Applied Biosystems)

1. Primer Express software (Applied Biosystems).
2. Unmodified PCR primers.
3. Dual-labeled fluorogenic probes.
4. ABI 7700, 7900, or 7000 Sequence Detection System.
5. Amplification plates and optical adhesive covers (Applied Biosystems).

3. Methods

Methods are provided below for genomic DNA isolation from human blood (**Subheading 3.1.**) and also genomic DNA isolation from mouse tail sections (**Subheading 3.2.**), whole genome SNP scan (by real-time PCR using SYBR® green dye) (**Subheading 3.3.**), resequencing of candidate genes (**Subheading 3.4.**), and allelic discrimination by the TaqMan method (**Subheading 3.5.**).

3.1. Genomic DNA Isolation From Human Blood

1. Collect two 8-mL blood samples per human subject. Collection of a second, independent sample provides greater overall yield and serves as a backup for the DNA isolation protocol.
2. Spot blood cards from each sample, prelabeled with sample ID, study name, and date. Genomic DNA can be isolated from blood cards should the wet samples become depleted or destroyed, and can serve as a reference standard if sample mix-ups occur.
3. Allow blood cards to air dry completely, then store in a notebook in a cool dry place.
4. Genomic DNA from blood samples collected in purple cap tubes can be isolated by the Gentra PUREGENE™ method (Gentra Systems, Minneapolis MN) according to the manufacturer's protocol. Samples collected in purple top tubes should be stored at 4°C and processed within 48 hours of collection. Samples collected in PAXgene tubes can remain at room temperature, and should be isolated using PAXgene reagents as per protocol.
5. Quantify genomic DNA samples by UV spectrophotometry. Typical yield is 18 to 25 μg per mL of whole blood.
6. Prepare working dilutions of DNA samples in water at a concentration of 10 ng/μL.
7. To permit high-throughput genotyping, store the working dilutions in sample tube racks that are compatible with a 96-well format automatic liquid handling robot. Racks are resealed with reusable mat caps.
8. Store concentrated DNA stocks in 1.5-mL screw-cap tubes with o-rings at –20°C. Working dilutions can be stored at 4°C and dispensed into assay plates as needed.

3.2. Genomic DNA Isolation From Mouse Tail Sections

1. Cut a 3 to 6 mm long piece of tissue from the end of the tail of each mouse using sharp dissecting scissors. For more efficient digestion, it is best to cut this piece in half.
2. With tweezers, place tail sections in a labeled 1.5-mL microcentrifuge tube. Sections can be stored at 4°C if genomic DNA will be isolated within 2 wk. For longer storage, freeze the tissue at –20°C.
3. Isolate genomic DNA from the tail sections as per kit instructions.
4. Quantify genomic DNA samples by UV spectrophotometry.
5. Store concentrated DNA stocks in polypropylne 1.5-mL screw-cap tubes with o-rings at –20°C.
6. Prepare working dilutions of DNA samples in water at a concentration of 10 ng/µL.
7. To permit high-throughput genotyping, store the working dilutions in sample tube racks compatible with a 96-well format automatic liquid handling robot. Racks are sealed with reusable mat caps.
8. Store concentrated DNA stocks in 1.5-mL screw-cap tubes with o-rings at -20°C. Working dilutions can be stored at 4°C.

3.3. Whole Genome SNP Scan

This protocol can be used on all or part of the mouse genome to detect QTL in animals resulting from an F2 cross. It is much faster and far less labor-intensive than microsatellite marker screening.

1. Determine a quantitative fibrosis phenotype for individual F2 mice resulting from a cross between differentially susceptible strains.
2. Obtain a tail clipping from each animal, and isolate genomic DNA by the DNeasy method, according to the manufacturer's specifications.
3. Measure DNA concentration by UV spectrophotometry, and store samples in X1 Tris-HCl/EDTA (TE) buffer at –70°C.
4. Prepare separate pools of genomic DNA from F2 mice at the highest 10% and lowest 10% of the quantitative phenotype. Combine equal quantities of DNA from each mouse to create pools.
5. Order approx 300 strain-specific SNP allele assay primer sets for genome-wide analysis. Sequences corresponding to parental strain allele-specific primers are available on the Roche Mouse SNP Database at http://mousesnp.roche.com/cgi-bin/msnp.pl.
6. Perform real-time PCR by the SYBR green method using an ABI model 7000, 7700, or 7900 Sequence Detection System, using standard conditions recommended by the manufacturer. Use 50 ng of genomic DNA per well, and include control samples of DNA derived from each parental strain, as well as a 1:1 mix of both parental strain DNAs.
7. Percentages of parental strain DNAs are calculated using the formula $\% = 100 \times 1/(1 + 2^{\Delta CT})$, where C_T is the PCR cycle number (C) at which the intensity of fluorescence crosses a set threshold ($_T$).

3.4. Resequencing of Candidate Genes

1. Obtain sequences for each exon of your candidate gene with flanking genomic sequence via genome browser. 500 nt of flanking genomic sequence is sufficient. Use repeat masker software to mask repetitive sequence elements in the region.
2. Use primer design software to design a 500nt amplicon surrounding each exon. For large exons, design overlapping fragments. Primers with 40 to 60% GC content, Tm of 60 to 62°C, and length of 20 nt or more are optimal.
3. Order primers.
4. Reconstitute dried primers with X1 TE to a stock concentration 1 mg/mL.
5. Prepare primer dilutions in water at 200 ng/μL, then mix the forward and reverse primers for each amplicon for a final concentration of 100 ng/μL (each primer).
6. Set up PCR reactions with 40 ng of template DNA using any brand of "hot start" Taq polymerase. Use of a hot start enzyme will greatly increase the specificity of your PCR reaction. Follow the enzyme manufacturer's instructions for preparation of the PCR cocktail (we use a dNTP of 0.2 m*M*, [Mg^{2+}] of 1.5 m*M* and 4 ng of each primer), and for the initial thermal cycling steps, which activate enzyme activity.
7. Perform the following steps after the activation steps:
   35 cycles of:
   95° 30 s
   Tm-2° 30 s
   72° 45 s
   Followed by:
   72° 10 min
   4° hold indefinitely
8. Run a check gel (1% agarose).
9. Purify PCR products with the QIAquick 96 PCR Purification Kit according to the manufacturer's instructions.
10. Follow the recommendation of your local sequencing facility for optimal primer and template concentrations for automatic sequencing.
11. View sequence chromatograms to assess sequence quality and read length (Chromas).
12. Upload sequence data in batches by exon into sequence analysis software to detect polymorphic loci (Polyphred).

3.5. Allelic Discrimination by the TaqMan Method

1. Paste sequence containing your polymorphism (including approx 100 nt of flanking sequence) into a non-rich-text format such as Notepad.
2. Design Assay using Primer Express software, following the guidelines in the User Manual.
3. Order primers and dual-labeled fluorescent probes (Applied Biosystems).
4. Set up PCR cocktail according to the instructions outlined in your sequence Detection System owner's manual.
5. Dispense DNA and PCR cocktail to plates, and cover plates with optical adhesive covers (Applied Biosystems).

6. Perform the thermal cycling step. Thermal cycling conditions for the MJ Tetrad thermal cycler (MJ Research, Waltham, MA) are as follows: initial cycles of 50°C for 2 min and 95°C for 10 min followed by 40 cycles of 95°C for 15 s and 60°C for 1 min, with a final holding cycle of 4°C (*see* **Note 7**).
7. Perform the allelic discrimination "plate read" step on an ABI Sequence Detection System (*see* **Note 8**).
8. Visualize the data as a scatter plot using SDS software (Applied Biosystems), and adjust allele calls manually as needed.
9. Export genotypes in Excel format for statistical analysis.

4. Notes

1. Depending on your study protocol, you may choose to collect blood in standard purple top tubes containing EDTA to prevent clotting, or you may find it more convenient to use Qiagen's PAXgene blood DNA isolation system, because their proprietary tubes maintain sample stability at room temperature for 14 d and even longer at 4°C. This allows for samples to be shipped without ice, which reduces shipping cost and makes collection, shipping, and processing less hectic. PAXgene collection tubes must be on hand at the collection site because blood samples are drawn directly into these tubes.
2. Traditionally, microsatellite marker screening was performed on standard denaturing acrylamide gels. Even with the inclusion of regularly spaced size standards, some miscalling of allele size is inevitable by this method as a result of irregularities in migration across the gel or "smiling" and human error. Microsatellite marker screening on a microcapillary platform is not only much less labor-intensive, it also produces more reliable allele calls by eliminating the possibility of smiling and by the inclusion of an internal electrophoresis size standard that is mixed with each sample prior to loading, permitting automated allele calling.
3. With traditional backcross methods it may take years to produce a congenic strain with more than 99% of the recipient (background) genotype. However, the selective breeding of individual animals with the greatest representation of background genome in each generation can accelerate the production of a congenic strain. This strategy is known as marker-assisted backcross, or accelerated backcross. The MAX-BAX program (Charles River Laboratories), at http://www.criver.com/ offers a range of products and services to assist the investigator with accelerated backcross projects.
4. The use of repeat masking software is essential in selecting good primers for genomic amplification. At the UCSC Web site, simply check the "repeat masker" box and indicate that you prefer that repeats are masked to "N." Primer prediction software will avoid regions containing Ns and resulting primer designs will be more specific.
5. Avoid runs of any nucleotide, particularly runs of four G's are to be avoided. Primers should also be screened to rule out secondary structure formation, and 3' end complementarity that could yield excessive formation of primer-dimer.

6. TaqMan assay optimization is simplified by the use of control sequences for each allele. Allele-specific long oligo control sequences corresponding to the entire assay amplicon can be ordered from Integrated DNA Technologies (www.idtdna.com), and diluted to a concentration of 200 fg/μL for use (in place of genomic DNA at 10 ng/μL) as control template. The PCR fragment that is amplified from human subjects in each assay can also be gel purified and either diluted to 200 fg/μL or ligated into the pCRII cloning vector (Invitrogen) to serve as control DNA for subsequent assays. Individual plasmid clones are sequenced to confirm that both the Allele 1 and Allele 2 constructs are obtained. Plasmids diluted to a concentration of 20 fg/μL substitute well for genomic DNA at 10 ng/μL in most PCR-based assays. These plasmids are a renewable and consistent assay standard. The PCR amplicon from individuals with a known genotype can also be used as control template without subcloning. Simply gel purify the fragment and dilute the DNA to 200 fg/μL for use in place of genomic DNA in TaqMan assays. This is particularly useful when you plan to genotype a fairly rare SNP as it is difficult to optimize the assay unless all three genotype clusters are well represented.
7. Although Applied Biosystems Sequence Detection Systems are thermal cyclers, use of this instrument for thermal cycling that does not require fluorescent detection is inefficient. To increase throughput of SNP genotyping, run the thermal cycling protocol of the TaqMan assay on other thermal cyclers, and perform only the plate read (allelic discrimination) step on the Sequence Detection System.
8. BioRad's iCycler is another platform for fluorescent sequence detection, and is offered in a price range that is affordable to an individual investigator.

References

1. Dahlquist K. D., Salomonis N., Vranizan K., Lawlor S. C., and Conklin B. R. (2002) GenMAPP, a new tool for viewing and analyzing microarray data on biological pathways. *Nat. Genet.* **31(1),** 19–20.
2. Doniger S. W., Salomonis N., Dahlquist K. D., Vranizan K., Lawlor S. C., and Conklin B. R. (2003) MAPPFinder: using Gene Ontology and GenMAPP to create a global gene-expression profile from microarray data. *Genome Biol.* **4(1),** R7.
3. Hosack D. A., Dennis G. Jr., Sherman B. T., Lane H. C., and Lempicki R. A. (2003) Identifying biological themes within lists of genes with EASE. *Genome Biol.* **4(10),** R70.
4. Grupe, A., Germer, S., Usuka, J., et al. (2001) In silico mapping of complex disease-related traits in mice. *Science* **292(5523),** 1915–1918.
5. Wiltshire, T., Pletcher, M. T., Batalov, S., et al. (2003) Genome-wide single-nucleotide polymorphism analysis defines haplotype patterns in mouse. *Proc Natl Acad Sci USA* **100(6),** 3380–3385.
6. Williams, R. W., Gu, J., Qi, S., and Lu, L. (2001) The genetic structure of recombinant inbred mice: High-resolution consensus maps for complex trait analysis. *Genome Biol.* **2(11),** RESEARCH0046.
7. Lynch, M. and Walsh, B. (1998) *Genetics and Analysis of Quantitative Traits.* Sinauer Associates, Sunderland, MA.

8. Zeng Z. B., Kao C. H., and Basten C. J. (1999) Estimating the genetic architecture of quantitative traits. *Genet. Res.* **74(3),** 279–289.
9. Manly, K. F., Cudmore, R. H., Jr., and Meer, J. M. (2001) Map Manager QTX, cross-platform software for genetic mapping. *Mammalian Genome* **12,** 930–932.
10. Germer, S., Holland, M. J., and Higuchi, R. (2000) High-throughput SNP allele-frequency determination in pooled DNA samples by kinetic PCR. *Genome Res.* **10,** 258–266.
11. Supplement to *Nature Genetics.* (2002) User's guide to the human genome. *Nature Genetics* **32,** 1–79.
12. Silver, L. M. (1995) *Mouse Genetics.* Oxford University Press, NY.
13. Rozen, S. and Skaletsky, H. J. (2000) Primer3 on the WWW for general users and for biologist programmers, in: *Bioinformatics Methods and Protocols: Methods in Molecular Biology.* (Krawetz, S. and Misener, S., eds.), Humana, Totowa, NJ, pp. 365–386.
14. Ewing, B., Hillier, L., Wendl, M. C., and Green, P. (1998) Base-calling of automated sequencer traces using phred. I. Accuracy assessment. *Genome Res.* **8(3),**175–185.
15. Ewing B. and Green P. (1998) Base-calling of automated sequencer traces using phred. II. Error probabilities. *Genome Res.* **8(3),** 186–194.
16. Gordon D., Abajian C., and Green P. (1998) Consed: a graphical tool for sequence finishing. *Genome Res.* **8(3),** 195–202.
17. Nickerson D. A., Tobe V. O., and Taylor S. L. (1997) PolyPhred: automating the detection and genotyping of single nucleotide substitutions using fluorescence-based resequencing. *Nucleic Acids Res.* **25(14),** 2745–2751.
18. Mural, R. J., Adams, M. D., Myers, E. W., et. al. (2002) A comparison of whole-genome shotgun-derived mouse chromosome 16 and the human genome. *Science* **296**, 1661–1671.
19. Brudno, M., Do, C.,Cooper,G., et al. (2003) LAGAN and Multi-LAGAN: efficient tools for large-scale multiple alignment of genomic DNA, *Genome Res.* **13(4),** 721–731.
20. Bray, N., Dubchak, I., and Pachter, L. (2003) AVID: a global alignment program. *Genome Res.* **13(1),** 97–102.
21. Dubchak I., Brudno M., Loots G. G., Mayor C., Pachter L., Rubin E. M., and Frazer, K. A. (2000) Active conservation of noncoding sequences revealed by 3-way species comparisons. *Genome Res.* **10,** 1304–1306.
22. Mayor C., Brudno M., Schwartz J. R., et al. (2000) VISTA: visualizing global DNA sequence alignments of arbitrary length. *Bioinformatics* **16,** 1046–1047.
23. Loots, G. G., Ovcharenko, I., Pachter,L., Rubin, E., and Dubchak, I., (2002) rVISTA: a high throughput comparative approach to identifying eukaryotic transcriptional regulatory elements in noncoding genomic sequences. *Genome Res.* **12**, 832–839.
24. Nebert, D. W., Dalton, T. P., Stuart, G. W., and Carvan, M. J., 3rd (2000) Gene-swap "knock-in cassette in mice to study allelic differences in human genes. *Ann. NY Acad. Sci.* **919,** 148–170.

25. McManus M. T. and Sharp P. A. (2002) Gene silencing in mammals by small interfering RNAs. *Nat Rev Genet.* **3(10),** 737–747.
26. Shi Y. (2003) Mammalian RNAi for the masses. *Trends Genet.* **19(1),** 9–12.

19

Genetic Studies to Identify Hepatic Fibrosis Genes and SNPs in Human Populations

Christopher Paul Day

Summary

Increasing evidence suggests that non-sex-linked genetic factors play a role in determining both susceptibility to, and progression of, liver fibrosis. The elucidation of these factors will have many potential benefits in the management of patients with chronic liver disease. A variety of approaches can be used to look for genetic factors playing a role in liver fibrosis. In the future, genome-wide single nucleotide polymorphism (SNP) scanning of cases and controls may become feasible; however, to date, studies have relied on candidate-gene, case–control, allele-association methodology. This section will focus on the design and interpretation of case–control association studies in liver disease using non-alcoholic fatty liver disease (NAFLD) to illustrate the key issues and potential pitfalls of this approach.

Key Words: Association studies; haplotypes; linkage disequilibrium; polymorphism; fibrosis.

1. Introduction

Increasing evidence suggests that, in addition to the undoubted influence of gender *(1)*, non-sex-linked genetic factors play a role in determining both susceptibility to, and progression of, liver fibrosis attributable to toxic, viral, and immune etiologies *(2)*. The elucidation of these factors will have many potential benefits in the management of patients with chronic liver disease. First, it may lead to an improved understanding of disease pathogenesis and, accordingly, the identification of new therapeutic targets. Second, it may enable patients with apparently the same disease phenotype to be categorized according to specific disease mechanisms amenable to specific treatment strategies. Third, identifying genetic factors that increase the risk of progressive fibrosis may allow better determination of prognosis, which may affect patient management, for example in the timing of liver transplantation or entry into therapeutic trials. Finally, in diseases where the environmental or

From: *Methods in Molecular Medicine, Vol. 117: Fibrosis Research: Methods and Protocols*
Edited by: J. Varga, D. A. Brenner, and S. H. Phan © Humana Press Inc., Totowa, NJ

exogenous factor is known, such as alcohol- or drug-induced liver disease, the identification of genetic factors determining fibrosis risk offers opportunities for prevention.

In light of these potential benefits, it is perhaps not surprising that journals are increasingly bombarded with studies purporting to show evidence for genetic factors involved in the development and progression of various liver diseases *(3)*. Unfortunately, the majority of common liver diseases are examples of so-called "complex traits" that do not exhibit classical Mendelian recessive or dominant inheritance attributable to a singe gene locus *(4)*. In complex traits, disease risk is determined by the interaction of several different gene loci with environmental factors that are often unknown. Identifying genetic factors with small effects on risk in complex traits is considerably more difficult than identifying genes responsible for rare single-gene disorders such as Wilson's disease. Studies are subject to a variety of potential pitfalls that often limit the significance of reported data. As a result, and as is the situation with many other diseases, the number of genetic reports in the hepatological literature that stand up to close scrutiny, and are therefore likely to influence clinical practice, are limited.

It is therefore clear in this "post-genome" era that both clinical and "basic" hepatologists either designing genetic studies or reading/reviewing papers require some knowledge of the methods available with which to study genetic factors in liver disease and an understanding of the pitfalls of study design. Without changes in current practice aided by collaboration between hepatologists and genetic epidemiologists, there is a real danger that much scientific effort will continue to be wasted, that our journals will be full of meaningless genetic data, and that our ability to exploit the benefits offered by the sequencing of the human genome will remain limited *(5)*. This chapter is focused on the methods available for studying genes involved in chronic liver diseases, with particular emphasis on the design of candidate-gene, case–control association studies using non-alcoholic fatty liver disease (NAFLD) to illustrate the key issues. The important pitfalls of this methodology will be illustrated with good and bad examples from the hepatological literature. Finally, recommendations for the design of future association studies in liver disease will be given.

2. Methodology for Studying Genes Involved in Liver Disease

Available methods for detecting genes contributing to complex traits, including most of the common liver diseases, fall into three broad and overlapping categories: family-based allele-sharing methods (linkage analysis), candidate-gene studies, and genome-wide, single nucleotide polymorphism (SNP) scanning.

2.1. Family-Based Linkage Studies

Allele-sharing methods involve studying affected relatives in a pedigree to determine how often a particular copy of a chromosomal region is shared identical-by-descent (IBD). The frequency of IBD sharing at a particular locus can then be compared with random expectation (reviewed in **ref. *4***). Typically, this has involved linkage analysis in large cohorts of affected sibling pairs, using widely spaced multiallelic markers such as microsatellites to identify chromosomal regions. Unfortunately, linkage analysis, which has been so successful in identifying genes responsible for single-gene disorders, has (with few notable exceptions; *see* **ref. *6***) been generally disappointing when applied to polygenic diseases, probably because of its limited power to detect genes of moderate effect ***(7)***.

2.2. Candidate-Gene Studies

An alternative methodological approach involves the study of candidate genes. In this method, a polymorphism (or polymorphisms) is identified by various means in a candidate gene—a gene whose product is considered to play a role in disease pathogenesis. The polymorphism is then examined for association with disease using one of two approaches, intra-familial allelic association studies and case–control association studies. The most commonly used test for familial association is the transmission disequlibrium test (TDT) which compares the frequency with which the allele under study is transmitted to affected offspring by each parent with the frequency expected by random transmission ***(8)***. The major limitation of TDT testing is that the index case must have at least one surviving parent (and preferably two) from whom to collect DNA. This clearly poses particular problems for studies looking for genes determining susceptibility to advanced liver disease. Variations on the TDT using siblings of affected individuals (discordant sibship) have recently been proposed ***(9)***; however, as with the TDT, when the allele frequency is low, achieving statistical significance requires a very large number of families. In view of these difficulties, it is perhaps not surprising that studies using the candidate-gene approach to look for genetic factors influencing the progression of liver diseases have thus far relied almost entirely on case–control methodology ***(10)***. In this method, the frequency of the polymorphism(s) under study is compared in cases and controls to see whether it is associated with disease. The details of this methodology along with its pitfalls will be discussed in the next section.

2.3. Whole-Genome Scanning

An alternative to this "hypothesis-driven" methodology based on the selection of potential candidate genes is the possibility of looking for disease associations in polygenic diseases by performing a genome-wide survey utilizing the recently available human SNP map *(11,12)*. At present, genome-wide scanning is extremely expensive, but costs may fall in the future as more efficient genotyping technologies are developed and the number of SNPs requiring genotyping falls as a result of the availability of haplotype maps *(13,14)*. Haplotypes are defined by multiple SNPs that co-segregate (are inherited together more often than expected by chance) and are in so-called linkage disequlibrium (LD). Recent studies of haplotype structure in the human genome have shown that the genome consists of discrete "haplotype blocks" separated by recombination hotspots *(13,14)*. There appears to be a limited number of haplotypes within each block; therefore, they can be defined by the analysis of relatively small numbers of diagnostic SNPs known as haplotype-tagging (ht) SNPs *(15)*.

3. Design of Case–Control Association Studies in Liver Fibrosis

Because candidate-gene case–control studies have been, and seem likely to continue to be, the principal methodology used in studies aimed at elucidating genetic factors involved in the development and progression of liver fibrosis, this section will focus on the design and interpretation of case–control association studies, using NAFLD to illustrate the key issues and illustrating the potential pitfalls with examples from the hepatological literature.

3.1. Choice of Candidate Gene

A candidate gene being chosen for a case–control association study for a variety of reasons (**Table 1**):

1. *The gene product is considered to play an important role in disease pathogenesis.* The product may be important in determining susceptibility to the etiological factor, to the development of early or advanced liver injury, or to progression to cirrhosis. As an illustration, in NAFLD this could include genes encoding products involved in: (a) the development of obesity and insulin resistance; (b) the accumulation of fat within the liver; (c) progression to steatohepatitis (cytokines and oxidative stress); and (d) fibrogenesis (**Table 2**).
2. *The gene is known to be altered in a familial form of the disease.* In NAFLD, this would include the microsomal triglyceride transfer protein (MTP) gene which is known to be mutated in congenital abetalipoproteinemia, which is associated with hepatic steatosis and cirrhosis *(16)*.
3. *Under ("knockout")- or over ("transgenic")-expression of the gene in animal models influences disease development* **(2)**. For example, in NAFLD, a role for the leptin gene in disease susceptibility is suggested by studies in the leptin knockout (Ob/Ob) mouse, which develops spontaneous fatty liver and steatohepatitis *(17)*.
4. *The gene lies within a chromosomal region associated with disease in a genome-wide linkage study.* A recent genome-wide analysis of liver fibrosis in inbred

Table 1
Reasons for Selecting a Gene As a Candidate in an Association Study

Gene product considered to play a role in disease pathogenesis
Gene is known to be mutated in a familial form of the disease
Gene knockout/overexpression in animal models influences disease development
Gene lies in a chromosomal region associated with disease in a linkage study
Gene expression is altered in microarray studies of tissue from patients with disease
Gene is identified in a phenotype-driven mouse mutagenesis study

Table 2
Potential Candidate Genes in Nonalcoholic Fatty Liver Disease

Category of genes	Example(s)
Genes determining the magnitude and pattern of fat deposition	11β-HSD-1, lipodystrophic genes
Genes determining insulin sensitivity	Adiponectin, HFE, insulin receptor genes, PPARγ, Resistin
Genes involved in hepatic lipid storage and export	Apolipoprotein E, MTP, Leptin, SCD-1
Genes involved in hepatic fatty acid oxidation	PPARα, Acyl-CoA oxidase, CYP2E1, CYP4A family members
Genes influencing the generation of oxidant species	HFE, TNF-α
Genes encoding proteins involved in the response to oxidant stress	SOD2, UCP2
Cytokine genes	IL-10, TNF-α
Genes encoding endotoxin receptors	CD14, NOD2, TLR4
NAFLD-related fibrosis genes	CTGF, Leptin

11β-HSD-1, 11β hydroxysteroid dehydrogenase type 1; CTGF, connective tissue growth factor; CTLA-4, cytotoxic T-lymphocyte antigen-4; SOD2, superoxide dismutase-2; MTP, microsomal triglyceride transfer protein; PPAR, peroxisomal proliferator receptor; SCD-1, stearoyl CoA desaturase-1; TLR4, toll-like receptor-4; UCP2, uncoupling protein-2; TNF-α, tumor necrosis factor α; IL-10, interleukin 10; NOD2, nucleotide oligomerization domain 2.

mice has identified two susceptibility loci that suggest a number of novel fibrosis genes worthy of study in humans, including complement factor 5 ***(18)***.

5. *The gene is up- or downregulated in oligonucleotide microarray ("chip") studies of liver tissue from patients with disease* ***(19)***. Whether changes in gene expression are a primary phenomenon (therefore contributing to disease susceptibility) or secondary to disease onset (contributing to disease phenotype) may be difficult to determine, however, this methodology has the potential to identify novel candidate genes worthy of subjection to proximal promoter SNP screening strategies.

6. *The gene is identified in a phenotype-driven mouse mutagenesis study **(20)***. In this technique, male mice are treated with the mutagen ethyl nitrosourea, and their progeny are screened for dominant mutations giving rise to the phenotypic change of interest. The mutation is then mapped to a specific gene, and finally the human homolog is screened for SNPs which are subsequently tested for disease association using standard case–control methodology.

3.2. Choice of Polymorphism

Once a candidate gene has been selected, the particular polymorphism or combination of polymorphisms to be studied must be determined. This is particularly important given the increasing number of SNPs being reported ***(11)***. In the past, many of the polymorphisms studied were those that gave rise to restriction fragment length polymorphisms (RFLPs) that were discovered by hybridization rather than by sequencing or mutation-scanning studies. This almost certainly led to functionally significant polymorphisms in candidate genes being ignored, and to the publication of many negative studies looking for associations between liver diseases and polymorphisms that were neither functional nor linked with a functionally significant polymorphism ***(21)***. Ideally, the functional significance of a polymorphism or linked set of polymorphisms (haplotype) should be established both in vitro and in vivo prior to performing association studies. However, because the acquisition of this data can often be difficult, costly, and time-consuming, on a practical basis these studies are often performed after an allele–disease association has been observed, both to provide supportive evidence that the association is valid and to gain further insight into disease pathogenesis. In the absence of strong *a priori* evidence that a particular SNP has a significant functional effect, it is important that all of the common (occurring in at least 1 in 20 of the normal population) haplotype-defining SNPs within a candidate gene are examined together for disease association, because studies limited to only a few SNPs could miss a real association if the particular SNPs studied are either unlinked or only weakly linked to the true disease-causing polymorphism. Unfortunately, at present, with the exception of studies on major histocompatibility complex (MHC) genes in autoimmune liver disease and interleukin (IL)-10 polymorphisms in chronic hepatitis C virus (HCV) infection ***(22)***, virtually no studies on the genetics of liver disease have focused on common haplotypes of candidate genes.

3.3. Selection of Cases and Controls

The selection of cases and controls is crucial to study design in terms of: (a) minimizing the chance that any difference in allele frequency observed between cases and controls is spurious; (b) maximizing the chances of detecting a real association; and (c) the specific hypothesis to be tested. For example, in NAFLD, case and control selection in a study aimed at identifying genes involved in the development of steatosis will differ completely from that in a study aimed at identifying genes involved in the progression from steatohepatitis to fibrosis.

3.3.1. Population Stratification

When the population under study consists of a mixture of two or more subpopulations that have different allele frequencies and disease risk (for environmental or genetic reasons unrelated to the allele under study) associations between genotype and outcome can be confounded by population stratification. This confounding could give rise to spurious "false-positive" associations of disease with genotype at loci that are unlinked to any locus that affects disease susceptibility. Even if no difference in disease frequency between subpopulations are present, spurious associations can arise if the chance of a case or control being selected into the study is not independent of the subpopulation of origin ***(5)***. It is therefore important to ensure that cases and controls are derived from the same demographic background. Although this may appear obvious, there are numerous examples in the liver literature of genetic studies in which allele frequencies in cases from the author's unit have been compared with "control" allele frequencies from another geographically remote and ethnically different population ***(23)***. However, in the absence of such obvious errors in study design, it has recently been calculated that when reasonable attempts are made at demographic matching, population stratification is unlikely to be a significant problem ***(24)***. When population stratification cannot be controlled for by demographic matching, techniques are now available to assess the degree of stratification using a panel of unlinked ("anonymous") genetic markers with adjustments made for any association observed between the disease and the candidate gene under study ***(25,26)***. The TDT and related tests of interfamilial association previously referred to were designed principally to overcome population stratification; however, for reasons already discussed, these tests are often not possible in patients with late-onset liver disease.

3.3.2. Controlling for Confounding Factors

When the exogenous etiological factor for a liver disease is known—for example, excessive alcohol intake in alcoholic liver disease (ALD), HCV infection for chronic HCV disease, or a particular medication in drug-induced liver disease—it is clearly desirable that the controls are individuals that have been exposed to this factor. Without this proviso, potential "cases" may be misclassified as "controls," thereby weakening the power of the study to detect a real effect. In addition to the primary etiological factor, there may be several other confounding factors that influence the development and severity of liver disease and which, if not accounted for, may significantly reduce the chances of detecting a real association. Gender and alcohol intake in chronic HCV disease are an obvious example of "confounding" factors. In practice, it is often impractical to match cases and controls for all possible confounding factors. However, information on these factors should be collected and accounted for; this is most commonly done with a logistic regression model in which the number of copies of a particular allele (0, 1, 2) in an individual's genotype is entered as a covariate along with the potential confounding factors, which can be both quantitative and qualitative traits ***(27)***. This approach has recently been successfully applied in two studies examining the influence of HFE genotype on the severity of fibrosis in patients with chronic HCV ***(28,29)***. After duration of infection, age, gender, HCV genotype, and histological inflammation score were controlled for, the presence of the two common HFE mutations, C282Y and H63D, was significantly associated with advanced fibrosis in both studies, resolving 5 yr of controversy since the initial report ***(30)***. Failure to account for confounding factors may also lead to "false-positive" disease associations if the confounding factor is under genetic control. An example of this pitfall is the recently reported association between homozygosity for CCR5Δ32, a defective allele of the chemokine/human immunodeficiency virus (HIV) co-receptor CCR5, and susceptibility to HCV infection ***(31)***. In the initial study, more than 80% of the HCV infected patients were HIV-seronegative hemophiliacs; however, because the CCR5Δ32 mutation is associated with resistance to HIV infection, it is not surprising that the frequency of this allele was higher than in controls. A subsequent study in HCV-infected patients without hemophilia showed no association ***(32)***.

3.3.3. Studies Designed to Look for Genes Involved in Susceptibility to Early Disease

Although much has been made of the division between "susceptibility" and "progression" genes in liver disease ***(2)***, this distinction is rather arbitrary because genetic factors involved in any stage of disease development, from susceptibility to an etiological factor through to susceptibility to fibrosis, clearly influence the risk of disease progression. Accordingly, the identification of any of these factors is likely to improve our understanding of disease pathogenesis and potentially aid the identification of novel treatment targets and/or strategies. Until recently, studies examining genetic factors in liver disease have traditionally compared allele frequencies in patients with established liver disease with those in healthy controls. With this type of study design it is often impossible to know if any association observed is with the etiological factor(s) or with disease mechanisms *per se* ***(33,34)***, even though this is clearly important in terms of the implications of the association for pathogenesis. To overcome this problem, the selection strategy for cases and controls must be designed to address specific hypotheses appropriate to the genes being studied. Studies looking for genetic factors involved in susceptibility to etiological factors such as alcoholism and obesity are clearly out of the realms of hepatologists. However, included in this category are studies that have investigated genes involved in susceptibility to persistent HCV infection, with a consensus emerging that possession of the HLA allele DQB1*0301 is associated with self-limiting infection and is therefore a protective factor for the development of chronic HCV disease ***(35)***. To look for genes involved in susceptibility to the initial development of liver disease, allele frequencies should be compared in patients with "early" disease (e.g., steatosis in ALD and NAFLD) and controls with no liver disease exposed to the etiological factor where this is known. A particular problem with this type of study is the correct assignment of "exposed" patients to the control group without disease, because the absence of clinical signs and normal liver biochemistry is not a guarantee of normal histology in chronic HCV disease, ALD, or NAFLD ***(36)***. In practice, the "best" controls are likely to be patients with established risk factors (e.g., heavy drinkers, obese, or HCV polymerase chain reaction [PCR] positive individuals) and found to have normal or near normal histology on liver biopsy. As a minimum requirement, however, controls should be "exposed" subjects with normal liver biochemistry and a normal appearance on some type of liver imaging. This problem is less of an issue with rare liver diseases in which the etiological factor is unknown, such as the autoimmune liver diseases, because it is highly unlikely that healthy controls will either have or go on to develop these diseases.

3.3.4. Studies Designed to Look for Genes Involved in Susceptibility to Advanced Disease

The simplest way to look for genes involved in susceptibility to more advanced forms of liver disease is to compare allele frequencies in "cases" with late forms of the disease with "controls" with less severe disease, ideally matched for duration and magnitude of exposure to any known etiological factor. In these studies it is important that appropriate and uniform diagnostic criteria are used for diagnosis and histological staging of disease. For example, in NAFLD, allele frequencies could be compared in patients with steatohepatitis and fibrosis and patients with steatosis only, with potential confounding factors accounted for either by matching or by logistic regression. Similarly, in HCV disease, allele frequencies could be correlated with fibrosis severity in patients "matched" for duration of infection or the duration of infection, could be included along with other potential confounders in a logistic regression model ***(29)***. In view of the problem of ascertaining the timing of disease onset in cross-sectional studies, in the future it is likely that studies looking for liver disease progression genes will categorize patients as "rapid" or "slow" fibrosers based on serial biopsies *(37)*. Because the final pathways to hepatic inflammation and fibrosis appear to converge for most liver diseases, it seems likely that, in contrast with "early" susceptibility genes influencing susceptibility to disease-specific mechanisms of liver injury, many "late" susceptibility genes will be common to different liver diseases. This implies that when a polymorphism has been associated with advanced liver disease of one etiology, it becomes a potential candidate for association studies in other liver diseases. An exception to this may be genes influencing response to disease-specific therapy that can also be considered as susceptibility genes for disease progression. A study design considering responders and nonresponders to treatment as "cases" and "controls" can be used to test for "treatment response" genes; using this approach, two independent groups have recently reported an association between a "low expression" IL-10 haplotype and response to antiviral therapy in patients with chronic HCV infection *(22,38)*. It must be noted, however, that one of these studies included only 43 patients *(38)*.

3.4. Statistical Issues

Having selected an appropriate candidate gene/polymorphism combination and designed a suitable and robust recruitment strategy, researchers must also tackle the increasingly complex statistical issues inherent in designing and interpreting disease association studies. These issues can be considered in terms of the appropriate strategies designed to minimize the risks of a type II error (accepting the null hypothesis when it is false) and a type I error (rejecting the null hypothesis when it is true).

3.4.1. Statistical Power

The risk of a study being subject to a type II error depends on the whether or not the study is adequately powered to detect the small effects (genotype relative risk or odds ratio) expected in liver diseases which typically have only modest familial aggregation (sibling recurrence risk ratios [λs] of 10 or less *[39]*). For diseases with such a low λs, it can be predicted that only a few common polymorphisms of large effect (genotype risk ratio >2) will exist, along with many polymorphisms of smaller effect (genotype risk ratios <1.5) *(5)*. With risk ratios of this magnitude (risk ratio = 1.5), even for relatively common polymorphisms (allele frequency approx 20%), more than 400 patients and controls are required to give a study 90% power to detect a significant effect at the 5% level. Studies in which more than one outcome is studied simultaneously (e.g., fibrosis and inflammation) or where there are significant gene–environment interactions, require even larger numbers to ensure that individual subgroups retain adequate power to detect significant associations with narrow confidence intervals ***(40)***. Even these conservative estimates of the numbers required are significantly higher than almost all reported studies in the current hepatological literature, suggesting that at least some of the few reports of negative associations that make it to publication may have missed significant, albeit small, effects of the candidate genes studied.

3.4.2. Exclusion of "Chance" Findings

Because of the undoubted bias favoring the publication of positive associations, the exclusion of results seen by chance is a much more significant problem for interpreting genetic association studies in liver disease than false-negative reports ***(5)***. Chance findings arise from a combination of small sample sizes prone to random error, usually overestimating the size of any genetic effect ***(40,41)***, and multiple tests for association with both multiple alleles and subgroup analysis. Clearly, the more tests of association that are performed, the greater the likelihood of finding an association significant at the 5% level by chance alone. The most appropriate way of excluding chance as an explanation for genetic associations is a matter of considerable debate, but it is clear that some strategy is required ***(5)***. The simplest (and most commonly used) strategy is to reduce the p value at which significance is declared for multiple tests, rejecting the null hypothesis only when this is less than $0.05/n$ when n tests of association are being performed. Alternatively, using a Bayesian approach aimed at achieving a ratio of true-positive to false-positive associations of 20:1, it has recently been suggested that a p value of 5×10^{-5} should be the standard required for declaration of statistical evidence in association studies ***(5)***. These stringent criteria for studies with no pre-established hypothesis can be relaxed somewhat for studies in which there are good functional data on the polymorphism under study and a plausible *a priori* hypothesis linking this functional effect with disease pathogenesis ***(5,42)***. The liver literature contains several examples of studies that have tested multiple alleles for association with disease and declared evidence of genetic association on the basis of relatively high (>0.01) and unadjusted p values ***(43)***, and even more examples of studies with extremely small sample sizes often compounded by subgroup analysis ***(38,44,45)***. These studies, which often quote *post hoc* biological plausibility for the reported association, are highly likely to have reported chance observations.

3.4.3. Replication Studies

The sample size needed to maintain statistical power to detect a given association at these stringent p values is in the range of 5000 to 10,000 for the size of effect expected in the majority of complex diseases ***(5)***. As an alternative to

Table 3
Independently Replicated Associations of Major Histocompatibility Complex (MHC) Polymorphisms and Susceptibility to Autoimmune Liver Diseases

	MHC alleles	Odds ratios	Ref.
AICAH	DRB1*0301,	3.39	***47***
	DRB1*0401	3.35 (in DRB1*0301 negative patients)	
PSC	DRB3*0101-DRB1*0301 -DQA1*0501-DQB1*0201	2.69	***48***
	DRB1*1301-DQA1*0103-DQB1*0603	3.8	
DRB1*04-DQB1*0302		0.26 (protective)	
PBC	DRB1*0801	3.3–15.3 (Northern Europe/USA)	***49***
	DRB1*0803	2.2–12 (Japan)	

AICAH, autoimmune chronic active hepatitis; PSC, primary sclerosing cholangitis; PBC, primary biliary cirrhosis.

focusing entirely on SNPs with well-defined functional effects, investigators with access to considerably smaller DNA collections have relied on replication of associations in independent collections as supportive evidence of a true association. This approach, which has gained increasing acceptance ***(46)***, is particularly important when the initial association was observed after subgroup analysis ***(40)***. Despite the fact that liver disease is perfectly suited to replication studies, with the exception of MHC genes in autoimmune liver diseases ***(47–49)*** (**Table 3**), HCV infection ***(35)***, and, most recently, HFE mutations and progression of HCV ***(28,29)***, the literature contains almost no examples of associations that have been replicated in independent studies and only one example of a study that has attempted to replicate its initial findings in a second data set ***(45)***. This general failure to replicate positive results in subsequent studies, which has led to increasing scepticism about the value of genetic association studies ***(50)***, has been attributed largely to the failure of the initial study to exclude chance as an explanation for the apparent association ***(5)***. This problem is compounded by publication bias in which negative studies are often not submitted, let alone published, limiting the value of systematic reviews of the published literature ***(51)***. This implies that, with few notable exceptions ***(52,53)***, initial chance observations often remain unchallenged in the literature despite the probable existence of several subsequent unpublished negative studies.

Table 4
Recommendations for Design and Interpretation of Association Studies in Liver Disease

Candidate gene	Is there a sound rationale for the choice of candidate genes included in the study?
Polymorphism	Are there data on the functional significance of the polymorphism(s) studied and does this lead to a plausible *a priori* hypothesis? In the absence of functional data, have all the common haplotype-defining single nucleotide polymorphisms been studied?
Case and control selection	Does the phenotype method ensure robust classification of cases? Are cases and controls likely to come from similar genetic backgrounds and, if not, have steps been taken to adjust for population stratification? Are cases and controls matched for exposure to known etiological factors and, if so, has significant disease been excluded in the controls? Have confounding factors been accounted for in study design, either in the matching of cases and controls or included in the analysis of the gene effect? To what stage of disease is the study designed to detect susceptibility genes?
Statistical analysis	For positive studies, is the evidence strong enough to exclude chance? Is the study large enough to exclude random error? How low is the p value for the association? Can the association be explained by the functional effect of the polymorphism and is there a dose–response effect? For studies with no *a priori* hypothesis for a link between a single nucleotide polymorphism and disease or subgroup, is the p value in the order of 5×10^{-5} or at least $0.05/n$ where n = the number of associations (alleles and sub groups) tested, or is there replication of the association in an independent set of cases and controls? For negative replication studies, was the study sufficiently powered to exclude a significant effect?

4. Overview of Published and Future Association Studies in Liver Disease

Unfortunately, based on the recommendations shown in **Table 4** and highlighted in a recent review *(2)*, at present the hepatological literature contains very few examples of genetic associations that stand up to any degree of scrutiny. In particular, with the exception of MHC genes in autoimmune liver disease and HCV and HFE mutations in HCV, there are few examples of associations that have replicated in more than one well designed study. Given the size of the odds ratios observed for the MHC associations in autoimmune liver diseases, the most likely reason why reproducible results have been reported from relatively small studies is that, compared with the more common liver diseases ALD, NAFLD, and chronic HCV, these diseases are likely to have a stronger genetic component *(39)* and, accordingly, susceptibility genes with greater effects. The early adoption of the study of haplotypes in these MHC studies is a further reason why they were more likely to detect significant associations than non-MHC studies relying on SNPs, which were often in weak LD with the true disease-causing polymorphism. For the more common liver diseases, two complementary approaches can be taken. First, individual groups with well-characterized case–control DNA collections of reasonable size (500–1000 of each) can focus on liver diseases likely to have a significant genetic component such as autoimmune diseases. For more common but less "genetic" diseases, studies of this order of magnitude should focus on polymorphisms for which the functional effect is established and leads to a plausible link to disease pathogenesis or, where the functional effect is less clear, seek replication in an independent case–control set. Second and more importantly, considerable efforts should be made toward establishing multicenter/multinational DNA banks of patients with similar disease phenotypes as has been achieved for nonliver diseases *(5)*. The collection of samples from patients enrolled in large multicenter clinical trials may be one way to organize and fund these collections. This approach will allow the hepatological community to exploit the rapidly growing amount of information on variations within the human genome *(11)*, along with recent advances in high-throughput genotyping technology, by enabling the performance of adequately powered studies that minimize the risk of spurious associations. With these combined approaches, much currently wasted research effort may eventually be transformed into significant benefits for patients with liver disease both in terms of prevention and targeted therapeutic and management strategies.

References

1. Poynard, T., Mathurin, P., Lai, C.-L., et al., for the PANFIFBROSIS Group. (2003) A comparison of fibrosis progression in chronic liver diseases. *J. Hepatol.* **38,** 257–365.
2. Bataller, R., North, K. E., and Brenner, D. A. (2003) Genetic polymorphisms and the progression of liver fibrosis: a critical appraisal. *Hepatology* **37,** 493–503.

3. Montgomery, H. and Dansek, A. H. (2003) In search of genetic precision. *Lancet* **361,** 357.
4. Lander, E. S. and Schork, N. J. (1994) Genetic dissection of complex traits. *Science* **265,** 2037–2048.
5. Colhoun, H. M., McKeigue, P. M., and Davey Smith, G. (2003) Problems of reporting genetic associations with complex outcomes. *Lancet* **361,** 865–872.
6. Hugot, J.-P., Chamaillard, M., Zouali, H., et al. (2001) Association of NOD2 leucine-rich repeat variants with susceptibility to Crohn's disease. *Nature* **411,** 599–603.
7. Risch, N. and Merikangas, K. (1996) The future of genetic studies of complex human diseases. *Science* **273,** 156–157.
8. Speilman, R. S. and Ewens, W. J. (1996) The TDT and other family-based tests for linkage disequlibrium. *Am. J. Hum. Genet.* **59,** 983–989.
9. Speilman, R. S. and Ewens, W. J. (1998) A sibship test for linkage in the presence of association: the sib transmission/disequilibrium test. *Am. J. Hum. Genet.* **62,** 450–458.
10. Daly, A. K. and Day, C. P. (2001) Candidate gene case-control association studies: advantages and potential pitfalls. *Br. J. Clin. Pharmacol.* **52,** 489–499.
11. The International SNP Map Working Group. (2001) A map of human genome sequence variation containing 1.42 million single nucleotide polymorphisms. *Nature* **409,** 928–933.
12. Judson, R., Salisbury, B., Schneider, J., Windemuth, A., and Stephens, J. C. (2002) How many SNPs does a genome-wide haplotype map require? *Pharmacogenomics* **3,** 379–391.
13. Patil, N., Berno, A. J., Hinds, D. A., et al. (2001) Blocks of limited haplotype diversity revealed by high resolution scanning of human chromosome 21. *Science* **294,** 1719–1723.
14. Daly, M. J., Rioux, J. D., Schaffner, S. F., Hudson, T. J., and Lander, E. S. (2001) High resolution haplotype structure in the human genome. *Nat. Genet.* **29,** 229–232.
15. Johnson, G. C., Esposito, L., Barrat, B. J., et al. (2001) Haplotype tagging for the identification of common disease genes. *Nat. Genet.* **29,** 233–237.
16. Partin, J. S., Partin, J. C., Schubert, W. K., and McAdams, A. J. (1974) Liver ultrastructure in abetalipoproteinemia: evolution of micronodular cirrhosis. *Gastroenterology* **67,** 107–118.
17. Yang, S. Q., Lin, H. Z., Lane, M. D., et al. (1997) Obesity increases sensitivity to endotoxin liver injury: implications for the pathogenesis of steatohepatitis. *Proc. Natl. Acad. Sci. USA* **94,** 2557–2562.
18. Hillebrandt, S., Goos, C., Matern, S., and Lammert, F. (2002) Genome-wide analysis of hepatic fibrosis in inbred mice identifies the susceptibility locus Hfib1 on chromosome 15. *Gastroenterology* **123,** 2041–2051.
19. Shackel, N. A., Gorrell, M. D., and McCaughan, G. W. (2002) Gene array analysis and the liver. *Hepatology* **36,** 1313–1325.
20. Justice, M., Noveroske, J. K., Weber, J. S., Zheng, B., and Bradley, A. (1999) Mouse ENU mutagenesis. *Hum. Mol. Genet.* **8,** 1955–1963.

21. Daly, A. K. (2003) Candidate gene case-control studies. *Pharmacogenomics* **4,** 1–13.
22. Yee, L. J., Tang, J., Gibson, A. W., Kimberly, R., Van Leeuwen, D. J., and Kaslow, R. A. (2001) Interleukin 10 polymorphisms as predictors of sustained response in antiviral therapy for chronic hepatitis C infection. *Hepatology* **33,** 708–712.
23. Bonkovsky, H. L., Jawaid, Q., Tortorelli, K., et al. (1999) Non-alcoholic steatohepatitis and iron: increased prevalence of mutations of the HFE gene in non-alcoholic steatohepatitis. *J. Hepatol.* **31,** 421–429.
24. Wacholder, S., Rothman, N., and Caporaso, N. (2000) Population stratification in epidemiological studies of common genetic variants and cancer: quantification of bias. *J. Natl. Cancer Inst.* **92,** 1151–1158.
25. Pritchard, J. K. and Rosenberg, N. A. (1999) Use of unlinked genetic markers to detect population stratification in association studies. *Am. J. Hum. Genet.* **65,** 220–228.
26. Bacanu, S.-A., Devlin, B., and Roeder, K. (2000) The power of genomic control. *Am. J. Hum. Genet.* **66,** 1933–1944.
27. Sasieni, P. D. (1997) From genotypes to genes: doubling the sample size. *Biometrics* **53,** 1253–1261.
28. Erhardt, A., Maschner-Olberg, A., Mellenthin, C., et al. (2003) HFE mutations and chronic hepatitis C: H63D and C282Y heterozygosity are independent risk factors for liver fibrosis and cirrhosis. *J. Hepatol.* **38,** 335–342.
29. Tung, B. Y., Emond, M. J., Bronner, M. P., Raaka, S. D., Cotler, S. J., and Kowdley, K. V. (2003) Hepatitis C, iron status, and disease severity: relationship with HFE mutations. *Gastroenterology* **124,** 318–326.
30. Smith, B. C., Grove, J., Guzail, M. A., et al. (1998) Heterozygosity for hereditary haemochromatosis is associated with more fibrosis in chronic hepatitis C. *Hepatology* **27,** 1695–1699.
31. Woitas, R. P., Ahlenstie, G., Iwan, A., et al. (2002) Frequency of the HIV-protective CC chemokine receptor 5-Delta32/Delta32 genotype is increased in hepatitis C. *Gastroenterology* **122,** 1721–1728.
32. Promrat, K., McDermott, D. H., Gonzalez, C. M., et al. (2003) Association of chemokine system polymorphisms with clinical outcomes and treatment responses of chronic hepatitis C. *Gastroenterology* **124,** 352–360.
33. Day, C. P., Bashir, R., James, O. F. W., et al. (1991) Investigation of the role of polymorphisms at the alcohol and aldehyde dehydrogenase loci in genetic predisposition to alcohol related end-organ damage. *Hepatology* **14,** 798–801.
34. Valenti, L., Fracanzani, A. L., and Dongiovanni, P. (2002) Tumour necrosis factor a promoter polymorphisms and insulin resistance in nonalcoholic fatty liver disease. *Gastroenterology* **122,** 274–280.
35. Thursz, M. (2001) MHC and the viral hepatitides. *Quart J. Med.* **94,** 287–291.
36. Pouneh, M., Contos, M. J., Haque, M., et al. (2003) Clinical and histologic spectrum of nonalcoholic fatty liver disease associated with normal ALT values. *Hepatology* **37,** 1286–1292.
37. Rosenberg, W. M. C. (2003) Rating fibrosis progression in chronic liver diseases. *J. Hepatol.* **38,** 357–360.

38. Edwards-Smith, C. J., Jonsson, J. R., et al. (1999) Interleukin-10 promoter polymorphism predicts initial response of chronic hepatitis C to interferon alfa. *Hepatology* **30,** 526–530.
39. Jones, D. E. J., Watt, F. E., Metcalf, J. V., Bassendine, M. F., and James, O. F. W. (1999) Familial primary biliary cirrhosis reassessed: a geographically-based population study. *J. Hepatol.* **30,** 402–407.
40. Cardon, L. R. and Bell, J. I. (2001) Association studies designs for complex diseases. *Nat. Rev.* **2,** 91–99.
41. Ioannidis, J. P. A., Trikalinos, T. A., Ntzani, E. E., and Contopoulos-Ioannidis, D. G. (2003) Genetic associations in large versus small studies: an empirical assessment. *Lancet* **361,** 567–571.
42. Perneger, T. V. (1998) What's wrong with Bonferroni adjustments? *Br. Med. J.* **316,** 1235–1237.
43. Powell, E. E., Edwards-Smith, C. J., Hay, J. L., et al. (2000) Host genetic factors influence disease progression in chronic hepatitis C. *Hepatology* **31,** 828–833.
44. Degoul, F., Sutton, A., Mansouri, A., et al. (2001) Homozygosity for alanine in the mitochondrial targeting sequence of superoxide dismutase and risk for severe alcoholic liver disease. *Gastroenterology* **120,** 1468–1474.
45. Satsangi, J., Chapman, R. W. G., Haldar, N., et al. (2001) A functional polymorphism of the stromelysin gene (MMP-3) influences susceptibility to primary sclerosing cholangitis. *Gastroenterology* **121,** 124–130.
46. Editorial. (1999) Freely associating. *Nat. Genet.* **22,** 1–2.
47. Donaldson, P. T. (2002) Genetics in autoimmune hepatitis. *Semin. Liver Dis.* **22,** 353–363.
48. Donaldson, P. T. and Norris, S. (2002) Evaluation of the role of MHC Class II alleles, haplotypes and selected amino acid sequences in primary sclerosing cholangitis. *Autoimmunity* **35,** 555–564.
49. Jones, D. E. J. and Donaldson, P. T. (2003) Genetic factors in the pathogenesis of primary biliary cirrhosis. *Clin. Liver Dis.* **7,** 841–864.
50. Gambaro, G., Anglani, F., and D'Angelo, A. (2000) Association studies of genetic polymorphisms and complex disease. *Lancet* **355,** 308–311.
51. Egger, M., Davey Smith, G., Schneider, M., and Minder, C. (1997) Bias in meta-analysis detected by a simple graphical test. *Br. Med. J.* **315,** 629–634.
52. Borràs, E., Coutelle, C., Rosell, A., et al. (2000) Genetic polymorphism of alcohol dehydrogenase in Europeans: the ADH2*2 allele decreases the risk for alcoholism and is associated with ADH3*1. *Hepatology* **31,** 984–989.
53. Stewart, S. F., Leathart, J. B., Chen, Y., et al. (2002) The valine-alanine manganese superoxide dismutase polymorphism is not associated with increased oxidative stress or susceptibility to advanced alcoholic liver disease. *Hepatology* **36,** 1355–1360.

20

Analysis of Microarray Experiments for Pulmonary Fibrosis

Nilesh B. Davé and Naftali Kaminski

Summary

Microarray technology allows the investigator to examine the simultaneous expression of thousands of genes in a given cell or tissue. Such experiments that probe tens of thousands of genes produce immense amounts of information. In recent years, there has been a steady increase in the availability of tools for analysis of microarray data. Although many commercial tools are being aggressively marketed, we mostly use shareware tools. In this chapter, we present our approach to the analysis of microarray data mainly using tools that were generated by our collaborators or that are freely available. Step-by-step explanations of software operation are provided.

Key Words: Microarrays; gene expression; multiple sampling; bioinformatics; clustering; Scoregene; GeneXpress; GenMapp; functional analysis.

1. Introduction

Microarrays enable the simultaneous profiling of complete genomes. Since their introduction a decade ago, microarrays have been applied to all fields of biology, the most successful and applied are in cancer research *(1–4)*.

There have been only a few reports of the use of microarrays in the analysis of nonmalignant lung diseases, three of them in pulmonary fibrosis and recently reviewed by us *(5)*. Using microarray technology, we have gained insight into the molecular mechanisms of this disease. Osteopontin and the chemokine C10 have been implicated in pulmonary fibrosis based on data from microarray based analysis of murine lungs exposed to bleomycin. Analyzing human samples on microarrays, we identified matrix metalloproteinase (MMP)-7 as a potential regulator of pulmonary fibrosis in humans *(5)*. With the introduction of whole genome arrays for human, rat, and mouse, microarray data from animal models of idiopathic pulmonary fibrosis and microarray data from humans afflicted with this disease allow cross-species comparison. The goal of this

From: *Methods in Molecular Medicine, Vol. 117: Fibrosis Research: Methods and Protocols*
Edited by: J. Varga, D. A. Brenner, and S. H. Phan © Humana Press Inc., Totowa, NJ

type of comparison is to use microarray data to find a core group of genes that are conserved through evolution and are important for disease pathogenesis.

The challenge most often complained about by scientists using microarrays is the immense amount of information generated by these experiments. An important feature of this information is its complexity. For instance, for every experimental point in our dataset, we can have expression levels for 20,000 or more transcripts, but we can also have additional information that relates to the experimental attribute. For example, in the analysis of a clinical human sample, we will have epidemiological and clinical information, whereas for a mouse experiment, we will have the mouse strain and experimental setting. We may also have technical information about the experiments. To address this challenge, we need tools that allow us to perform several tasks including scoring genes for relevance, classifying genes and samples, compensating for multiple testing, visualizing data in an intuitive fashion, and loading the results with biological information. After a brief period characterized by a lack of analytical tools, multiple applications have been developed. **Table 1** provides a list of some of the commercially available applications, whereas **Table 2** provides a list of some of the publicly available software applications.

In our view, successful analysis of microarray data requires careful consideration and knowledge of the biological questions and depends on insight into the best microarray study design to help answer these questions. Moreover, having a solid and fundamental understanding of microarray analysis helps the researcher plan the experiment more efficiently. This serious and careful planning must occur so that proper statistical analysis of the microarray data can be performed. In fact, we have even run microarray experiments on "exciting" samples only to realize, after much time and money was spent, that the experiment needs to be repeated because of poor study design. Once the initial planning is done and the microarrays have been hybridized, the exciting steps of microarray analysis can be initiated.

Microarray experiments commonly result in large data files (often more than 10 megabytes in size!) and subsequent use of computer memory. This data must be carefully and systematically mined and analyzed using various computational tools and approaches. Generally, the data set must be pared to a reasonable number of genes from 10,000 to 55,000 using various filtering criteria. Once this filtering has occurred, more critical analyses can be started. We will not deal herein with normalization or filtering techniques, as these are highly variable and beyond the scope of this chapter. Rather, we will describe our approach to microarray data analysis using various freeware programs available through the Internet, some of them developed by our collaborators. All of these programs are freely available and are commonly used in our laboratory and by researchers using microarrays.

Table 1
Commercial Comprehensive Software Packages

Company	Web site	Analysis	Visualization	Annotations	Data storage
Silicon Genetics	http://www.silicangenetics.com/cgi/SiG.cgi/index.smf	X	X	X	X
Spotfire	http://www.spotfire.com/	X	X	X	X
Biodiscovery	http://www.biodiscovery.com/	X	X	X	X
Iobion	http://www.iobion.com/products/products_GENETRAFFIC.html	X	X	X	X
Partek	http://www.partek.com/index.html	X	X		X
Genesifter	http://www.genesifter.net/	X	X	X	
Ocimum Biosolutions	http://www.ocimumbio.com/web/default.asp	X	X	X	X
Rosetta Biosoftware	http://www.rosettabio.com/	X	X	X	
Strand Genomics	http://avadis.stradgenomics.com/	X	X	X	

Table 2
Freely Available Comprehensive Software Packages

Lab/institute	Name	Web site (http://)	Analysis	Visualization	Annotations	Data storage
Bioinformatics/ Gratz University	Genesis	www.genome.turgaz.at/Software	X	X	X	
TIGR/The Institute for Genome Research	TM4	www.tigr.org/software/tm4/mev.html	X	X	X	X
Open Source	Microarray Explorer	www.maexplorer.sourceforge.net/	X	X	X	
Computer Science/ Stanford University	GeneXpress	www.genexpress.stanford.edu/	X	X	X	
Bioinformatics/ Spanish Cancer Center	GEPAS	www.gepas.bioinfo.cnio.es/	X	X	X	
University of Pittsburgh Cancer Institute	GEDA	www.bioinformatics.upmc.edu/GE2/GEDA.html	X	X		
NCI/Biometric Research Branch	BRB Array Tools	www.linus.nci.nih.gov/BRB-ArrayTools.html	X	X	X	
Biostatistics/Dana Farber Institute/Harvard	Bioconductor	www.bioconductor.org/	X	X	X	
Center for Genome Research/MIT	GeneCluster	www.broad.mit.edu/cancer/software/software.html	X	X		

2. Materials: Hardware/Software

1. PC with high-end processor and at least 1 gigabyte random access memory (RAM).
2. Microsoft Excel and Access.
3. An Updated Java Virtual Machine (http://java.sun.com/j2se/1.4.2/download.html).
4. Scoregenes (http://www.cs.huji.ac.il/labs/compbio/scoregenes/).
5. Treeview/Cluster (http://rana.lbl.gov/EisenSoftware.htm).
6. GeneXpress (http://genexpress.stanford.edu/).
7. GeneMAPP (http://www.genmapp.org/).
8. Cancer gene expression data analysis tool (caGEDA)/SAM (http://bioinformatics.upmc.edu/GE2/GEDA.html).

3. Methods

The methods below describe our approach to analyzing microarray data after the data has been filtered and normalized. The programs that will be discussed are programs we commonly use. They are free for academic users. Filtering and normalization may vary depending on the platform being used. Because of this variability, we will not discuss the methods to filter and normalize data *(6)*. We will discuss steps of the analysis based on a final Excel table with expression values that have already been filtered and normalized. The programs that will be subsequently discussed require specific file formats for the data. The user must convert the Excel file into the appropriate format prior to loading the data into a specific program. We have mentioned this step where appropriate. The basic structure of our Excel database file with gene expression data has "GeneID" as the header in the first column with GeneBank Accession or LocusLink gene identification numbers as the column entries. The second column contains a description of the gene. Subsequent columns are experimental groups with names to help identify the experiment. The first row contains column headers such as GeneID, Description, Experiment 1, Experiment 2, etc. Header rows should not have symbols such as asterisks and exclamation points. Underscores are acceptable. Subsequent rows are identified as individual genes (**Fig. 1**).

We use Excel to modify our "master table." That is, we use Excel to remove columns or reformat data into files to be used in the analytical programs. The data files are not only saved in the Excel format (.xls). We also save these files as "Text-Delimited (.txt)" files. This file option can be seen when using the "Save As" option in Excel.

3.1. Scoregenes

Scoregenes *(7,8)* is a collection of programs that was developed by Nir Friedman's team at the Hebrew University in Jerusalem, Israel. This program

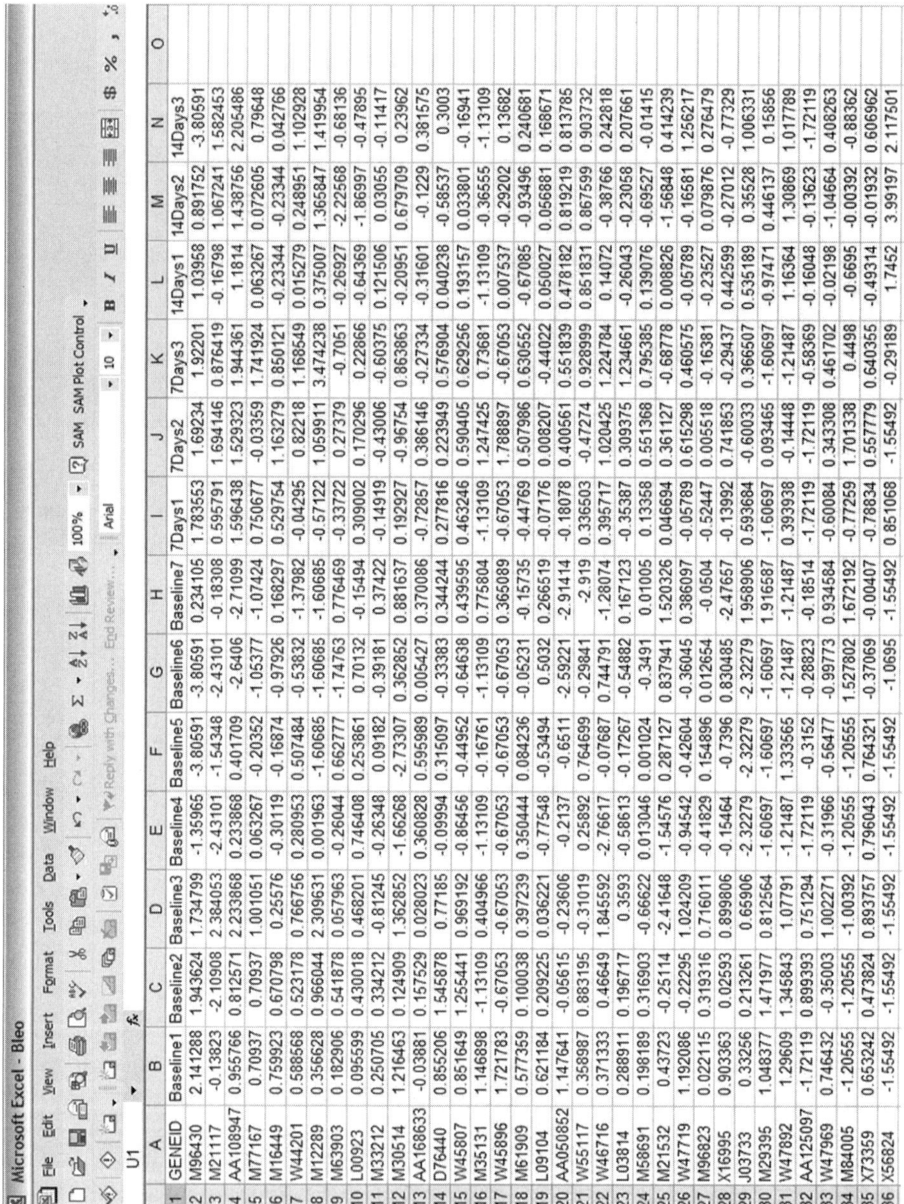

	A	B	C	D	E	F	G	H	I	J	K	L	M	N
1	GENEID	Baseline1	Baseline2	Baseline3	Baseline4	Baseline5	Baseline6	Baseline7	7Days1	7Days2	7Days3	14Days1	14Days2	14Days3
2	M96430	2.141288	1.943624	1.734799	-1.35965	-3.80591	-3.80591	0.234105	1.783553	1.69234	1.92201	1.03958	0.891752	-3.80591
3	M21117	-0.13823	-2.10908	2.384053	-2.43101	-1.54348	-2.43101	-0.18308	0.595791	1.694146	0.876419	-0.16798	1.067241	1.582453
4	AA108947	0.955766	0.812571	2.233868	0.233868	0.401709	-2.6406	-2.71099	1.596438	1.529323	1.944361	1.1814	1.438756	2.205486
5	M77167	0.70937	0.70937	1.001051	0.063267	-0.20352	-1.05377	-1.07424	0.750677	-0.03359	1.741924	0.063267	0.072605	0.79648
6	M16449	0.759923	0.670798	0.25576	-0.30119	-0.16874	-0.97926	0.168297	0.529754	1.163279	0.850121	-0.23344	-0.23344	0.042766
7	W44201	0.588568	0.523178	0.766756	0.280953	0.507484	-0.53832	-1.37982	-0.04295	0.82218	1.168549	0.015279	0.248951	1.102928
8	M12289	0.356628	0.966044	2.309631	0.001963	-1.60685	-1.60685	-1.60685	-0.57122	1.059911	3.474238	0.375007	1.365847	1.419954
9	M63903	0.182906	0.541878	0.057963	-0.26044	0.662777	-1.74763	0.776469	-0.33722	0.27379	-0.7051	-0.26927	-2.22568	-0.68136
10	L00923	0.095599	0.430018	0.468201	0.746408	0.253861	0.70132	-0.15494	0.309002	0.170296	0.22866	-0.64369	-1.86997	-0.47895
11	M33212	0.250705	0.334212	-0.81245	-0.26348	0.09182	-0.39181	0.37422	-0.14919	-0.43006	-0.60375	0.121506	0.03055	-0.11417
12	M30514	1.216463	0.124909	1.362852	-1.66268	-2.73307	0.362852	0.881637	0.192927	-0.96754	0.863863	-0.20951	0.679709	0.23962
13	AA168633	-0.03881	0.157529	0.028023	0.360828	0.595989	0.005427	0.370086	-0.72857	0.386146	-0.27334	-0.31601	-0.1229	0.381575
14	D76440	0.855206	1.545878	0.77185	-0.09994	0.315097	-0.33383	0.344244	0.277816	0.223949	0.576904	0.040238	-0.58537	0.3003
15	W45807	0.851649	1.255441	0.969192	-0.86456	-0.44952	-0.64638	0.439595	0.463246	0.590405	0.629256	0.193157	0.033801	-0.16941
16	M35131	1.146898	-1.13109	0.404966	-1.13109	-0.16761	-1.13109	0.775804	-1.13109	1.247425	0.73681	-1.13109	-0.36555	-1.13109
17	W45896	1.721783	-0.67053	-0.67053	-0.67053	-0.67053	-0.67053	0.365089	-0.67053	1.788897	-0.67053	0.007537	-0.29202	0.13682
18	M61909	0.577359	0.100038	0.397239	0.350444	0.084236	-0.05231	-0.15735	-0.44769	0.507986	0.630552	-0.67085	-0.93496	0.240681
19	L09104	0.621184	0.209225	0.036221	-0.77548	-0.53494	0.5032	0.266519	-0.07176	0.008207	-0.44022	0.050027	0.056881	0.168671
20	AA050852	1.147641	-0.05615	-0.23606	-0.2137	-0.6511	-2.59221	-2.91414	-0.18078	0.400561	0.551839	0.478182	0.819219	0.813785
21	W55117	0.358987	0.883195	-0.31019	0.25892	0.764699	-0.29841	-2.919	0.336503	-0.47274	0.928999	0.851831	0.867599	0.903732
22	W46716	0.371333	0.46649	1.845592	-2.76617	-0.07687	0.744791	-1.28074	0.395717	1.020425	1.224784	0.14072	-0.38766	0.242818
23	L03814	0.288911	0.196717	0.3593	-0.58613	-0.17267	-0.54882	0.167123	-0.35387	0.309375	1.234661	-0.26043	-0.23058	0.207661
24	M58691	0.198189	0.316903	-0.66622	0.013046	0.001024	-0.3491	0.01005	0.13358	0.551368	0.795385	0.139076	-0.69527	-0.01415
25	M21532	0.43723	-0.25114	-2.41648	-1.54576	0.287127	0.837941	1.520326	0.046694	0.361127	-0.68778	0.008826	-1.56848	0.414239
26	W47719	1.192086	-0.22295	1.024209	-0.94542	-0.42604	-0.36045	0.386097	-0.05789	0.615298	0.460575	-0.05789	-0.16581	1.256217
27	M96823	0.022115	0.319316	0.716011	-0.41829	0.154896	0.012654	-0.0504	-0.52447	0.005518	-0.16381	-0.23527	0.079876	0.276479
28	X16995	0.903363	0.02593	0.899806	-0.15464	-0.7396	0.830485	-2.47657	-0.13992	0.741853	-0.29437	0.442599	-0.27012	-0.77329
29	J03733	0.33256	0.213261	0.65906	-2.32279	-2.32279	-2.32279	1.958906	0.593684	-0.60033	0.366507	0.535189	0.35528	1.006331
30	M29395	1.048377	1.471977	0.812564	-1.60697	-1.60697	-1.60697	1.916587	-1.60697	0.093465	-1.60697	-0.97471	0.446137	0.15856
31	W47892	1.29609	1.345843	1.07791	-1.21487	1.333565	-1.21487	-1.21487	0.393938	-0.14448	-1.21487	1.16364	1.30869	1.017789
32	AA125097	-1.72119	0.899393	0.751294	-1.72119	-0.3152	-0.28823	-0.18514	-1.72119	-1.72119	-0.58369	-0.16048	-0.13623	-1.72119
33	W47969	0.746432	-0.35003	1.002271	-0.31966	-0.56477	-0.99773	0.934584	-0.60084	0.343308	0.461702	-0.02198	-1.04664	0.408263
34	M84005	-1.20555	-1.20555	-1.00392	-1.20555	-1.20555	1.527802	1.672192	-0.77259	1.701338	0.4498	-0.6695	-0.00392	-0.88362
35	X73359	0.653242	0.473824	0.893757	0.796043	0.764321	-0.37069	-0.00407	-0.78834	0.557779	0.640355	-0.49314	-0.01932	0.606962
36	X56824	-1.55492	-1.55492	-1.55492	-1.55492	-1.55492	-1.0695	-1.55492	0.851068	-1.55492	-0.29189	1.7452	3.99197	2.117501

Fig. 1. Excel file of data used in this analysis. Note column headers and general format. Data has been normalized and transformed into log base 2 format. GENEID are Genbank Accession numbers.

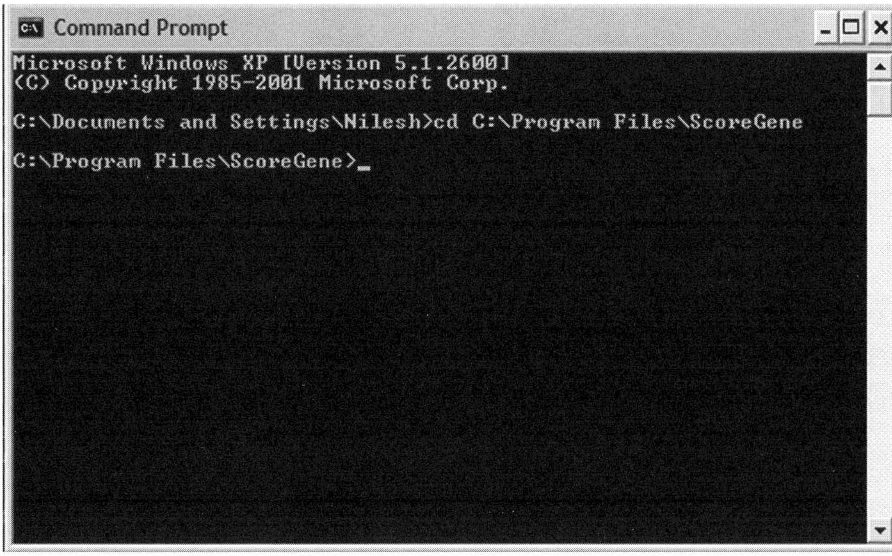

Fig. 2. DOS command to change to the file directory containing Scoregenes program.

covers several aspects of microarray data analysis including scoring genes for relevance, leave-one-out cross-validation (LOOCV), and clustering. It also generates visualization files that can be viewed in Treeview. Using Scoregenes requires some knowledge of Microsoft DOS with regard to command entry. In DOS, syntax is very important, because a typographical error in file name can result in error messages and subsequently, errant output or failure of command execution. Before this program can be used, the user must activate the "Command Prompt" window which is typically found under the "Accessories" folder using the "Start" menu in Windows. Alternatively, one can select the "RUN" option and type "cmd" to activate DOS. Using DOS syntax, the user must access the folder containing the Scoregenes files (**Fig. 2**). Another option is to put Scoregenes in the path statement in the environment variables in the advanced settings of the systems settings window (consult your Windows manual for more details). Every order in Scoregenes is a single-word operator.

This program requires the use of a data file and a label file. The purpose of the label file is to help categorize the experiments, usually by experimental condition. Data and label files used in this program are in the "Tab-Delimited (.txt)" format, a file format option in Excel that can be chosen when a file is saved. These label files are made in Excel and contain the names of the experi-

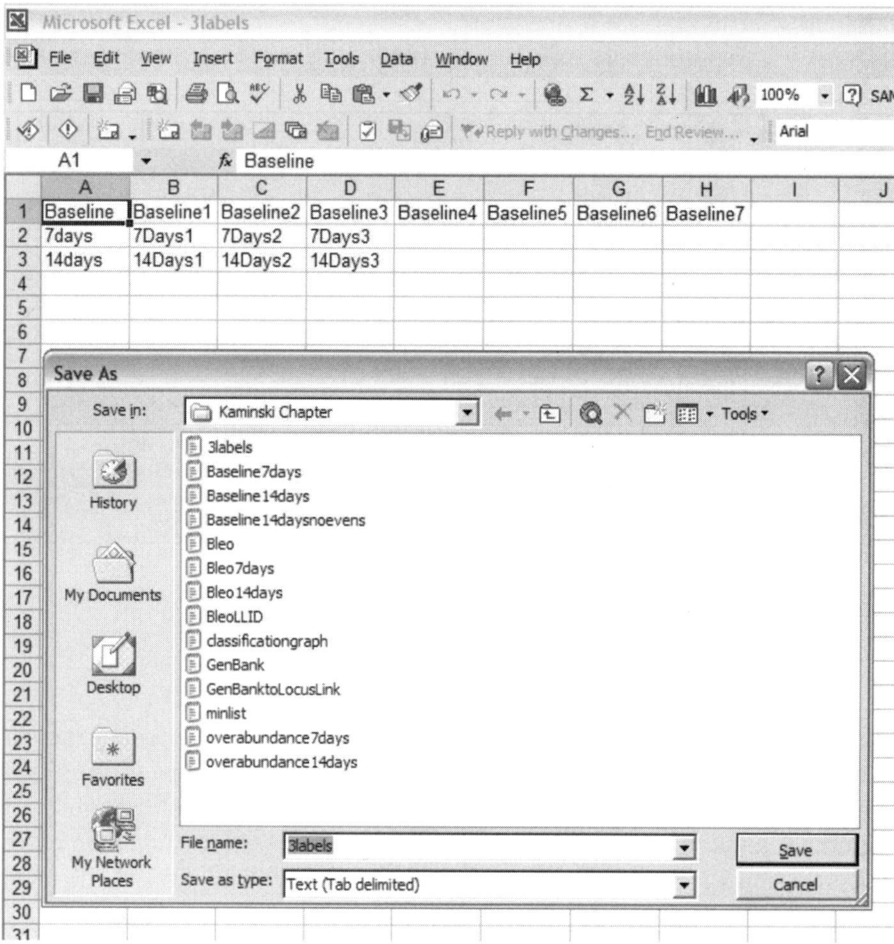

Fig. 3. Label file in Excel with "Save As" box showing "Text (Tab-delimited)" option. Column A contains row labels. Subsequent columns contain experiment names.

ments as they exactly appear in the data file. **Figure 3** is an example of a label file. The first column contains a "group name" and subsequent entries in each row have the exact experimental names. If the experimental names are not exact, errors will occur or the resulting analysis may be severely flawed. In **Fig. 3**, note the categorization and exactness of the names of the experiments as seen in a prior diagram.

It is best to store these files in a primary folder in the main hard drive (e.g., C:\) rather than within multiple subfolders. Fewer subfolders will result in easier and shorter command entry, which will be shown in subsequent examples. Data files must also be exported from Excel into "(.txt) Tab-Delimited" file form. For further information, the user can access the Scoregenes Help Manual available on the Internet at http://www.cs.huji.ac.il/labs/compbio/scoregenes/ScoreGenesManual.html.

3.2. Scoring Genes for Relevance

Using the command "Scoregene" the user can have the software analyze the data set and rank genes based on *p* value. Various scoring methods like TNOM, Info, *t*-test, and Komagorov-Smirnov can be used to score the genes ***(9)***. The output of this command is a Tab-Delimited text file that can be opened in Excel as a spreadsheet. The options for the "Scoregene" command include (note the default options for this command):

-m	Compute TNOM score
-i	Compute Info score
-w	Compute Wilcoxon score
-l	Compute logistic score
-g	Compute Gaussian overlap score
-t	Compute t-test score
-k	Compute Komogorov-Smirnov score (KS)
-n	Compute n-1 fold change
-f	Compute fold change
-F	Compute fold change in logarithmic data
-V	Computer intersection of tTest, KS
-v	Compute intersection of tTest, TNoM, Info
-p <target>	Compute Pearson correlation to target
-d	Print gene descriptions in report

The default options are "-f -d -w -g -i -n -m"

The command structure and example are as follows:

Structure:	Scoregene [options] Datafile Labelfile Outputfile
Example:	Scoregene –m –i –t –f "C:\My Documents\Data\Bleomycin.txt" "C:\MyDocuments\Data\labeldata.txt" "C:\MyDocuments\Data\scoregeneanalysis.txt"

The "scoregeneanalysis.txt" file can then be imported into Excel to examine the list of significant genes based on *p* value. Genes with *p* values less than 0.05 are considered significant. This list can be used to gain insight into the experimental question by sorting genes (in Excel) according to their *p* values, TNOM scores, Info scores, or *t*-test scores. Top scoring genes may help add insight to the biological process under investigation, and the activation of these genes can be verified with proteomic methods.

3.3. Compensating for Multiple Testing

The asymmetry between the number parameters (genes) measured and the number of samples is a cause for concern in statistical analysis of microarray data. This multiple testing phenomenon predicts that a number of significant *p* values will always be spurious. One approach is the *Bonferroni threshold*, a *p* value threshold that is the significance level divided by the number of genes measured. In most cases, this threshold is too stringent and leads to elimination of multiple biologically meaningful genes. We often use the *False Discovery Rate* (FDR) method that relaxes the Bonferroni threshold. An additional approach that we use is to determine the surprise contained in the dataset. In this approach, we examine the number of genes at different *p* values and compare them to the *expected* number under the null hypothesis (the assumption that the separation of the samples is random). The difference between the expected and observed number in each significant *p* value is an estimate of the *overabundance of information* and the surprise in the analyzed dataset.

3.4. Overabundance Order

Overabundance analysis, one function of Scoregenes software, assesses the number of genes, or abundance of genes, that are significant between groups in a data set. This function measures the number of genes at various levels of significance or *p* values against the null hypothesis which assumes that the samples are randomly different from each other. By graphing the observed number and expected number of genes at various *p* values, we can see if the experimental groups are different. We look at the number of genes at *p* values less than and equal to 0.05. This output file is visualized in Excel. The "overabundance" command can analyze the data using various options:

-m	Compute TNOM score
-i	Compute Info score
-w	Compute Wilcoxon score
-l	Compute logistic score
-g	Compute Gaussian overlap score
-k	Compute Kolmogorov-Smirnov score (KS)
-t	Compute t-test score
-n	Compute n-1 fold change
-f	Compute fold change
-v	Compute Intersection of tTest, TNoM, and Info
-V	Computer intersection of tTest and KS
-p <target>	Compute Pearson Correlation to target
-s <sig>	Set significance level

The default option is "-m"

The data file is again a Text delimited file that has only two different experimental groups. In other words, if an experiment is looking at the effect of Condition 1 and Condition 2 vs control, then the data file should have the control group and one of the condition groups. A separate data file can be made with the control and the condition group not included in the first analysis. The label file should contain the names of the experiments in the data file. There is no limit to the number of arrays included in each of the two groups; the limiting step is that there can only be two groups. The structure and sample command lines for this analysis are as follows:

Structure: Overabundance [options] Datafile Labelfile Outputfile
Example: Overabundance –m –i –t "C:\MyDocuments\Data\Bleomycin.txt" "C:\MyDocuments\Data\labeldata.txt" "C:\MyDocuments\Data\overabundance.txt"

After successful execution of this command, the output file can be found in the designated folder and can be opened by Excel. Using the X-Y scatter graphing option with smoothing lines in Excel, the output can be graphically visualized. (Please note that by using Excel, we merged two overabundance graphs into one in order to have both experimental groups on the same plot. This merging is done using Excel and not Scoregenes.) We can now begin to see the overabundance of informative genes at a given p value that are significant compared with an expected number of genes (**Fig. 4**).

In **Fig. 4**, the 14-d group has over 400 genes from a possible 2500 with $p < 0.05$ that are not a result of random variability as designated by the "Expected" line. The 7-d group has about 275 genes with $p < 0.05$. Therefore, it is unlikely that the differences in gene expression are a result of random separation of the groups. An additional output of overabundance order is the number of genes that pass Bonferroni and FDR and a measure of maximum surprise.

3.5. Visualization and Estimating Classification Efficiency

3.5.1. PlotTopGenes Order

One common approach to estimate the ability of the top scoring genes to serve as classifiers is using LOOCV. "PlotTopGenes," a command in Scoregenes, provides a combination of classifying genes using LOOCV and an intuitive visualization tool. Essentially, this command uses a set of enriched genes in the experiments to predict whether an array is a control or an experimental group. This iterative prediction model is grounded in the behavior of the genes. For a given group of arrays, "PlotTopGenes" removes one array and examines the expression of each gene across the remaining arrays. Using the other samples as a training set, the software will predict if the removed array is "control" or "experiment." The sample will be assigned a classification score

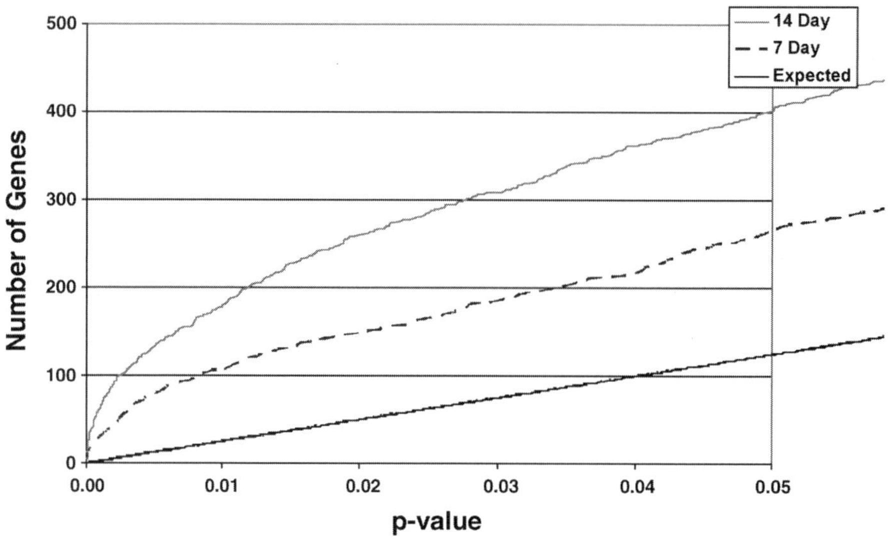

Fig. 4. Overabundance analysis graph showing the observed number of genes at 7 and 14 d compared with the expected number of genes at $p \leq 0.05$.

that is is the sum of the probabilities assigned by the genes involved in the classification process. This process is iterative in that every array is removed and the expression of all genes among the remaining arrays is analyzed to predict the characteristic of the removed array. One can repeat this process for genes with different *p* values or even all of the genes. There are several options for the "PlotTopGenes" command:

-T <threshold>	Threshold for choosing genes
-F <sig>	Choose genes that pass FDR
-B <sig>	Choose genes that pass Bonferroni
-s	Scale to std = 1
-L	Print logarithms of expression values
-M <min>	Min value to truncate with
-N	Normalized with respect to training class
-C	Do not classify
-O	Omit non-labeled genes
-m	Compute TNOM score
-i	Compute Info score
-w	Compute Wilcoxon score
-l	Compute logistic score
-g	Compute Gaussian overlap score
-t	Compute t-test score

-n	Compute n-1 fold change
-b	Classify with AdaBoost
-a	Classify with Naive Bayes (NB)
-c	Classify with Gaussian NB

The default option is "-m".

The output of this command results in a .cdt file (data file for cluster image). The organization of this output is different than the output from a clustering algorithm. **Figure 5** is an example of a "PlotTopGenes" cluster diagram.

The heat-map from this command shows a "checkerboard" pattern which is the typical output for the "PlotTopGenes" command. The output can be divided in the middle with a horizontal line. The top half, with light grey towars the top right corner and black at the bottom left corner, lists the genes that are upregulated in the experiment but downregulated in the control group. The most significant gene is listed first. The "bottom" half, with light grey at top left and black at bottom right, ranks genes most upregulated in the control and downregulated in the experimental group.

3.5.2. ClassificationGraph

ClassificationGraph is based on similar principles using LOOCV. The difference is that the program counts the number of errors generated when using different numbers of genes and *p* value thresholds. The options are:

-m	Compute TNOM score
-i	Compute Info score
-w	Compute Wilcoxon score
-l	Compute logistic score
-g	Compute Gaussian overlap score
-t	Compute t-test score
-n	Computer n-1 fold change
-k	Compute Komogorov-Smirnov score (KS)
-s	Do not perform gene selection within iterations
-T	Define test set labels
-C	Labels file for Leave-Class-Out procedure
-b	Classify with AdaBoost
-a	Classify with Naïve Bayes
-U	Classify with TAN
-u	Classify with TAN using continuous attributes only
-d	Classify with TAN using discrete attributes
-f	Skip first iterations

The default options are "-m -a".

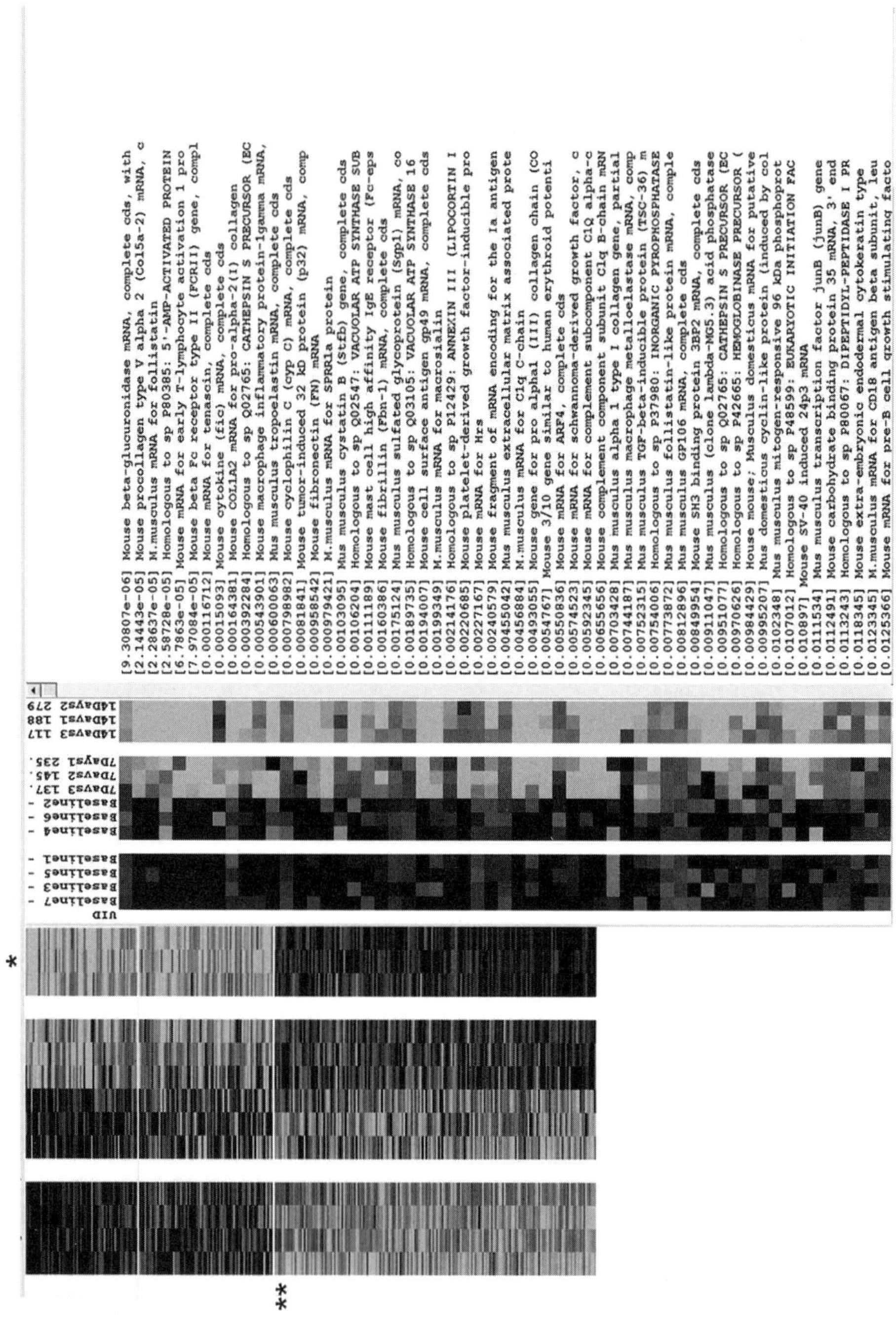
*
**
UID
Baseline7 -
Baseline3 -
Baseline5 -
Baseline1 -
Baseline4 -
Baseline6 -
Baseline2 -
7Davs3 137.
7Davs2 145.
7Days1 235.
14Davs3 117
14Davs1 188
14Days2 279
[9.30807e-06] Mouse beta-glucuronidase mRNA, complete cds, with
[2.14443e-05] Mouse procollagen type V alpha 2 (Col5a-2) mRNA, c
[2.28637e-05] M.musculus mRNA for follistatin
[2.58728e-05] Homologous to sp P80385: 5'-AMP-ACTIVATED PROTEIN
[6.7863e-05] Mouse mRNA for early T-lymphocyte activation 1 pro
[7.97084e-05] Mouse beta Fc receptor type II (FCRII) gene, compl
[0.000116712] Mouse mRNA for tenascin, complete cds
[0.00015093] Mouse cytokine (fic) mRNA, complete cds
[0.000164381] Mouse COL1A2 mRNA for pro-alpha-2(I) collagen
[0.000392284] Homologous to sp Q02765: CATHEPSIN S PRECURSOR (EC
[0.000543901] Mouse macrophage inflammatory protein-1gamma mRNA,
[0.000600063] Mus musculus tropoelastin mRNA, complete cds
[0.000798982] Mouse cyclophilin C (cyp C) mRNA, complete cds
[0.00081841] Mouse tumor-induced 32 kD protein (p32) mRNA, comp
[0.000958542] Mouse fibronectin (FN) mRNA
[0.000979421] M.musculus mRNA for SPRR1a protein
[0.00103095] Mus musculus cystatin B (Stfb) gene, complete cds
[0.00106204] Homologous to sp Q02547: VACUOLAR ATP SYNTHASE SUB
[0.00111189] Mouse mast cell high affinity IgE receptor (Fc-eps
[0.00160386] Mouse fibrillin (Fbn-1) mRNA, complete cds
[0.00175124] Mus musculus sulfated glycoprotein (Sgp1) mRNA, co
[0.00189735] Homologous to sp Q03105: VACUOLAR ATP SYNTHASE 16
[0.00194007] Mouse cell surface antigen gp49 mRNA, complete cds
[0.00199349] M.musculus mRNA for macrosialin
[0.00214176] Homologous to sp P12429: ANNEXIN III (LIPOCORTIN I
[0.00220685] Mouse platelet-derived growth factor-inducible pro
[0.00227167] Mouse mRNA for Hrs
[0.00240579] Mouse fragment of mRNA encoding for the Ia antigen
[0.00455042] Mus musculus extracellular matrix associated prote
[0.00456884] M.musculus mRNA for C1q C-chain
[0.00493055] Mouse gene for pro alpha1 (III) collagen chain (CO
[0.0054767] Mouse 3/10 gene similar to human erythroid potenti
[0.00550836] Mouse mRNA for ARF4, complete cds
[0.00574523] Mouse mRNA for schwannoma-derived growth factor, c
[0.00592345] Mouse mRNA for complement subcomponent C1Q alpha-c
[0.00655656] Mouse complement component subunit C1q B-chain mRN
[0.00703428] Mus musculus alpha 1 type I collagen gene, partial
[0.00744187] Mus musculus macrophage metalloelastase mRNA, comp
[0.00752315] Mus musculus TGF-beta-inducible protein (TSC-36) m
[0.00754006] Homologous to sp P37980: INORGANIC PYROPHOSPHATASE
[0.00773872] Mus musculus follistatin-like protein mRNA, comple
[0.00812896] Mus musculus GP106 mRNA, complete cds
[0.00849954] Mouse SH3 binding protein 3BP2 mRNA, complete cds
[0.00911047] Mus musculus (clone lambda-MG5.3) acid phosphatase
[0.00951077] Homologous to sp Q02765: CATHEPSIN S PRECURSOR (EC
[0.00970626] Homologous to sp P42665: HEMOGLOBINASE PRECURSOR (
[0.00984429] House mouse; Musculus domesticus mRNA for putative
[0.00995207] Mus domesticus cyclin-like protein (induced by col
[0.0102348] Mus musculus mitogen-responsive 96 kDa phosphoprot
[0.0107012] Homologous to sp P48599: EUKARYOTIC INITIATION FAC
[0.010897] Mouse SV-40 induced 24p3 mRNA
[0.0111534] Mus musculus transcription factor junB (junB) gene
[0.0112491] Mouse carbohydrate binding protein 35 mRNA, 3' end
[0.0113243] Homologous to sp P80067: DIPEPTIDYL-PEPTIDASE I PR
[0.0118345] Mouse extra-embryonic endodermal cytokeratin type
[0.0123345] M.musculus mRNA for CD18 antigen beta subunit, leu
[0.0125366] Mouse mRNA for pre-B cell growth stimulating facto

3.6. Clustering

Clustering is a mathematical approach to organizing the large amount of gene expression data into groups of similarly expressed genes. There are several types of clustering algorithms, such as k-means clustering and hierarchical clustering ***(10)***. "pcluster" is a command that uses a filtered and normalized set of data to create a file of clusters of genes based on Bayesian probability that can be visualized in Treeview, a software package that will be subsequently discussed. One unique feature of "pcluster" is an option that allows ordering the leaves in the hierarchical tree. This command also has various options for clustering:

-G	Use Gaussian model (default)
-Z	Use zero compression/Gaussian model
-B	Use Bernouli model (0/1 values only)
-M	Use Mixture of Dirichlet model (0/1 values only)
-l	Take log of expression values
-s	Scale each gene to have mean 0 and variance 1
-S	Scale only the output of the process
-b	Use marginal likelihood (instead of ML)
-L	Use leafs to determine order (default)
-T	Use trunks to determine order
-O	Use optimal leaf ordering
-o	Almost optimal leaf ordering
-g <Genes>	Work only on the genes listed in the attached file
-u	Do not introduce empty columns between classes
-d <file>	Output file to dump gene tree

The command can be written as below:

Structure: Pcluster [options] Datafile Labelfile Outputfile
Example: Pcluster–l "C:\MyDocuments\Data\datafile.txt" "C:\MyDocuments\Data\labeldata.txt" "C:\MyDocuments\Data\pclusterdata"

(Note that the output file does not require a file suffix [e.g., .cdt])

Once the command is entered, the process can take several minutes. When the process is nearly complete, a countdown will begin starting from the number of genes in the data set. For example, if there were 8000 genes in the data set, the countdown will start from 8000 and decrease until 10, when it will be

---

Fig. 5. *(opposite page)* PlotTopGenes heat map showing top genes in the 7- and 14-d experimental groups in the top half (*) and top genes in the control group in bottom half (**).

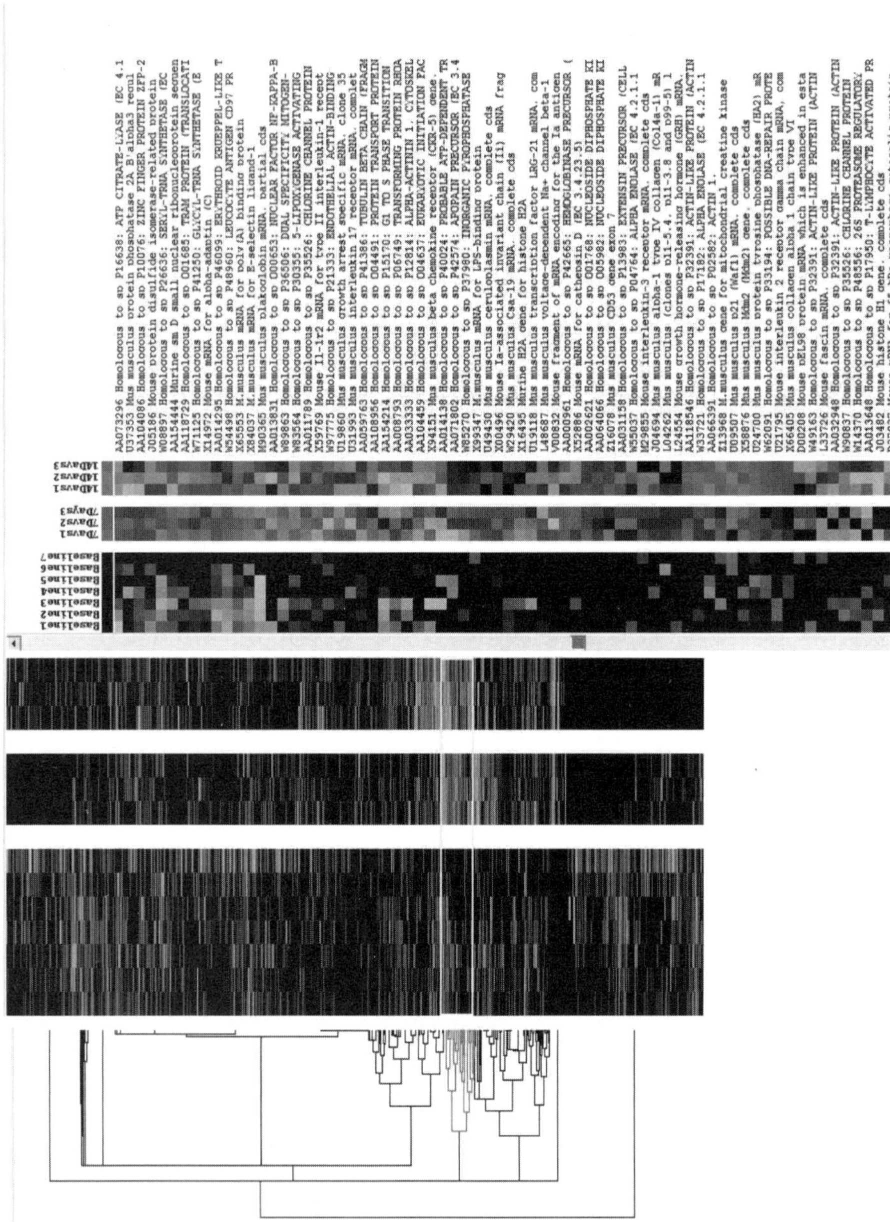

Fig. 6. Heat map of our dataset after using "pcluster" command. The vertical white columns separate the groups based on the label file groupings.

complete. Once this is done, a .cdt file with the name specified in the output file (pclusterdata.cdt) can then be loaded into Treeview to view the cluster diagram. The user can then examine genes in the various clusters and even search for specific genes (**Fig. 6**).

3.7. Treeview

Treeview is one of the most widely used visualization tools used to view heat maps ***(10)***. Treeview software enables the user to load cluster files and visualize clusters of genes. Cluster files are typically denoted as ".cdt" files. We typically use the "pcluster" feature of Scoregenes or a program called Cluster (which was developed by the same group that developed Treeview) ***(10)*** to make our cluster files. After loading the cluster file, Treeview displays the cluster diagram above. The Treeview program has defaults for size and color. Using the "Options" menu, pixel size, contrast, and color (note "Colors" tab) can be adjusted to size and desired color format to the user's preferences (**Fig. 7**).

When the "Image Contrast" is set to 1, subtle color changes will not be seen in genes with subtle expression changes. This lower image-contrast setting allows for more noticeable differences. Increasing this value will add gradation to the colors in the image. To fully understand how these options change the image, it is best to just experiment with stepwise settings changes. This image can be customized and then saved in bitmap form.

Cluster, which is bundled with Treeview, is a clustering program that uses the hierarchical clustering algorithm. The important aspect of this program is that the data file is essentially the same as the one used for Scoregenes. There is a file format help menu in Cluster to aid in properly formatting the file (**Fig. 8**).

3.8. GeneXpress

GeneXpress is a shareware program that features attribute analysis, expression analysis, and motif analysis developed by E. Segal, D. Koller, and N. Friedman in a collaborative effort of the departments of computer science at Stanford US and the Hebrew University, Jerusalem, Israel. Prior to using GeneXpress, data should already be clustered. The clustered heat-map can then be imported as a .cdt file and visualized in GeneXpress so that further analysis can be done. We commonly use the .cdt file format for importing the images, but there are options to load a .tab file (Tab-Delimited) or a .gxp file, the gene express file format. Below is our dataset seen in GeneXpress after the data set was clustered using the "plcuster" command in Scoregenes. Note the visual display and tree root display to allow localization of specific clusters (**Fig. 9**).

GeneXpress can perform attribute and experimental group analysis. In this analysis, each cluster can be analyzed for the presence of user-defined at-

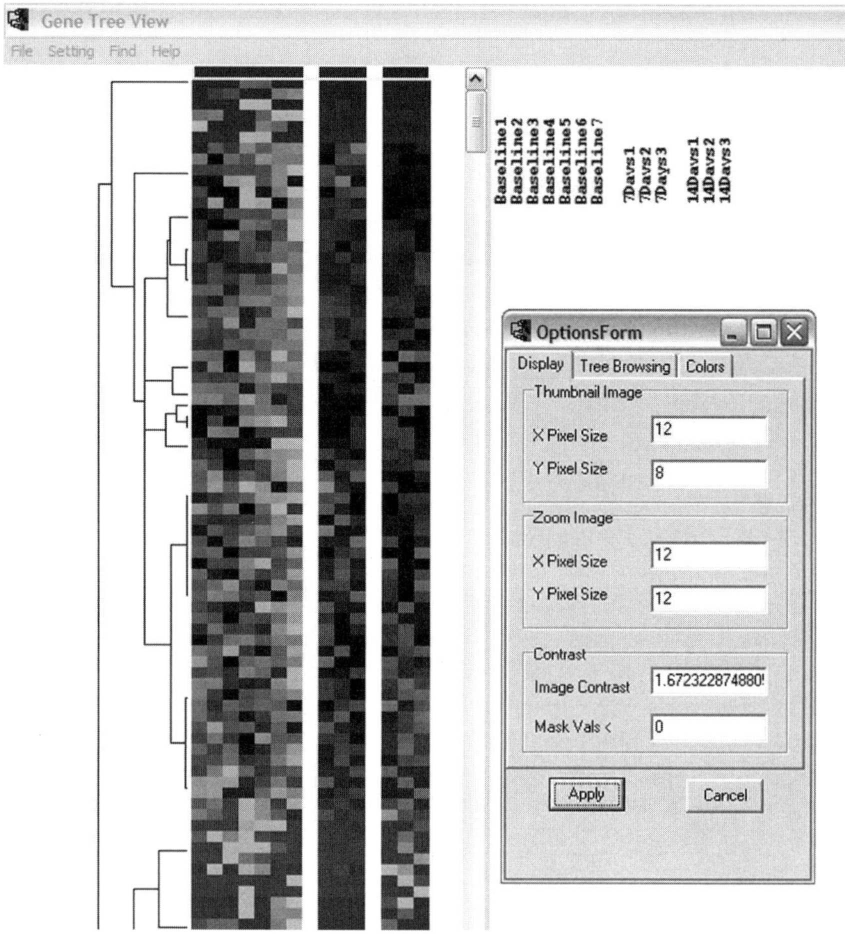

Fig. 7. Treeview is a widely used viewing program for CDT files. Display size, contrast of colors, and color choices can be adjusted by the user in the Options Form.

tributes. We commonly use this feature to characterize the data based on physiological function as defined by gene ontology (GO) annotations. This analysis' output is a graphical display that can be customized by color to reflect strong versus weak presence of a particular attribute.

To generate such a file for your genes, generate a file in which the first column is the gene ID list. (These files, called "dat" files, are simply tab separated text files with the suffix ".dat.") Subsequent columns contain attributes/annotations of interest (one attribute per column). Then, mark any gene that belongs to this annotation with 1, and all the genes that do not with 0. You can

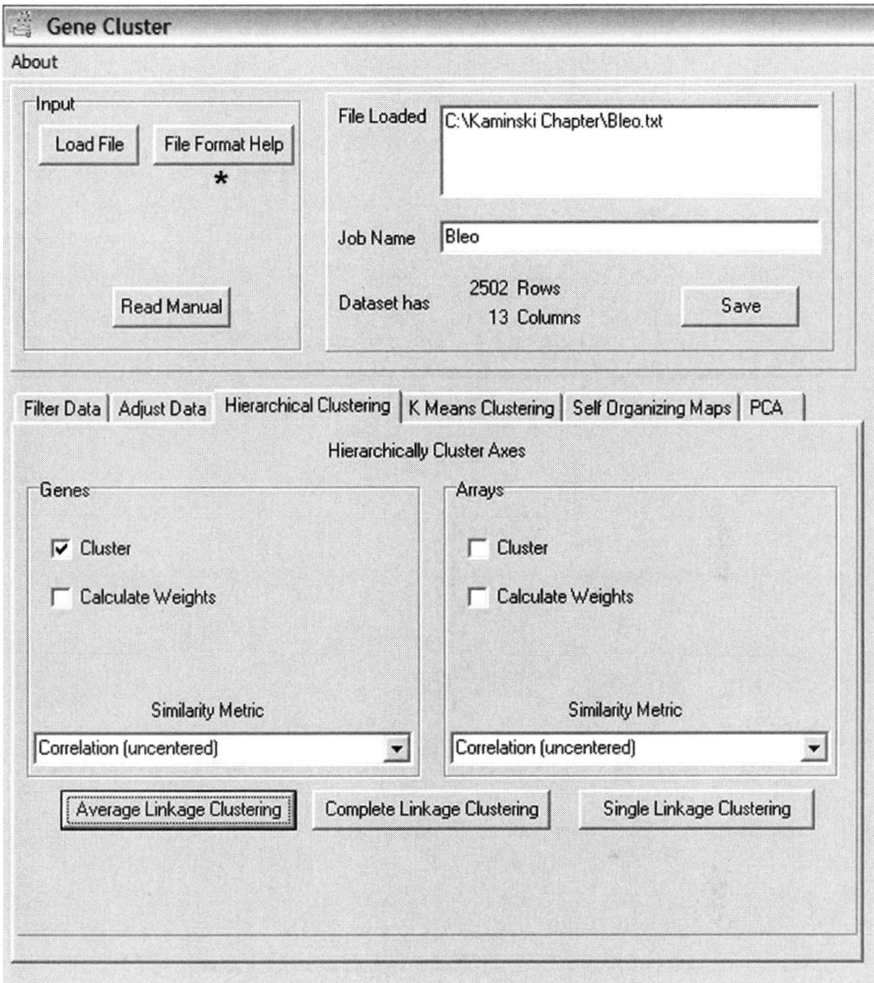

Fig. 8. Menu in Eisen's Cluster program. This program can filter and cluster data using various methods. Data files are similar to the one used in Scoregenes. Note the "File Format Help" button (*).

then load this file into your attribute or expression analysis. The same goes for experimental attribute. Generate a Tab-Delimited file in which the first column is the experiment headings and the next ones are experimental attributes. An experiment that belongs to a certain attribute will get the value 1 and the one that does not will get the value 0. Then this file can be loaded into the expression analysis as previously described.

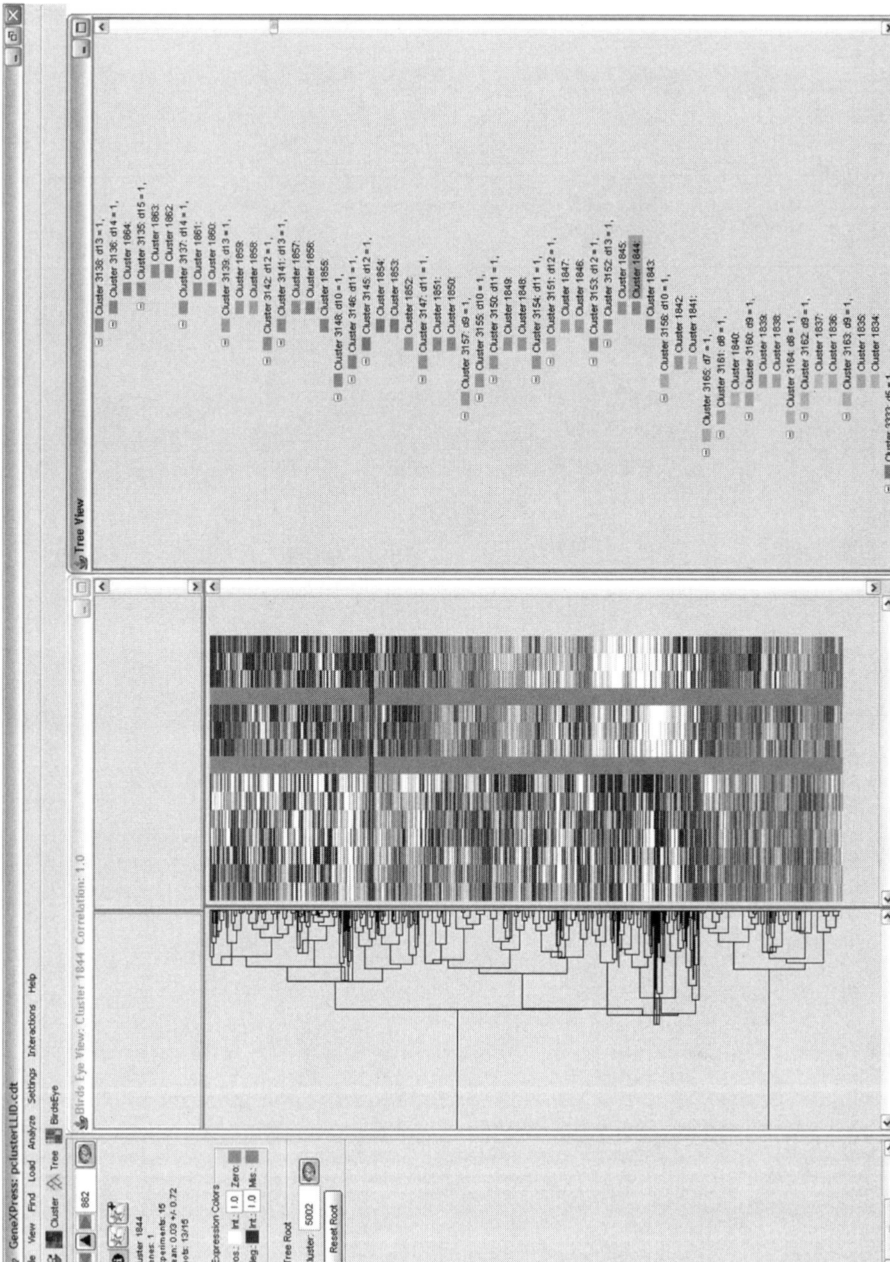

Fig. 9. Like Treeview, GeneXpress also allows visualization of the heat map with the added feature of visualizing the relationships of clusters using the tree root. Also, expression colors and heat-map size can be adjusted.

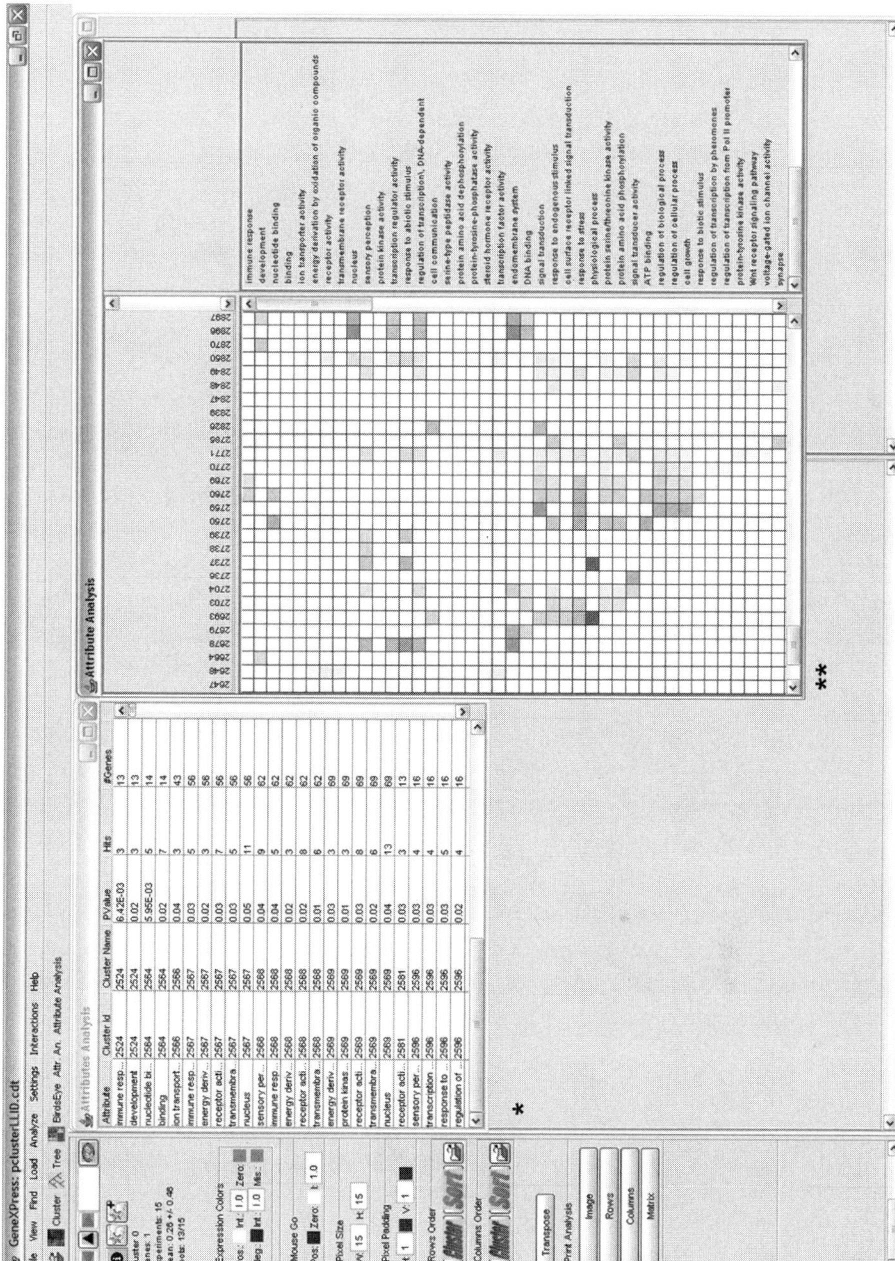

Fig. 10. Using a Mouse Go annotation file, an attribute analysis was done with our dataset using GeneXpress. Two outputs are displayed in spreadsheet form with attribute groups (*) and in graphic form with clusters in columns and attribute groups as rows (**). Color intensity reflects the degree of gene expression for that attribute.

In **Fig. 10**, each column is a cluster and each row is an attribute. The grid contains varying shades of black with the darkness of the square positively correlating with the degree of representation of the attribute. This analysis is limited by the completeness of the attributes; that is, GeneXpress will perform attribute analysis only for the attributes that are loaded by the user (**Fig. 11**).

3.9. GenMAPP

GenMAPP is a freeware program that enables the user to view gene expression data on MAPPs. MAPPs are graphical representations of various biological pathways that can be modified using the GenMAPP program. Because of the openness of the program, various groups of researchers can modify the MAPPs using a drawing tool and leave their identification information on the MAPP to foster open communication between researchers. Raw expression data is imported into GenMAPP, which then converts the raw data into a GenMAPP Expression Dataset using a GenMAPP database that can be downloaded from the GenMAPP website. The unique feature of this pathway visualization tool is that gene expression data can be seen on the pathway as shown in **Fig. 12**.

Each experimental group can be assigned a color and then visualized on the MAPP. Double-clicking on an element in the pathway will link it to functional information and also give the viewer a list of gene expression values sorted by experiment. This program allows the user to change the colors represented by each experimental group and to modify the expression criterion (e.g., fold change) of the expression data set (**Fig. 13**).

For example, the user can have only genes with greater than twofold in the experimental groups and less than 1.5-fold in the control experiments. It is likely that there will be a new version of GenMAPP at the time of this publication.

3.10. caGEDA

caGEDA (cancer gene expression data analysis tool) is a user-friendly Web-based tool that integrates various features of gene expression data analysis into one tool *(11)*. caGEDA is an open source tool that is continuously updated. It has a very good online manual with sample data files for tutorial purposes. Using this tool does not substitute the previously mentioned programs, but caGEDA does complement the analysis.

4. Conclusions

Microarray analysis involves a series of systematic steps using freely available tools described here. Using these tools, basic analysis can be performed

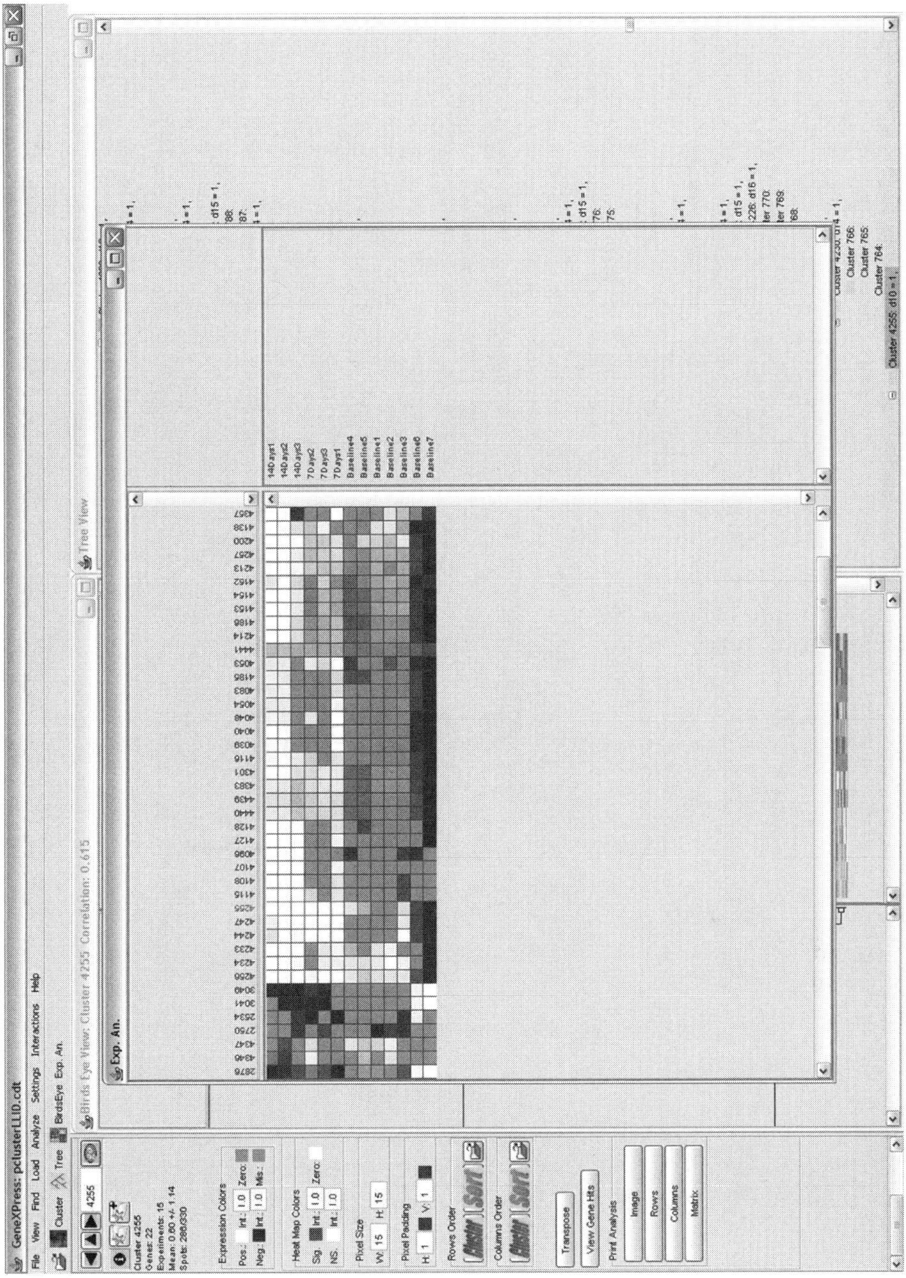

Fig. 11. GeneXpress can perform expression analysis in which columns are clusters and rows are experimental groups. This analysis allows the user to see the behavior of clusters across experimental conditions. This analysis is useful to find clusters of genes that behave very differently from control.

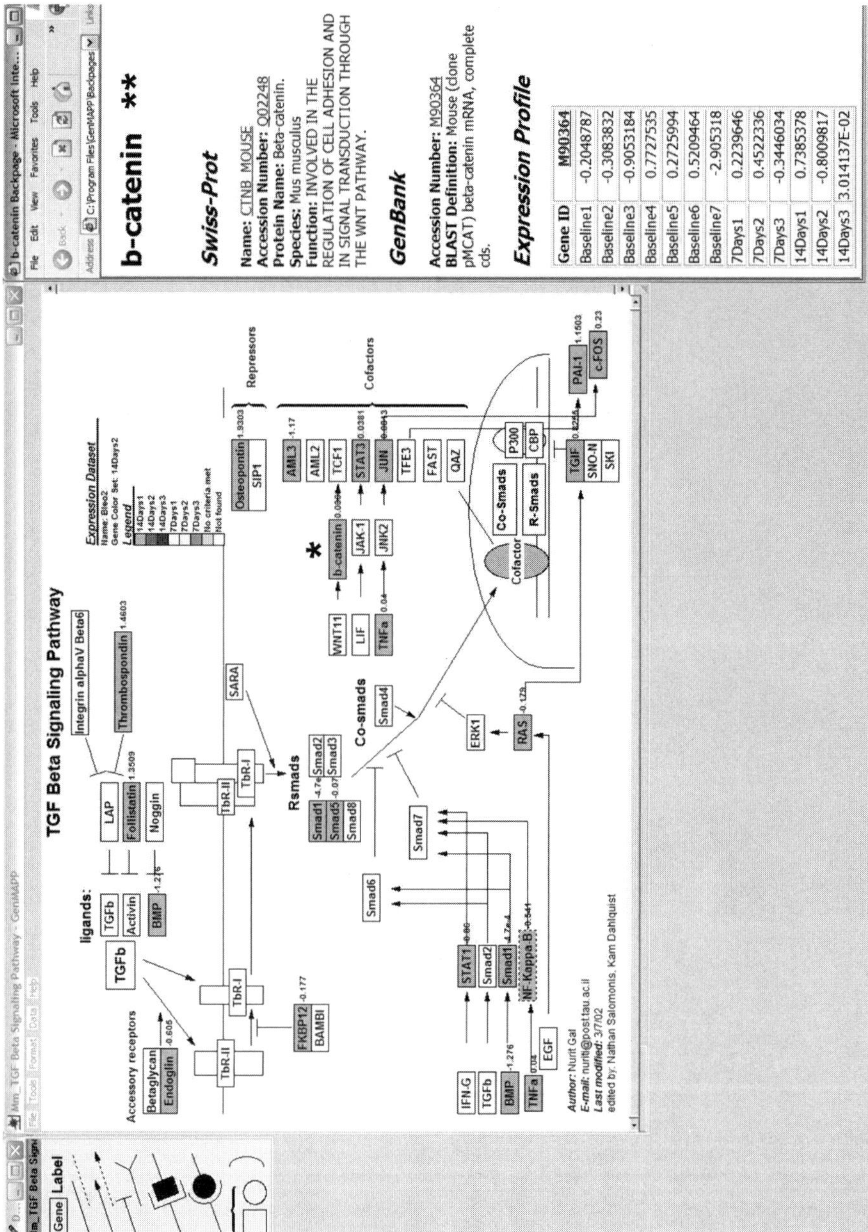

Fig. 12. GenMAPP display of transforming growth factor (TGF)-β pathway with highlighting of various mediators based on gene expression. β-catenin (*) is shown to be increased in the "14-d 1" experiment with associated expression value. Clicking on the "β-catenin" box reveals the panel on the right with annotation information and an expression profile from our experimental data.

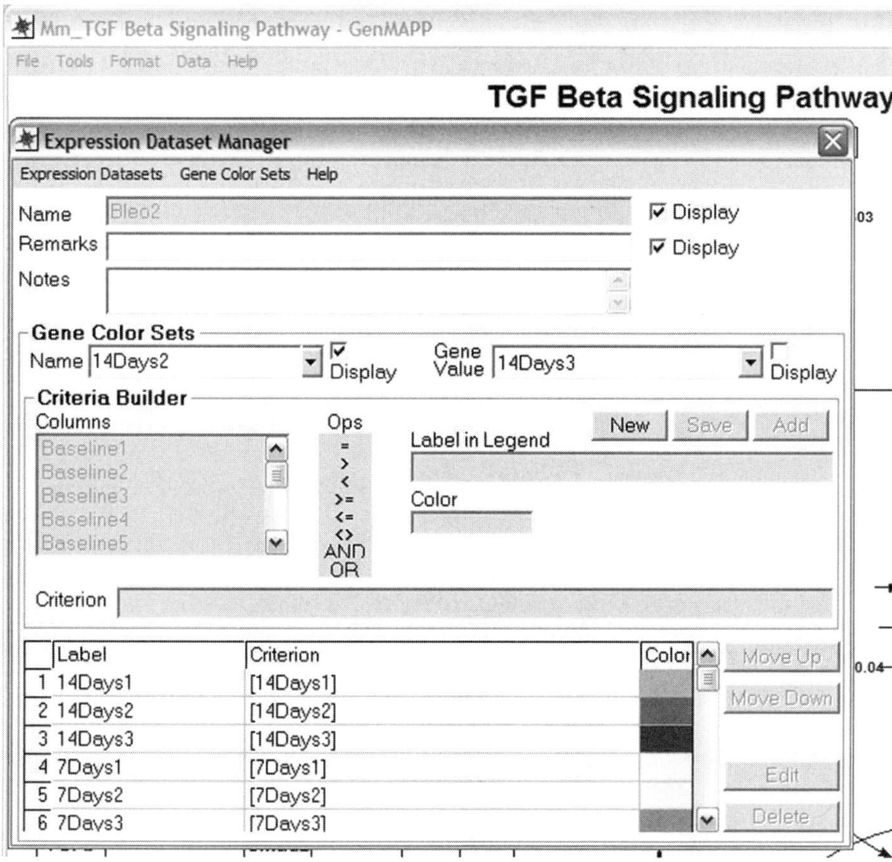

Fig. 13. GenMAPP Dataset Manager offers options to change colors in the signaling pathway map and to add criteria to limit the display of genes (e.g., fold change parameters) in the expression dataset.

by most people without the immediate need for computational biologists. As the analysis becomes more complicated, the services of computational biologists are indispensable. Microarrays are powerful tools that have changed our understanding of many diseases, and with their widespread application, exciting discoveries will continue. The "discovery" aspect of microarrays injects excitement into science, but only the astute scientist will be able to capture this in a mound of microarray data. As Louis Pasteur said: "Chance favors only the prepared mind" ***(12)***. We hope that readers of this chapter are able to follow our steps and begin to make scientific discoveries of their own.

References

1. Cojocaru, G., Friedman, N., Krupsky, M., et al. (2002) Transcriptional profiling of non-small cell lung cancer using oligonucleotide microarrays. *Chest* **121(3 Suppl),** 44S.
2. Cojocaru, G. S., Rechavi, G., and Kaminski, N. (2001) The use of microarrays in medicine. *Isr. Med. Assoc. J.* **3(4),** 292–296.
3. Bullinger, L., Dohner, K., Bair, E., et al. (2004) Use of gene-expression profiling to identify prognostic subclasses in adult acute myeloid leukemia. *N. Engl. J. Med.* **350(16),** 1605–1616.
4. Valk, P. J., Verhaak, R. G., Beijen, M. A., et al. (2004) Prognostically useful gene-expression profiles in acute myeloid leukemia. *N. Engl. J. Med.* **350(16),** 1617–1628.
5. Kaminski, N. (2003) Microarray analysis of idiopathic pulmonary fibrosis. *Am. J. Respir. Cell Mol. Biol.* **29(3 Suppl),** S32–36.
6. Quackenbush, J. (2002) Microarray data normalization and transformation. *Nat. Genet.* **32 (Suppl),** 496–501.
7. Zuo, F., Kaminski, N., Eugui, E., et al. (2002) Gene expression analysis reveals matrilysin as a key regulator of pulmonary fibrosis in mice and humans. *Proc Natl Acad Sci USA* **99(9),** 6292–6297.
8. Dekel, B., Burakova, T., Arditti, F. D., et al. (2003) Human and porcine early kidney precursors as a new source for transplantation. *Nat. Med.* **9(1),** 53–60.
9. Kaminski, N. and Friedman, N. (2002) Practical approaches to analyzing results of microarray experiments. *Am. J. Respir. Cell Mol. Biol.* **27(2),** 125–132.
10. Eisen, M. B., Spellman, P. T., Brown, P. O., and Botstein, D. (1998) Cluster analysis and display of genome-wide expression patterns. *Proc Natl Acad Sci USA* **95(25),** 14,863–14,868.
11. Patel, S., Bhattacharya, S., and Lyons-Weiler, J. (2003) GEDA: a web application for the integrated analysis of global gene expression patterns in cancer. *Applied Bioinformatics*, in press.
12. Pasteur, L. (1854) Lecture, University of Lille, December 7.

21

DNA Microarrays and Data Mining To Study Hepatic Fibrosis

Bernd Schnabl, Youkyung Hwang Choi, Curt H. Hagedorn, and Ramón Bataller

Summary

The pathogenesis of liver fibrosis has evolved dramatically in recent years. Hepatic stellate cells (HSCs) have been recognized as the main fibrogenic cells in the injured liver, and key fibrogenic cytokines have been identified. We propose the use of DNA microarrays to study changes in gene expression in activated HSCs and in fibrotic livers in order to identify key genes involved in liver fibrosis. For this purpose, RNA can be extracted from both cultured cells and liver tissue. The target RNA is hybridized to probes, which are gene-specific sequences immobilized on chips. The hybridization signal is assessed using a confocal laser scanner. Comparison of hybridization signals and patterns allows the identification of mRNAs that are differentially expressed. Statistical analysis enables classification and clustering of genes according to their up- or downregulation. By using this powerful technique, we have identified genes that are differentially regulated in both HSCs and the fibrotic human liver.

Key Words: Liver fibrosis; hepatic stellate cells; DNA microarray; gene expression analysis; genomics.

1. Introduction

Liver fibrosis is the common consequence of chronic liver injury of any cause. When advanced, it disrupts the normal liver architecture, causing portal hypertension and hepatic failure. In the last decade, remarkable progress has been made in the knowledge of the pathogenesis of liver fibrosis. In particular, hepatic stellate cells (HSCs) have been identified as the main fibrogenic cell type in the injured liver. These cells activate in response to paracrine stimuli from injured neighboring liver cells including hepatocytes as parenchymal cells, Kupffer cells as resident macrophages, hepatic endothelial cells, and

From: *Methods in Molecular Medicine, Vol. 117: Fibrosis Research: Methods and Protocols*
Edited by: J. Varga, D. A. Brenner, and S. H. Phan © Humana Press Inc., Totowa, NJ

inflammatory cells recruited during the host response to liver injury *(1)*. The activation of HSCs is characterized by the transdifferentiation of quiescent, vitamin A-storing cells into proliferative, myofibroblast-like cells that secrete large amounts of extracellular matrix proteins and release cytokines *(2)*. Therefore, activated HSCs exert profibrogenic and pro-inflammatory properties. Culturing quiescent HSCs on plastic results in a spontaneous activation resembling that observed in vivo *(3)*.

These dramatic phenotypic changes require a complete reprogramming of gene expression in HSCs. To understand the molecular basis for liver fibrosis, it is necessary to not only analyze the global changes of gene expression in HSCs, but also to define the coordinated changes in adjacent cells during the onset and progression of liver disease. For this purpose, DNA microarrays allow changes in the expression of thousands of genes to be determined simultaneously *(4)*. The first requirement for a microarray experiment is the ability to recover sufficient quantities of high quality RNA from cells or tissue—generally in the range of 10 to 30 μg of total RNA or approx 3 to 5 μg of purified mRNA. The use of purified mRNA frequently has the advantage of decreasing background noise levels in the final quantitative step of "reading" the array. mRNA is used to prepare cDNA and "labeled" cRNA is synthesized for hybridization to the array in one of the more frequently used systems (Affymetrix oligonucleotide arrays). Following hybridization of probes to the DNA array, which usually represent 10,000 to 20,000 eukaryotic genes to be assayed, the array is washed and the hybridization signal is quantitated using a confocal laser scanner. By comparing hybridization signals and patterns with controls, the quantity and identity of mRNAs are determined. Analysis of a complicated data set also enables the classification and clustering of up- and downregulated genes to be determined and programs of gene expression to be identified. Arrays generally need to be done in duplicate or triplicate to permit accurate statistical analysis, and verification studies of specific genes of interest, by Northern, reverse Northern, or real-time polymerase chain reaction (PCR) methods, are essential *(5,6)*.

Here we describe a detailed method for using oligonucleotide array technologies in the field of liver fibrosis research. We use commercially available Affymetrix GeneChips® (oligonucleotide arrays; Santa Clara, CA) to which fragments of biotinylated cRNA, which are representative of the initial mRNA population being analyzed, are hybridized. The cRNA probes are recognized by a Streptavidin R-Phycoerythrin (SAPE) conjugate and, following washing steps, a fluorescent image of the array is captured by a scanner. The protocols described have been optimized and used regularly in our laboratories *(5–7)*.

2. Materials

2.1. RNA Isolation and Quantification

1. Tissue was homogenized using a Polytron homogenizer (PowerGene 700, Fisher).
2. TRI Reagent (Molecular Research Center, Inc.), store at 4°C.
3. RNase-free deionized H_2O (either diethyl pyrocarbonate [DEPC]-treated Milli Q deionized H_2O or commercially available RNase-free deionized H_2O [Ambion or Biowhittaker]).

2.2. Preparation of cRNA

2.2.1. First-Strand cDNA Synthesis From Total RNA (see **Note 1**)

1. SuperScript II reverse transcriptase (RT; 200 U/μL) (Invitrogen, cat. no. 18064-071).
2. Oligo$(dT)_{24}$ primer containing a T7 RNA polymerase promoter (50 μ*M*) (Affymetrix, cat. no. 900375) (*see* **Note 2**).
3. 5X first-strand buffer (Invitrogen, cat. no. 18064-071).
4. 0.1 *M* dithiothreitol (DTT) (Invitrogen, cat. no. 18064-071).
5. 10 m*M* dNTP mix (dATP, dCTP, dGTP, dTTP) (Invitrogen, cat. no. 18427-013).

2.2.2. Second-Strand Synthesis

1. 5X second-strand buffer (Invitrogen, cat. no. 10812-014).
2. 10 m*M* dNTP mix (Invitrogen, cat. no. 18427-013).
3. *Escherichia coli* DNA ligase (10 U/μL) (Invitrogen, cat. no. 18052-019).
4. *E. coli* DNA polymerase I (10 U/μL) (Invitrogen, cat. no. 18010-025).
5. RNase H (2 U/μL) (Invitrogen, cat. no. 18021-071).
6. T4 DNA polymerase (5 U/μL) (Invitrogen, cat. no. 18005-25).
7. 0.5 *M* ethylenediamine tetraacetic acid (EDTA).

2.2.3. Cleanup of Double-Stranded cDNA

1. Phase Lock Gels (PLG) (Eppendorf, cat. no. 0032005152).
2. Phenol/chloroform (pH 7.9; Ambion, cat. no. 9730).

2.2.4. Preparation of cRNA

Enzo® BioArray™ HighYield™ RNA Transcript Labeling Kit (Enzo Diagnostics, cat. no. 42655-10).

2.2.5. Cleanup of Biotin-Labeled cRNA

RNeasy Mini Kit (Qiagen, cat. no. 74104).

2.3. Fragmentation of cRNA

5X fragmentation buffer: 200 m*M* Tris-acetate, pH 8.1, 500 m*M* KOAc, 150 m*M* MgOAc.

2.4. Hybridization

1. DNA arrays were purchased from Affymetrix (Santa Clara, CA). Arrays prepared on the basis of different genome databases are available (human, mouse, rat, or yeast). For details, check the Affymetrix website (www.affymetrix.com). We used Affymetrix human genome U95 (HGU95AV2) high-density oligonucleotide arrays containing probes for 12,000 genes.
2. 12X 2(*N*-morpholino)ethanesulfonic acid (MES) stock: for 1 L, add 70.4 g MES-free acid monohydrate (Sigma, cat. no. M5287), 193.3 g MES sodium salt (Sigma, cat. no. M5057). pH should be between 6.5 and 6.7. Filter through 0.2-μm filter. Store at 4°C in the dark.
3. 2X hybridization buffer: 8.3 mL 12X MES stock, 17.7 mL NaCl (5 *M*), 4 mL EDTA (0.5 *M*), 0.1 mL Tween-20 (10%), 19.9 mL H_2O. Store at 4°C in the dark.
4. Control oligonucleotide B2 (3 n*M*) (Affymetrix, cat. no. 900301).
5. Acetylated bovine serum albumin (BSA) solution (50 mg/mL) (Invitrogen, cat. no. 15561-020).
6. GeneChip Eukaryotic Hybridization Control Kit (Affymetrix, cat. no. 900299).
7. Herring sperm DNA (10 mg/mL) (Promega, cat. no. D1811).

2.4.1. Hybridization Washes and Staining

1. Fluidics Station 400 (Affymetrix).
2. 20X sodium chloride-sodium phosphate-EDTA (SSPE) (BioWhittaker Molecular Applications/Cambrex, cat. no. 51214).
3. Wash buffer A: 6X SSPE, 0.01% Tween-20. Filter through 0.2-μm filter.
4. Wash buffer B: 100 m*M* MES (*see* **Subheading 2.4.1.**), 0.1 *M* (Na^+), 0.01% Tween-20. Filter through 0.2-μm filter. Store at 4°C in the dark.
5. 2X stain buffer: 200 m*M* MES (*see* **Subheading 2.4.1.**), 2 *M* (Na^+), 0.1% Tween-20. Filter through 0.2-μm filter. Store at 4°C in the dark.
6. Streptavidin R-phycoerythrin (SAPE) (Molecular Probes, cat. no. S-866).
7. 10 mg/mL goat immunoglobulin (Ig)G stock (Sigma, cat. no. I5256): resuspend 50 mg in 5 mL phosphate-buffered saline (PBS) (Invitrogen, cat. no. 20012-027). Store at 4°C. Anti-streptavidin antibody (goat), biotinylated (Vector Laboratories, cat. no. BA-0500).
8. SAPE solution (1200 μL solution, sufficient for one array): 600 μL 2X stain buffer, 48 μL acetylated BSA (50 mg/mL), 12 μL streptavidin R-phycoerythrin (1 mg/mL), 540 μL H_2O. Store at 4°C in the dark (*see* **Note 3**).
9. Antibody solution (600 μL solution/array): 300 μL of 2X stain buffer, 266.4 μL of H_2O, 24 μL of acetylated BSA (50 mg/mL), 6 μL of normal goat IgG (10 mg/mL), 3.6 μL of biotinylated antibody (0.5 mg/mL).

2.5. Scanning

Hewlett-Packard G2500A Gene Array Scanner.

3. Methods

3.1. RNA Isolation and Quantitation

3.1.1. RNA Isolation From Cultured HSCs

Human HSCs are isolated and cultured as previously described *(5)*. Subconfluent HSCs in tissue culture dishes are washed once in cold PBS prior to harvesting. After aspiration of PBS, we recommend to directly harvesting cells with TRI Reagent (Molecular Research Center, Inc.) in the culture flak or dish.

1. Resuspend cells in TRI Reagent (1 mL/10 cm^2 culture dish area), harvest using a cell scraper and transfer HSCs in RNase-free tubes.
2. Incubate for 5 min at room temperature.
3. Add 0.2 vol of chloroform (0.2 mL/1 mL TRI reagent) and shake vigorously for 15 s.
4. Store the sample for 15 min at room temperature.
5. Centrifuge the tube at 12,000*g* for 15 min at 4°C.
6. Transfer the aqueous phase to a new tube.
7. For precipitation, add 0.5 vol isopropanol (0.5 mL/1 mL TRI reagent) and mix.
8. Store sample at room temperature for 10 min.
9. Centrifuge at 12,000*g* for 10 min at 4°C.
10. Remove supernatant and add 1 vol 75% ethanol (1 mL/1 mL TRI reagent) to wash RNA pellet.
11. Centrifuge at 7500*g* for 5 min.
12. Air dry RNA pellet for 5 min.
13. Dissolve the RNA pellet in approx 20 μL (for 10 cm^2 culture dish area) of DEPC-treated H_2O by pipeting to get an estimated RNA concentration of 5 μg/μL (*see* **Note 4**).
14. Quantitate the RNA by determining the absorbance at the wavelengths of 260 and 280 nm using a spectrophotometer (Beckman DU series). A260 × dilution factor × 40 equals the amount of RNA in μg/mL. The ratio OD260/OD280 should be close to 2.0 for pure RNA.
15. Store total RNA at –80°C and determine RNA integrity on a regular formamide agarose gel electrophoresis.

3.1.2. RNA Isolation From Human Liver Tissue

1. Starting material: human liver tissue that is frozen in sterile RNase-free tubes in liquid N_2 and stored at –80°C or liquid N_2.
2. Combine 0.8 to 0.9 g of human liver tissue with 10 mL TRI Reagent.
3. Homogenize the tissue with a Polytron homogenizer (PowerGene 700, Fisher) for 30 to 40 s and incubate homogenate at room temperature for 5 min.
4. Continue with **Subheading 3.1.1., step 4** analogous to the RNA preparation described for cultured cells.

3.2. Labeling of RNA

This procedure for the preparation of cRNA essentially follows the Affymetrix protocol (www.affymetrix.com).

3.2.1. First-Strand cDNA Synthesis From Total RNA

1. Prepare a RT-master mix: 4 μL 5X first-strand buffer, 2 μL DTT (100 m*M*), 1 μL dNTP mix (10 m*M*), 3 μL SuperScript II RT (200 U/μL), DEPC-treated H_2O to a final volume of 20 μL. The final volume includes the volume for RNA (*see* **step 2** below). Mix well and spin briefly (*see* **Note 5**).
2. Add the following to a tube: 30 μg of total RNA and 1 μL of oligo(dT)$_{24}$ primer containing a T7 RNA polymerase promoter (100 pmol/μL).
3. Incubate the tube at 70°C for 10 min to denature RNA.
4. Chill the sample on ice for 2 min.
5. Add the RT-mastermix to each tube.
6. Mix well, spin briefly, and incubate at 42°C for 60 min.

3.2.2. Second-Strand Synthesis

1. Add to the first-strand synthesis tube (final volume 150 μL): 91 μL DEPC-treated H_2O, 30 μL 5X second-strand buffer, 3 μL dNTP mix (10 m*M*), 1 μL *E. coli* DNA ligase (10 U/μL), 4 μL *E. coli* DNA polymerase I (10 U/μL), 1 μL RNase H (2 U/μL).
2. Mix well, spin briefly, and incubate at 16°C for 120 min.
3. Add 2 μL T4 DNA polymerase (5 U/μL) and mix well.
4. Incubate at 16°C for 5 min.
5. Add 10 μL EDTA (0.5 *M*).
6. Proceed or store the sample at –20°C.

3.2.3. Clean-Up of Double-Stranded cDNA

1. PLG-Phenol/Chloroform extraction according to the protocol of the manufacturer (*see* **Note 6**).
2. For ethanol precipitation, add 0.5 vol of 7.5 *M* NH_4Ac plus 2.5 vol of absolute ethanol to the sample and mix.
3. Store at –20°C for overnight.
4. Centrifuge at 12,000*g* at 4°C for 30 min.
5. Wash pellet with 0.5 mL of 80% ethanol.
6. Centrifuge at 12,000*g* at 4°C for 10 min.
7. Air-dry the pellet. Check pellet for dryness before processing.
8. Resuspend in 12 μL of RNase-free water.

3.2.4. Preparation of Biotin-Labeled cRNA

All reagents are part of the Enzo® BioArray™ HighYield™ RNA Transcript Labeling Kit.

1. Add to RNase-free tube at room temperature (final volume 40 µL): 12 µL template cDNA, 10 µL DEPC-treated H_2O, 4 µL 10X HY reaction buffer (Vial 1), 4 µL 10X biotin-labeled ribonucleotides (Vial 2), 4 µL DTT (Vial 3), 4 µL RNase inhibitor mix (Vial 4), 2 µL 20X T7 RNA polymerase (Vial 5) (*see* **Note 7**).
2. Mix well, spin briefly and incubate at 37°C for 4 to 5 h, gently mixing the contents of the tube every 30 to 45 min.

3.2.5. Clean-Up of Biotin-Labeled cRNA

Purification was performed using RNeasy spin columns from Qiagen.

1. Adjust the volume to 100 µL with DEPC-treated H_2O.
2. Add 350 µL of buffer RLT to the sample and mix thoroughly.
3. Add 250 µL of ethanol (96–100%) and mix by pipeting.
4. Apply the sample to RNeasy mini spin column sitting in a collection tube.
5. Centrifuge for 15 s at ≥8000*g* (≥10,000 rpm). Discard flow-through and transfer the column into a new 2-mL collection tube.
6. Pipet 500 µL of buffer RPE onto the spin column. Centrifuge as above and discard flow-through.
7. Add 500 µL of RPE buffer onto the spin column and centrifuge for 2 min at maximum speed.
8. Transfer the RNeasy column into a 1.5-mL collection tube and pipet 30 µL of RNase-free H_2O directly onto the RNeasy membrane. Incubate for 1 min at room temperature and centrifuge 1 min at ≥8000*g* (≥10,000 rpm).
9. Check an aliquot (1–10%) on a regular formamide gel and measure the optimal density (OD) to determine concentration and purity.

3.3. Fragmentation of cRNA

1. Incubate 1 to 32 µL of cRNA (20–30 µg) and 8 µL of 5X fragmentation buffer in a final volume of 40 µL at 94°C for 35 min.
2. Place on ice. Proceed or store the sample at –20°C.

3.4. DNA Array Hybridization

3.4.1. Hybridization

1. For standard array, prepare a hybridization mixture: 20 to 30 µg fragmented cRNA, 5 µL control oligonucleotide B2 (5 n*M*), 15 µL 20X hybridization controls (bioB, bioC, bioD, cre), 3 µL herring sperm DNA (10 mg/mL), 3 µL acetylated BSA (50 mg/mL), 150 µL 2X hybridization buffer, H_2O to a 300 µL final volume.
2. Adjust the array to room temperature immediately before use.
3. Heat the hybridization mixture to 99°C for 5 min and then place in a 45°C water bath for 5 min. Centrifuge at maximum speed for 5 min so that no insoluble material is applied to the chip.

4. Add 200 µL of 1X hybridization buffer to the chip and incubate at 45°C for 10 min with rotation.
5. Remove the buffer solution from the probe array cartridge and fill with 200 µL of the clarified hybridization cocktail.
6. Hybridize at 45°C for 16 h with rotation at 60 rpm (*see* **Note 8**).

3.4.2. Hybridization Washes and Staining

For washing and staining, we use a Fluidics Station 400 of Affymetrix with the recommended settings:

1. 10 cycles of 2 mixes/cycle at 25°C with wash buffer A.
2. 4 cycles of 15 mixes/cycle at 50°C with wash buffer B.
3. Stain the array for 10 min in SAPE solution at 25°C.
4. 10 cycles of 4 mixes/cycle with wash buffer A at 25°C.
5. Stain the array for 10 min in antibody solution at 25°C.
6. Stain the array for 10 min in SAPE solution at 25°C.
7. Final wash with 15 cycles of 4 mixes/cycle with wash buffer A at 30°C. The holding temperature is 25°C.
8. Check the array window for large bubbles or air pockets. If bubbles are present, return the array holder of Fluidics Station, fill it with a fresh volume of the last wash buffer used, and inspect it again for bubbles.

3.5. Scanning

We use a Hewlett-Packard G2500A Gene Array Scanner for scanning SAPE-stained gene arrays at a wavelength of 570 nm. Prior to scanning, the laser must warm up for at least 15 min. If the array was stored at 4°C, warm to room temperature before scanning. **Figure 1** shows an example of a scanned chip array hybridized with RNA from early passage human HSCs (passage 3 [**A**]) and in vitro aged, senescent HSCs (passage 15 [**B**]) *(7)*.

3.6. Analysis of Microarray Data

Because of the large amount of data and the complexity of the analysis, appropriate computing power and software packages are required. Appropriate packages are usually supplied by companies that manufacture microarrays for commercial use and are also available on the internet. The most commonly used package is provided by Affymetrix. Details on using the Affymetrix software are available in the software manual. Parameters can be adjusted for individual gene array experiment.

Methods of microarray data analysis include pairwise comparison analysis and clustering analysis. The pairwise comparison (**Fig. 1**) of the differential expression levels of specific genes in two relevant samples is the most straightforward and informative method of analyzing a microarray experiment when

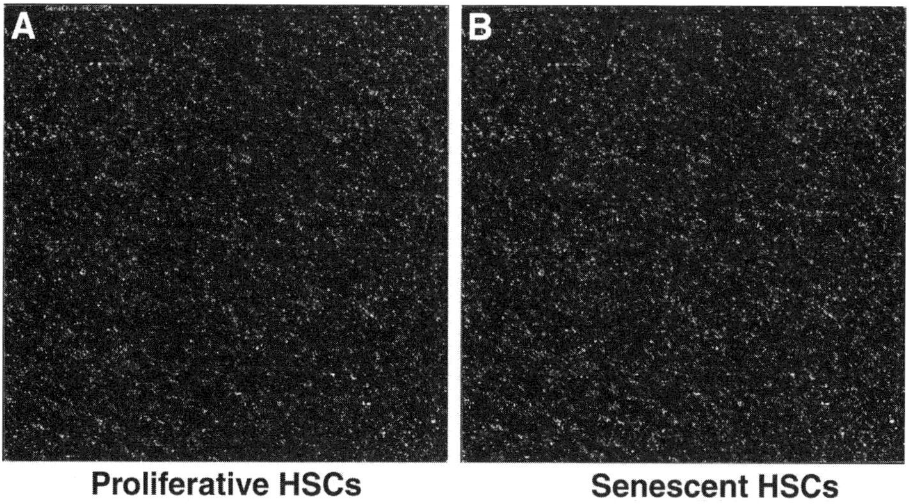

Fig. 1. Scanned images of a DNA microarray from proliferative, early passage human HSCs **(A)** and in vitro aged, senescent hepatic stellate cells **(B)**. Using the protocols described, 30 µg of total RNA was used to prepare cRNA and hybridized to an Affymetrix human genome U95 (HG-U95A) high density oligonucleotide array containing 12,000 genes.

the aim is to directly determine the effects of one type of treatment over another one. Pairwise comparison analysis can be used to compare diseased vs normal tissue, as well as to determine the effect of a particular treatment on a cell population such as viral or bacterial infection, gene transfection, or exposure to a biochemical substance of interest. The results are presented as relative differences of each gene.

When the expression of different genes is compared simultaneously in many samples, clustering analysis is of great interest. There are many types of so-called "clustering" algorithms including Self Organizing Maps. This type of analysis is especially valuable for following differential gene expression over a series of time points during in vivo or in vitro differentiation or development, or during a time-course of drug or other biochemical substance treatment. Finally, because there are limitations in the sensitivity and accuracy of microarray analysis, it is important to independently verify the differential gene expression data by alternative techniques (i.e., quantitative PCR, Northern blot, or RNase protection assay).

4. Notes

1. Background noise can be reduced by purifying mRNA using poly(A) or 5' cap-dependent purification methods *(6)*.

2. It is important to use a high-performance liquid chromatography purified primer.
3. SAPE should be stored in the dark at 4°C, either foil wrapped or kept in an amber tube. Remove SAPE from refrigerator and tap the tube to mix before preparing stain solution. Do not freeze concentrated or diluted SAPE solution. Always prepare SAPE stain solution immediately before use.
4. For better solubilization, RNA can be heated for 10 min at 70°C.
5. Adjust the amount of SuperScript II (200 U/μL) according to the total amount of RNA: 1 μL for 5 to 8 μg, 2 μL for 8.1 to 16 μg, and 3 μL for up to 40 μg of total RNA.
6. A standard phenol/chloroform extraction can be performed as an alternative to the PLG procedure.
7. Adjust the amount of template cDNA according to the total amount of RNA: 10 μL for 5 to 8 μg, 5 μL for 8.1 to 16 μg, and 3.3 μL for up to 40 μg of total RNA.
8. After 16 h of hybridization, remove the hybridization cocktail from the array and set it aside in a microcentrifuge tube. Store on ice during the procedure or at –20°C for long-term storage. Fill the array with an appropriate volume (i.e., 200 μL for standard array) of wash buffer A. With this condition, the array can be stored at 4°C for up to 3 h before proceeding with washing and staining.

Acknowledgments

This work was supported by a DFG-grant SCHN 620/3-1 (to B. Schnabl), a Judith Graham Pool Postdoctoral Fellowship from the National Hemophilia Foundation (to Y.H. Choi), and the National Institutes of Health (CA63640; to C.H. Hagedorn).

References

1. Bataller, R. and Brenner, D. A. (2001) Hepatic stellate cells as a target for the treatment of liver fibrosis. *Semin. Liver Dis.* **21,** 437–451.
2. Gressner, A. M. (1998) The cell biology of liver fibrogenesis - an imbalance of proliferation, growth arrest and apoptosis of myofibroblasts. *Cell. Tissue Res.* **292,** 447–452.
3. Rockey, D. C., Boyles, J. K., Gabbiani, G., and Friedman, S. L. (1992) Rat hepatic lipocytes express smooth muscle actin upon activation in vivo and in culture. *J. Submicrosc. Cytol. Pathol.* **24,** 193–203.
4. Schena, M., Shalon, D., Davis, R. W., and Brown, P. O. (1995) Quantitative monitoring of gene expression patterns with a complementary DNA microarray. *Science* **270,** 467–470.
5. Schnabl, B., Choi, Y. H., Olsen, J. C., Hagedorn, C. H., and Brenner, D. A. (2002) Immortal activated human hepatic stellate cells generated by ectopic telomerase expression. *Lab. Invest.* **82,** 323–333.
6. Choi, Y. H. and Hagedorn, C. H. (2003) Purifying mRNAs with a high-affinity eIF4E mutant identifies the short 3' poly(A) end phenotype. *Proc. Natl. Acad. Sci. USA* **100,** 7033–7038.

7. Schnabl, B., Purbeck, C. A., Choi, Y. H., Hagedorn, C. H., and Brenner, D. A. (2003) Replicative senescence of activated human hepatic stellate cells is accompanied by a pronounced inflammatory but less fibrogenic phenotype. *Hepatology* **37,** 653–664.

22

Analysis of Proteins Dominantly Expressed in Hepatic Stellate Cells of Activated Phenotype

The Molecular Approach for Liver Fibrosis

Norifumi Kawada

Summary

Stellate cells are principal producers of extracellular matrix proteins in the liver and play a major role in the development of liver fibrosis. Molecular basis of the cell activation has therefore been analyzed intensively during the past decade. Proteomics analysis is one of the most powerful tools with which to reveal the total protein synthesis in stellate cells, in particular the dynamic change in their expression level in response to activation. We have successfully analyzed over 300 stellate cell proteins by proteomics, several of which represented activation-associated change. Change in the level of some of these proteins was confirmed in liver tissue level. In addition, this approach led to the discovery of a novel globin in the vertebrate. Thus, proteomics is a research method for comprehensive understanding of the molecular basis of liver fibrosis.

Key Words: Stellate cell; liver fibrosis; proteomics; two-dimensional polyacrylamide gel electrophoresis; isoelectric focusing; mass spectrometry.

1. Introduction

1.1. The Stellate Cell As a Principal Player in Liver Fibrosis

Hepatic stellate cells play multiple roles in the pathophysiology of the liver *(1)*. Quiescent stellate cells represent a principal retinol-storing phenotype and metabolize a small amount of basement membrane-forming substrata. When liver injury occurs, they undergo transformation into myofibroblasts that show active proliferation, increased extracellular matrix (ECM) production, enhanced contractility, secretion of growth factors and chemotactic proteins, and retinoid loss. Stellate cell activation is initiated by oxidative stress from

From: *Methods in Molecular Medicine, Vol. 117: Fibrosis Research: Methods and Protocols*
Edited by: J. Varga, D. A. Brenner, and S. H. Phan © Humana Press Inc., Totowa, NJ

damaged hepatocytes, paracrine stimulation of cytokines and growth factors from Kupffer cells, endothelial cells, and infiltrating leukocytes, and early ECM changes including the production of a splice variant of cellular fibronectin (EIIIA isoform) ***(2–5)***. Activated stellate cells are highly responsive to growth factors such as platelet-derived growth factor (PDGF)-BB and insulin-like growth factor (IGF)-1; they induce the expression of receptors for individual growth factors, leading to the activation of intracellular signal cascade (mitogen-activated protein kinase [MAPK] pathway, phosphatidil inositol 3-kinase [PI3-K] pathway, etc.), and finally they are highly responsive to the DNA synthesis and proliferation ***(7,8)***. Transforming growth factor (TGF)-β is a key regulatory molecule for ECM metabolism. Increased contractility of activated stellate cell causes constriction of sinusoids, resulting in portal hypertension ***(11,12)***. Thus, analysis of the molecular mechanism underlying stellate cell activation is assumed to be indispensable for the establishment of a new therapy against liver fibrosis. An overall survey of molecular change associated with stellate cell activation is prerequisite for deeper knowledge of this subject.

1.2. Proteomics

About 5000 to 6000 proteins are likely expressed in one kind of cell and hence only a part of genes (number of genes encoding proteins is estimated to be about 39,000) on the genome are expressed in a cell- and tissue-specific manner. Therefore, analysis of cellular proteins, especially the change in their expression level and their post-transcriptional modification, is definitely required. The proteome (*pro*tein + gen*ome*), or proteomics, refers to the total protein profile of a given cell or tissue type. The proteomics research basically involves the following experimental steps (*see also* **Fig. 1**). First, proteins are separated in two-dimentional polyacrylamide gel electrophoresis (2D-PAGE) ***(13)***. This technique combines isoelectric focusing (IEF) in the first dimension with sodium dodecyl sulfate (SDS)-PAGE in the second dimension, and it is capable of separating several thousands of proteins on a single 2D gel. Second, identification and characterization of individual proteins by using mass spectrometric techniques such as matrix-assisted laser desorption ionization (MALDI) or electrospray ionization (ESI) mass spectrometry (MS) (**Fig. 1**) ***(14,15)***. Advancement in these techniques of protein analysis using MS has made it possible to increase the sensitivity of analysis (less than 100 fmol of proteins can be analyzed) and shorten the time for analysis (only 30 min is required for the partial sequencing of one protein spot). Moreover, the tandem mass (MS/MS) method represents directly the amino acid sequence of the protein spot analyzed without any prepurification, such as high-performance liquid chromatography (HPLC).

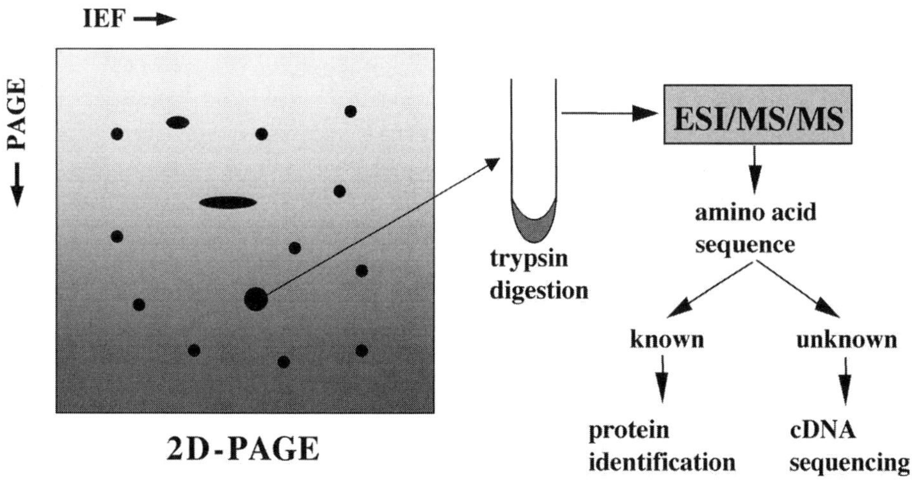

Fig. 1. Proteomics analysis. Stellate cell proteins are lysed and separated in two-dimentional (2D) polyacrylamide gel electrophoresis (PAGE), and then one protein spot is cut from the gel stained with silver staining. The protein is digested with trypsin and, after brief purification, the solution is applied to electrospray ionization/tandem mass spectrometry (ESI/MS/MS). The protein is identified by matching the obtained amino acid sequences against the SwissProt and GenBank databases using the Genome Net world-wide web server. In case unknown amino acid sequence is found, cDNA is cloned using degenerated polymerase chain reaction technique.

2. Materials

2.1. Animals

1. Male Wistar rats (about 300 g body weight, SLC, Shizuoka, Japan).
2. Animals should be housed at a constant temperature and supplied with laboratory chow and water *ad libitum*.

2.2. Chemicals

1. Pronase E (Merck, Darmstadt, FRG).
2. DNase (Boehringer Mannheim, Mannheim, FRG).
3. Collagenase and thioacetamide (Wako Pure Chemical Co., Osaka, Japan).
4. Nycodenz (Nycomed Pharmas, Oslo, Norway).
5. Dulbecco's modified Eagle's medium (DMEM) and fetal bovine serum (FBS) (Gibco-BRL, Gaithersburg, MD).
6. The other agents are basically obtained from Wako Pure Chemical Co. (Osaka, Japan) and Sigma Chemical Co. (Saint Louis, MO).

2.3. Isolation of Stellate Cells

Isolation procedure of stellate cells was previously described ***(16)***.

2.3.1. Liver Digestion and Purification of Stellate Cells

1. Perfusion of normal rat liver with a Ca^{2+}/Mg^{2+}-free buffer (8 g/L NaCl, 400 mg/L KCl, 88.17 mg/L $NaH_2PO_4 \cdot 2H_2O$, 120.45 mg/L Na_2HPO_4, 2380 mg/L *N*-2-hydroxyethylpiperazine-*N*'-2-ethansulfonic acid (HEPES), 350 mg/L $NaHCO_3$, 190 mg/L ehtyleneglycol-*bis*-(2-aminoethylether)-*N*-*N*-*N*'-*N*'-tetraacetic acid (EGTA), 900 mg/L glucose, pH 7.3) for 10 min at 37°C.
2. Perfusion-digestion of the liver by a buffer (8 g/L NaCl, 400 mg/L KCl, 88.17 mg/L $NaH_2PO_4 \cdot 2H_2O$, 120.45 mg/L Na_2HPO_4, 2380 mg/L HEPES, 350 mg/L $NaHCO_3$, 560 mg/L $CaCl_2 \cdot 2H_2O$, pH 7.3) containing 0.1% pronase and 0.04% collagenase for 40 min at 37°C.
3. Incubation-digestion of the excised liver in the identical buffer containing 0.08% pronase E, 0.08% collagenase, and 20 μg/mL of DNase at 37°C for 30 min.
4. Filtration of the digested resultants through a 150-μm mesh.
5. Centrifugation on an 8.2% Nycodenz cushion, which produces a stellate cell-enriched fraction in the upper-whitish layer.

2.3.2. Culture Medium of Isolated Stellate Cell

Cell culture medium: DMEM, 10% FBS, 10^5 U/L penicillin G, 100 mg/L streptomycin.

2.3.3. Plating of Isolated Stellate Cells

1. Plating of isolated stellate cells on noncoated plastic culture dishes (Falcon 3003, Beckton Dickinson, Franklin Lakes, NJ) at 5×10^6 cells/well.
2. Cell purity (more than 95% is required) should be assessed by a typical star-like configuration and by detecting vitamin A autofluorescence.

2.4. Preparation of Quiescent and Activated Stellate Cells

1. Allow stellate cells to attach to the culture dishes for 24 h in order to remove dead cells and debris after plating.
2. Change the culture medium every other day.
3. Quiescent stellate cells = stellate cells cultured for 1 d.
4. Activated stellate cells = stellate cells cultured for 7 d.

2.5. Lysis of Stellate Cells

Cell lysis buffer: 7 *M* urea, 2 *M* thiourea, 4% (w/v) 3-3-cholamidopropyl-dimethylammonio-1-propanesulfonate (CHAPS), 2% (v/v) ampholine, pH 3.5 to 10.0 (Pharmacia Hoefer, Upsala, Sweden), 1% dithiothreitol (DTT).

3. Methods

3.1. Sample Preparation

3.1.1. Cell Lysis

1. Wash the cell-attached culture plate at least four times with ice-cold phosphate-buffered saline (PBS) to remove culture medium, serum, and floating cells.
2. Add lysis buffer to the culture plate (e.g., 1 mL buffer against 10-cm plate [Falcon 3003]) and mix the cells using cell scraper.
3. Put the cell lysate into an Eppendorf tube.
4. Determine the protein concentration.

3.1.2. Storage of the Samples

Lysed materials can be stored at –80°C before electrophoresis.

3.2. 2D-PAGE

3.2.1. Electrophoresis

1. Apply protein samples (100 μg total) overnight to Immobiline DryStrips (pH 4.0–7.0, 18 cm, Pharmacia Hoefer, Uppsala, Sweden) by in-gel rehydration.
2. First dimension IEF, a Pharmacia Hoefer Multiphor II electrophoresis chamber (Uppsala, Sweden).
3. Second-dimension SDS-PAGE, 9 to 18% acrylamide gradient gels utilizing the Iso-Dalt system from Pharmacia Hoefer (Uppsala, Sweden).

3.2.2. Staining of Proteins and Identification of Protein Spots (see **Fig. 2**)

1. Silver staining.
2. Scanning the 2D gels on an Epson ES 8000 scanner (Seiko Epson Corporation, Suwa, Japan).
3. Image analysis, protein quantification, and 2D gel proteome database management, the Melanie 3 software package from GeneBio (Geneva, Switzerland).
4. The Melanie 3 software arbitrarily calculates the 2D spot intensity by integrating the optical density over the spot area (i.e., the spot "volume").
5. After scanning, the 2D gels can be dried between two cellophane sheets and stored at room temperature for further reference.

3.3. Tryptic In-Gel Digestion

3.3.1. In-Gel Digestion of 2D-PAGE-Resolved Proteins (**17**)

1. Excise protein spots of interest from the 2D gels and rehydrate them in 100 m*M* ammonium carbonate.
2. Wash the gel pieces twice in MilliQ water.
3. Incubate them in 15 m*M* potassium ferricyanide and 50 m*M* sodium thiosulfate for being destained.

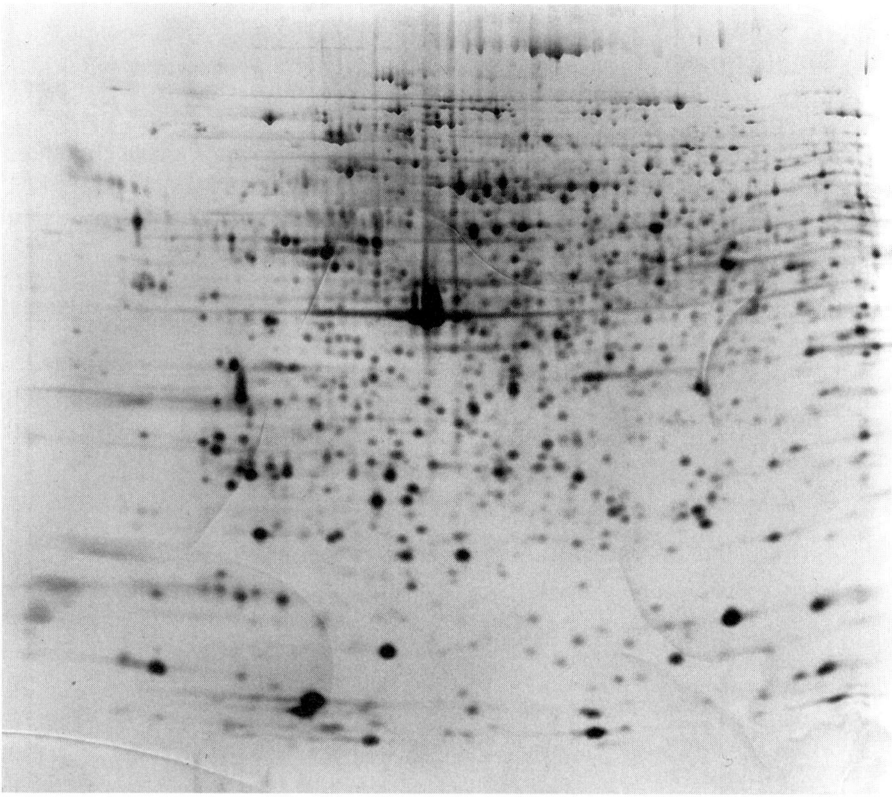

Fig. 2. Typical analysis of cell-associated proteins separated by 2D sodium dodecyl sulfate-polyacrylamide gel electrophoresis. Rat skin fibroblast. Silver Staining. This figure is kindly provided by Dr. Dan Bach Kristensen (MDS Denmark, Denmark).

4. Rinse them twice in MilliQ water and once in 100 m*M* ammonium bicarbonate and then dehydrate them in acetonitrile until they turn opaque white.
5. Dry them in a centrifugal vaporizer.
6. Rehydrate the gel pieces in a digestion buffer containing trypsin and digest them overnight at 37°C.
7. After digestion, add 5% trifluoroacetic acid (TFA) to terminate the reaction. Extract the peptides three times with 5% TFA in 50% acetonitrile.
8. Concentrate the extraction solutions in a centrifugal vaporizer, and then resuspend them in 1% formic acid in 4% methanol.
9. Load the solution to an OLIGO R3 column (PerSeptive Biosystems, Framingham, MA). Wash the column with 1% formic acid. The peptides can be eluted with 1% formic acid in 70% methanol.

3.4. ESI MS and Protein Identification

3.4.1. Identification of Amino Acid Sequence of the Peptide Fragments (17)

1. Load the eluted peptides into Au/Pd coated nanoelectrospray (ES) capillaries (Protana, Odense, Denmark), and then insert them into the nanoflow Z-spray source of a quadruple time-of-flight (Q-TOF) mass spectrometer (Micromass, Manchester, England).
2. Perform Q-TOF operation, data acquisition, and data analysis using MassLynx/BioLynx 3.2 software (Micromass, Manchester, England) on a Windows NT server.
3. Use the MS mode to scan samples for detectable peptides. Subsequently, use the MS/MS mode to fragment individual peptides.
4. Identify the proteins by matching the obtained amino acid sequences against the SwissProt and GenBank databases.

3.5. Current Status of Our Proteomics on Stellate Cells

We have analyzed 308 protein spots derived from stellate cells on 2D gels *(16)*. These include 225 protein spots derived from stellate cell lysate and 83 spots of secreted proteins. Among the identified proteins were Cu/Zn superoxide dismutase, plasminogen activator inhibitor (PAI)-1, ubiquitin, vimentin, and several heat-shock proteins. Several proteins whose expression levels were up- or downregulated in the course of stellate cell activation were identified. In particular, upregulation of galectin-1, calcyclin, and calgizzarin was reproduced in liver tissue level and the expression of their mRNAs was confirmed to increase in the process of stellate cell activation *(16)*. Recent further analysis demonstrated that galectin-1 acts as a novel mitogen against stellate cells by enhancing MAPK pathways *(18)*. In addition, our proteomics analysis has contributed in the discovery of a fourth globin of vertebrate, which is now named "cytoglobin/STAP" *(19,20)*.

4. Notes

1. *Recent methodological progress of proteomics.* Although we have utilized "classical" 2D-PAGE for the separation of cell-associated proteins, this technique has several disadvantages. First, only a few thousands of proteins are separated in one gel whereas more than 10,000 proteins are expected to express in any cells indicating that low abundant proteins, which include molecules involved in signal transduction and transcription factors, are overlooked. Second, basic membranous proteins and high molecular weight proteins are usually difficult to be separated by 2D-PAGE.

   Protein separation by liquid chromatography (LC) overcomes this problem. In addition, LC can be connected directly to MS/MS, resulting in the automatic, high-throughput and speedy determination and identification of proteins. Direct nanoflow liquid LC-MS/MS system will identify more than 100 proteins within 1 h *(21)*.

2. *Detection of protein modification by proteomics*. Function of proteins is regulated by posttranslational modification, i.e., phosphorylation, glycation, ubiquitination, etc. For instance, in stellate cells, phosphorylation of mitogen activated protein kinase and Akt is a key step for the cell proliferation and survival. Protein phosphorylation has been detected by labeling the cells with ^{32}P-ATP or by using phospho-specific antibodies. However, peptide mass fingerprint technique is a tool with which to identify phospho-protein without these conventional methods; increase in the molecular weight of 80 Da (HPO_3) indicates the occurrence of phosphorylation. Our preliminary data indicates that the number of phosphorylated proteins increase in accordance with stellate cell activation.

Acknowledgments

The author thanks Prof. Katsutoshi Yoshizato (Hiroshima University, Japan), Dr. Dan Bach Kristensen (MDS Denmark, Denmark), Drs. Naoto Maeda and Yukihiro Imanishi (Osaka City University, Japan), and Miss Hiroko Matsui (Osaka City University, Japan) for their co-working, comments, and discussion.

References

1. Blomhoff, R. and Wake, K. (1994) Perisinusoidal stellate cells of the liver; important roles in retinol metabolism and fibrosis. *FASEB J.* **5,** 271–277.
2. Friedman, S. L. (1993) The cellular basis of hepatic fibrosis. *N. Engl. J. Med.* **328,** 1828-1835.
3. Gressner, A. M. and Bachem, M. G. (1995) Molecular mechanism of liver fibrosis-a homage to the role of activated fat-storing cells. *Digestion* **56,** 335–346.
4. Olaso, E. and Friedman, S. L. (1998) Molecular regulation of hepatic fibrogenesis. *J. Hepatol.* **29,** 836–847.
5. Kawada, N. (1997) The hepatic perisiunusoidal stellate cell. *Histol. Histopathol.* **12,** 1069–1080.
6. Kim, Y., Ratziu, V., Choi, S. G., et al. (1998) Transcriptional activation of transforming growth factor beta1 and its receptors by the Kruppel-like factor Zf9/core promoter-binding protein and Sp1. Potential mechanisms for autocrine fibrogenesis in response to injury. *J. Biol. Chem.* **273,** 33,750–33,758.
7. Marra, F., Gentilini, A., Pinzani, M., et al. (1997) Phosphatidylinositol 3-kinase is required for platelet-derived growth factor's actions on hepatic stellate cells. *Gastroenterology* **112,** 1297–1306.
8. Kawada, N., Ikeda, K., Seki, S., and Kuroki, T. (1999) Expression of cyclins D1, D2 and E correlates with proliferation of rat stellate cells in culture. *J. Hepatol.* **30,** 1057–1064.
9. Hellerbrand, C., Stefanovic, B., Giordano, F., Burchardt, E. R., and Brenner, D. A. (1999) The role of TGF beta1 in initiating hepatic stellate cell activation in vivo. *J. Hepatol.* **30,** 77–87.

10. George, J., Roulot, D., Koteliansky, V. E., and Bissell, D. M. (1999) In vivo inhibition of rat stellate cell activation by soluble transforming growth factor beta type II receptor: a potential new therapy for hepatic fibrosis. *Proc. Natl. Acad. Sci. USA* **96,** 12,719–12,724.
11. Kawada, N., Tran-Thi, T. A., Klein, H., and Decker, K. (1993) The contraction of hepatic stellate (Ito) cells stimulated with vasoactive substances. Possible involvement of endothelin 1 and nitric oxide in the regulation of the sinusoidal tonus. *Eur. J. Biochem.* **213,** 815–823.
12. Rockey, D. C. and Weisiger, R. A. (1996) Endothelin induced contractility of stellate cells from normal and cirrhotic rat liver: implications for regulation of portal pressure and resistance. *Hepatology* **24,** 233–240.
13. O'Farrell, P. H. (1975) High resolution two-dimentional electrophoresis of proteins. *J. Biol. Chem.* **250,** 4007–4021.
14. Roepstorff, P. (1997) Mass spectrometry on protein studies from genome to function. *Curr. Opin. Biotechnol.* **8,** 6–13.
15. Yates, J. R. (1998) Mass spectrometry and the age of the proteome. *J. Mass. Spectrom.* **33,** 1–19.
16. Kristensen, D. B., Kawada, N., Imamura, K., et al. (2000) Proteome analysis of rat hepatic stellate cells. *Hepatology* **32,** 268–277.
17. Kristensen, D. B., Imamura, K., Miyamoto, Y., and Yoshizato, K. (2000) Mass spectrometric approaches for the characterization of proteins on a hybrid quadrupole time-of-flight (Q-TOF) mass spectrometer. *Electrophoresis* **21,** 430–439.
18. Maeda, N., Kawada, N., Seki, S., et al. (2003) Stimulation of proliferation of rat hepatic stellate cells by galectin-1 and galectin-3 through different intracellular signaling pathways. *J. Biol. Chem.* **278,** 18,938–18,944.
19. Kawada, N., Kristensen, D. B., Asahina, K., et al. (2001) Characterization of a stellate cell activation-associated protein (STAP) with peroxidase activity found in rat hepatic stellate cells. *J. Biol. Chem.* **276,** 25,318–25,323.
20. Sawai, H., Kawada, N., Yoshizato, K., Nakajima, H., Aono, S., and Shiro, Y. (2003) Characterization of the heme environmental structure of cytoglobin, a fourth globin in humans. *Biochemistry* **42,** 5133–5142.
21. Natsume, T., Yamauchi, Y., Nakayama, H., et al. (2002) A direct nanoflow liquid chromatography-tandem mass spectrometry system for interaction proteomics. *Anal. Chem.* **74,** 4725–4733.

Index

R

S